LARGE ANIMAL NEUROLOGY:

A Handbook for

Veterinary Clinicians

LARGE ANIMAL NEUROLOGY

A Handbook for

Veterinary Clinicians

I. G. MAYHEW, BVSc, DipOVC, PhD, MRCVS,

Diplomate ACVIM, Internal Medicine and Neurology
Professor, Department of Medical Sciences
College of Veterinary Medicine,
University of Florida
Gainesville, Florida, USA,
Currently,
Head, Department of Clinical Studies,
Animal Health Trust,
Newmarket, Suffolk, UK

Lea & Febiger · *Philadelphia* · *London* · *1989*

Lea & Febiger
600 South Washington Square
Philadelphia, Pa.   19106-4198
U.S.A.
(215) 922-1330

Lea & Febiger (UK) Ltd.
145a Croydon Road
Beckenham, Kent BR3 3RB
U.K.

Library of Congress Cataloging-in-Publication Data

Mayhew, Ian G.
    Large animal neurology: a handbook for veterinary clinicians /
I.G. Mayhew.
        p.   cm.
    Includes index.
    ISBN 0-8121-1183-4
    1. Veterinary neurology.   I. Title.
SF895.K43   1989
636.098′68—dc19
                                                            88-34037
                                                                CIP

Printed in the United States of America

Print Number: 5   4   3   2   1

To all the patients that, through their misfortune, taught me neurology.

PREFACE

"As a rule, the scientist takes off from the manifold observations of his predecessors, and shows his intelligence, if any, by selecting here and there the significant stepping stones that will lead across difficulties to new understanding. The one who places the last stone and steps across to terra ferma of accomplished discovery gets all the credit. Only the initiated know and honour those whose patient integrity and devotion to exact observation have made the last step possible."

Hans Zinsser (1878–1940)

The writing of this handbook will have been worthwhile if it fills the role of being a small, instructional stepping stone for other clinicians interested in diseases involving the nervous system of domestic large animals.

Over the years, considerable fear and anguish have been experienced by people observing animals suffering from neurologic diseases. Possibly because of these fears and the gloomy outlook cast upon neurologic disease, initial studies in veterinary neurology were primarily composed of morbid descriptions. Based on such early, masterful studies made by neuroanatomists, neurophysiologists, and neuropathologists, several pioneering veterinarians in Europe and the United States promoted comparative neuropathology and developed the clinical discipline of small animal neurology, which has since flourished. Only recently has the clinical specialty of large animal neurology received emphasis in veterinary degree curricula, graduate specialty courses, applied research, and continuing education programs. LARGE ANIMAL NEUROLOGY: A HANDBOOK FOR VETERINARY CLINICIANS is presented in response to this educational trend within our profession. It is intended principally for veterinarians to use as a reference and to guide them in handling large animal neurologic cases that they encounter. Additionally, veterinary students in clinical training and graduates in programs that encompass the discipline of neurology may find the book useful.

The approach I have used in this book is a practical one, and one that is based on the instructional course "Problems in Neurology," developed by Cheryl Chrisman and myself at the University of Florida. The content is divided into two parts: the first presents information needed by the clinican to approach large animal neurologic cases; the second is a clinical discussion of the diseases of the nervous system grouped under the syndromes that clinicians are presented with frequently. An attempt is made to cover diseases occurring in the western world, but this text is only based on experience gained in America, Australia, and Britain.

A great amount of my enthusiasm for and understanding of neurology has come from my association with Dr. Laura Smith-Maxie, Dr. Blakemore, my mentor Dr. Sandy de Lahunta, and my special friend Dr. Cheryl Chrisman. This book would not have been published if not for the expert assistance of Linda

Siedzik, Linda Rose, and Beth Senn at the University of Florida, and Lesley Kramer and Ray Kersey of Lea & Febiger.

Finally, my thanks are given to Rachel, Karen, Paul, and Chris for their patience, which I have tried.

Newmarket, Suffolk   I.G. Mayhew, DVM

CONTENTS

PART I

EVALUATION OF THE LARGE ANIMAL NEUROLOGIC PATIENT

CHAPTER 1

Clinical Neuroanatomy

Some of the most exciting aspects of clinical neurology involve being able to relate observed signs and syndromes with neuroanatomic sites of the lesions. This may be experienced when recognizing a syndrome of ataxia in a purebred animal and relating it to a particular familial cerebellar disorder for a client. Or one may be able to explain to a client how a certain lesion, detected at postmortem examination, can cause the particular clinical syndrome observed in the animal. The basic requirement for achieving this degree of diagnostic acumen is an understanding of applied neuroanatomy.

This chapter provides the basic information necessary to allow the clinician to appreciate the fundamentals of a neurologic examination and to interpret, accurately, the results of such an examination. As the clinician becomes adept at these tasks, further anatomic details may be sought. These can be found in the texts listed in the bibliography.

BASIC DESCRIPTIVE TERMINOLOGY

The following is a review of basic descriptive terminology. Note the derivation, abbreviation, combining form, synonym, or explanation is given in parenthesis.

The central nervous system (CNS) consists of the brain (encephalo) and spinal cord (myelo). It contains collections of neuronal cell bodies or somata in layers (laminae), nuclei, and columns of gray matter (polio). Tracts, sheets, and pathways of dendritic (afferent) and particularly axonal (efferent) processes of these cell bodies make up the white matter (leuko). These processes make up the majority of the CNS along with their fatty, myelin (myelino) coats. In the horse, some of these neuronal fibers extend 2 to 3 m and many exit and enter the CNS via the cranial and spinal nerves of the peripheral nervous system (PNS).

Both the cerebrum (cerebro) and cerebellum (cerebello) have an outer (cortex) and middle (medulla) portion. The remainder of the brain makes up the brainstem consisting of a thalamus, midbrain, pons, and medulla oblongata.

The spinal cord has enlargements at the levels of the thoracic and the pelvic limbs. This is the result of a higher density of neurons in the gray matter at these sites. They are called the brachial intumescence and the lumbosacral intumescence, respectively.

The entire CNS is protected within the bony cranium and vertebral column and is covered by meninges consisting of the thick (pachy) dura mater and thin (lepto) arachnoid and pia mater. Between the latter two membranes is the cerebrospinal fluid (CSF). This fluid also fills the cavities within the brain (ventricles) and spinal cord (spinal canal), which are lined by ciliated ependymal cells.

As well as meningeal cells, ependymal cells, neurons (somata and their axons and dendrites), and blood vessels, several types of supporting, protective, and nutritive ("glue") cells (neuroglia) make up a large part of the CNS. The largest of these glial cells are called astrocytes because of their star-shaped processes. These cells basically act to support the CNS, which has little cytoskeletal framework. Originally, the processes of other small glial cell types were thought to be few (oligo); these were named oligodendrocytes. We now know that their processes are extensive and extend to and maintain all the myelin sheaths of CNS axons. The small microglial cells appear to be the tissue macrophages of the reticuloendothelial system within the CNS.

The neuronal processes in the PNS, with their myelin sheaths, are called nerve fibers and make up the peripheral nerves. Some neurons, particularly those in the autonomic nervous system, and sensory neurons have their cell bodies in aggregations known as ganglia. Several networks of interwoven nerves (plexuses) occur in the PNS, the largest of which are the brachial plexus and the lumbosacral plexus. These supply the thoracic and pelvic limbs, respectively.

The cells that ensheath PNS nerve fibers are Schwann cells. These assist in maintaining a framework for nerves, as well as producing the myelin that surrounds all the larger fibers. The PNS has a fibrous connective tissue cytoskeleton that consists of the epineurium, which wraps around a nerve, the perineurium, which surrounds a bundle or fascicle of fibers, and the endoneurium, which separates the individual fibers.

FUNCTIONAL NEUROANATOMY

Probably, the most important structural and functional unit of the nervous system is the simple reflex pathway (Fig. 1–1). A neurologic examination basically involves testing simple and complex reflex pathways and interpreting the effected reflex activity and complex responses (see Chapter 2).

A simple spinal reflex pathway, depicted as a tendon stretch reflex in Figure 1–1, is composed of three neurons. Stimulation of a sensory stretch receptor in a tendon, and its sensory neuronal cell body in the dorsal root ganglion, stimulates an internuncial neuron that effects contraction of the limb muscle via a lower motor neuron (LMN). The LMN has its cell body in the ventral gray matter of the spinal cord. Reflex motor response to sensory stimuli will occur without any ascending or descending connections within the CNS as long as these three neurons and the sensory nerve ending, the neuromuscular junction, and the effector muscle all are intact.

The various reflex pathways, with their respective LMNs throughout the brainstem and spinal cord, are controlled for voluntary movement by higher motor centers—the upper motor neurons (UMN). Figure 1–2 depicts some of the UMN pathways. Corticospinal motor pathways are very important in primates but do not appear to be as important in large animals. Large lesions destroying the cerebrocortical motor centers (Fig. 1–2A) do not cause perma-

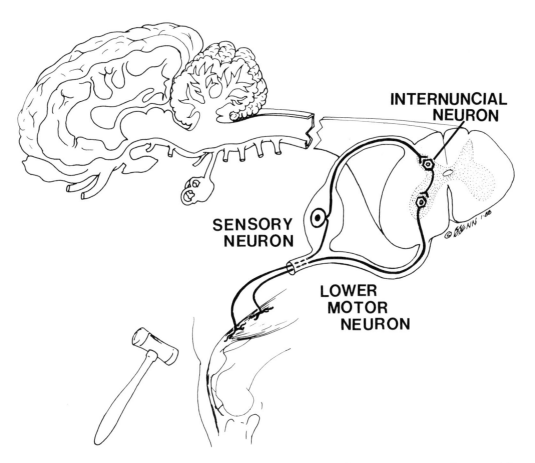

Figure 1–1. Simple reflex pathway (patellar reflex), showing the sensory neuron, internuncial neuron, and lower motor neuron in relation to the rest of the nervous system.

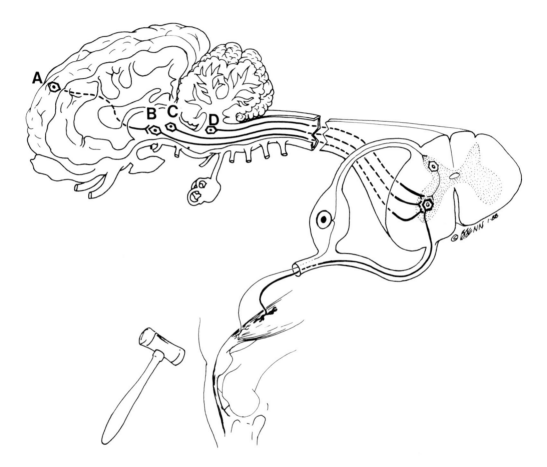

Figure 1–2. Motor pathways, showing several descending upper motor neuron pathways synapsing on the lower motor neuron of the reflex pathway. These descending pathways include cortico(rubro)spinal (A), rubrospinal (B), reticulospinal (C), and vestibulospinal (D) tracts.

nent abnormality in gait. After the acute effects of such lesions have resolved there can be deficits in subtle motor functions, such as jumping high fences and hopping on the thoracic limb opposite the side of the lesion. In contrast, brainstem lesions in the midbrain and medulla oblongata usually result in hemiparesis or tetraparesis because of damage to UMN centers and tracts, such as the rubrospinal and reticulospinal pathways. These UMN pathways tend to have a calming effect on reflexes, particularly those involved with supporting the body against gravity, such as the patellar reflex. Their major role, however, is to direct the various LMNs in voluntary movement.

Just as higher centers help control the LMN within the reflex arcs, the sensory inputs to these arcs are relayed to higher centers to give feedback on position sense (proprioception), and touch and pain perception (nociception) (Fig. 1–3). Ascending pathways travel to the thalamus and probably the sensory cerebral cortex for the perception of pain. These pathways are primarily multisynaptic and contain small fibers, which makes them resistant to interruption. Proprioceptive pathways, which are presumed to be consciously perceived, travel to thalamic and cerebral, conscious proprioceptive centers. Other unconscious proprioceptive information is contained in spinocerebellar tracts that ascend directly to the cerebellum.

Damage to the spinal cord at the level of a reflex arc and its LMN will denervate the effector muscle, resulting in flaccid paralysis with atonia and areflexia at the level of the lesion. In contrast, a similar severe lesion cranial to a reflex arc will result in spastic paralysis. This is characterized by a similar loss of voluntary motor function, but the reflex is unaffected. Indeed, the reflex may be released from the calming influence of its UMN and be hyperactive with concomitant spasticity or stiffness in the part (limb). When a UMN lesion causes a degree of spastic paralysis, involvement of adjacent proprioceptive and nociceptive pathways also results in ataxia and possibly hypalgesia, respectively.

The cerebellum is the major coordinating center for voluntary movement (Fig. 1–4). It synthesizes impulses received from the cerebral cortex, the brainstem UMN centers, and spinocerebellar proprioceptive pathways, and provides feedback impulses to the UMN centers to coordinate all motor function.

Cranial nerves, numbering I through XII, leave the forebrain and brainstem (Fig. 1–5). Some are involved with specialized modalities, such as smell (I), sight (II), and balance and hearing (VIII). Some innervate eyeball muscles (III, IV, VI), muscles of facial expression (VII), pharynx and larynx (IX, X), and tongue (XII). Others are involved with reflex function, such as facial reflexes (V, VII) and the gag reflex (IX, X). These cranial LMNs have UMN centers controlling them. They can be paralyzed by a lesion at the level of the cranial nerve or its nucleus (LMN lesion), or by a lesion affecting the descending motor pathways (UMN lesion). As with spinal reflexes, in the latter case the structure (e.g., face) shows spastic paralysis with intact or hyperactive reflexes.

Consciousness or mental awareness must be maintained for neurologic functions to occur. Numerous sensory inputs, including light, sound, touch, and metabolic and endocrine factors, interact on an area of the brainstem known as the reticular activating system (Fig. 1–6). This system, by relaying impulses to the cerebral hemispheres, maintains higher centers in this state of awareness and activity.

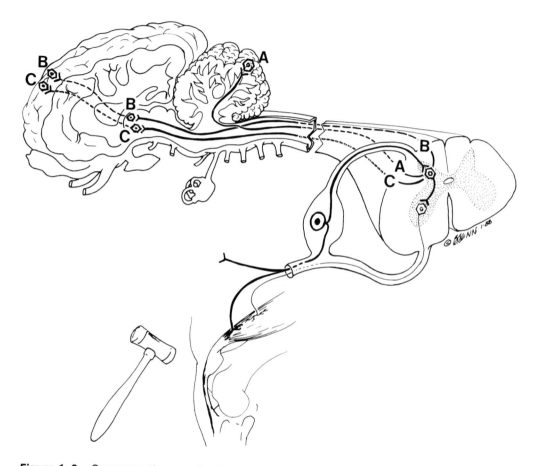

Figure 1–3. Sensory pathways, showing sensory neuron and ascending unconscious (A) and conscious (B) proprioceptive pathways, and nociceptive/pain (C) pathways.

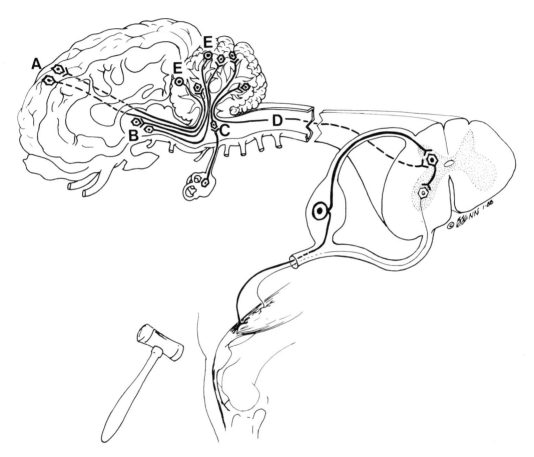

Figure 1–4. Important cerebellar connections. These include afferent input from cerebrocortical (A) and brain stem (B) motor areas, vestibular centers (C), and spinocerebellar pathways (D). Efferent cerebellar pathways from Purkinje neurons (E) connect to brain stem (B) and cerebrocortical (A) motor areas.

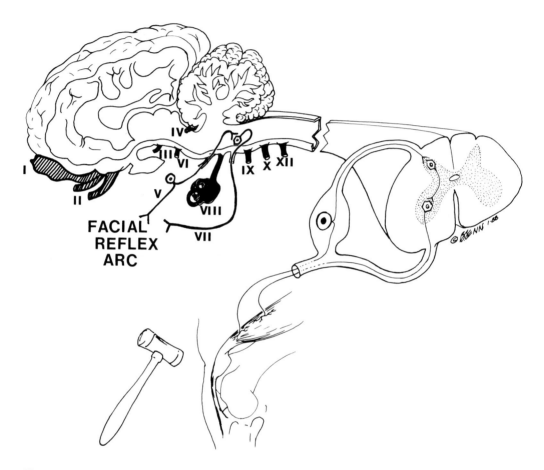

FACIAL REFLEX ARC

Figure 1–5. Cranial nerves. Some are involved with specialized modalities such as smell (I), sight (II), and balance and hearing (VIII). Others innervate eyeball muscles (III, IV, VI), facial muscles (VII), pharynx and larynx (IX, X), and the tongue (XII), while some are involved with reflex function, such as facial reflexes (V-VII), similar to spinal reflex arcs.

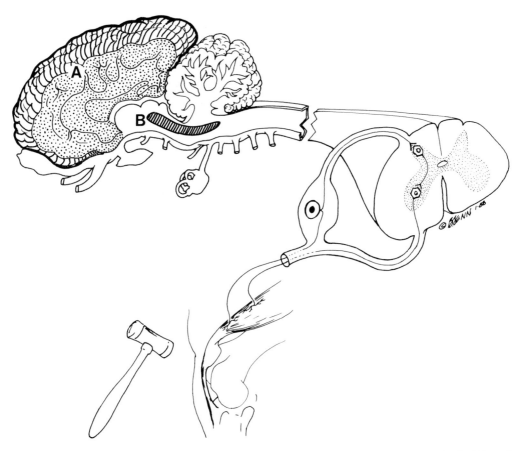

Figure 1–6. Areas maintaining consciousness or a state of alertness are the forebrain (A) and particularly the brain stem reticular activating system (B). Both areas receive input from many parts of the nervous system and are interconnected.

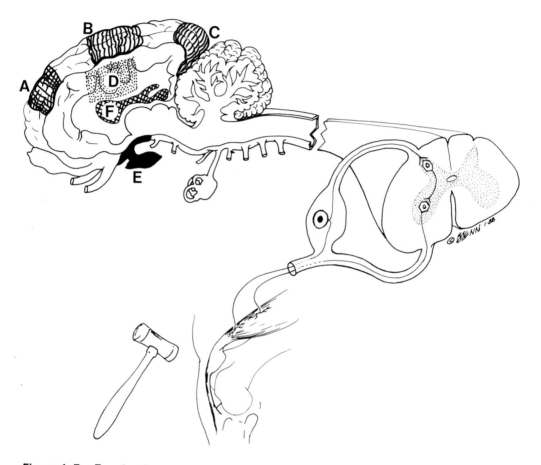

Figure 1–7. Functional areas of the forebrain include: the frontal cortex (A) involved with mentation, behavior, and fine motor activity; the parietal cortex (B) involved in pain perception and conscious proprioception; the occipital cortex (C) involved in vision; the temporal cortex (D) involved in behavior and hearing; the hypothalamus and pituitary (E) involved with autonomic and endocrine functions; and the deep-seated limbic system (F) involved with inherent behavior.

Finally, specialized areas of the higher functional centers exist in the forebrain, some of which have been introduced above (Fig. 1–7). The frontal and prefrontal cerebral lobes are involved with mentation, behavior, and fine motor activity. As in humans, the parietal lobes synthesize conscious proprioceptive and nociceptive input in the large animal species. Certainly, vision appears to require an intact occipital cortex in large animals. Control of normal (learned) behavior and perception of sound may be functions of the temporal lobes, whereas the deeper, old part of the brain, known as the limbic system, may be involved with inherent behavior patterns. Lastly, the hypothalamus and pituitary control autonomic and endocrine functions of the body.

With this understanding of functional neuroanatomy and a little practice, a neurologic examination can be performed and interpreted simply. An outline of such a neurologic examination is given in the next chapter.

BIBLIOGRAPHY

Crosby EC, Humphrey T, Lauer EW. *Correlative Anatomy of the Nervous System.* New York: Macmillan, 1962.
de Lahunta A. *Veterinary Neuroanatomy and Clinical Neurology.* 2nd Ed. Philadelphia: WB Saunders, 1983.
Jenkins TW. *Functional Mammalian Neuroanatomy.* 2nd Ed. Philadelphia: Lea & Febiger, 1978.
Peele TL. *The Neuroanatomic Basis of Clinical Neurology.* 3rd Ed. New York: McGraw-Hill, 1977.

CHAPTER 2

Neurologic Evaluation

A. OVERVIEW

Traditionally, a detailed neurologic examination follows the collection of information on a patient's signalment and history, an evaluation of the environment, and a complete physical examination. However, during evaluation of a large animal suspected of having a neurologic disorder, most busy practitioners include several components of a neurologic examination during the general physical examination. These should include observation of behavior, mental status, head posture, vision, pupillary light reflexes, structures of the eye, and inspection for facial symmetry, and inspection of the oral cavity. A laryngeal adductor response should be performed on horses, and evaluation of posture and gait while walking, trotting, and turning quickly ought to be included. Inspection and palpation for muscle mass, bony integrity, and patches of sweating over the body and limbs (horse) are also easily incorporated into this examination. Tail and anal tone and reflexes can be evaluated when the rectal temperature is recorded.

Usually, this examination allows the practitioner to decide whether a more detailed neurologic examination, as outlined below, is required.

Sometimes enough evidence is available from this examination to make a fairly accurate anatomic diagnosis. Thus, a differential diagnosis and initial plan can be developed. If this cannot be done, especially if a thorough case work-up is indicated, then a complete neurologic examination should be undertaken, which will probably uncover further neurologic findings helpful to case work-up.

B. SIGNALMENT

The age, breed, gender, use, and value of a patient all are important considerations in the diagnosis and prognosis of many neurologic conditions. Several diseases are age-dependent. Certain diseases are associated with particular breeds (see Appendix I). Only a few neurologic diseases depend upon gender. Certain uses to which animals are put can be associated with certain diseases, and this impacts considerably on the prognosis that accompanies the diagnosis. Because many large animals are kept for economic purposes, the value of the patient must always be kept in mind with respect to the depth of evaluation, cost of therapy, and future productivity; the survival of its herdmates must also be considered.

C. HISTORY

In addition to taking a general history of the patient, questioning of the client should focus on the primary complaint. Information concerning the precise circumstances of the environment, other animal contacts, and the nature of the first signs observed ought to be sought first. Further questioning is aimed at defining a relationship between the severity of the syndrome and the passage of time.

Most congenital and familial diseases begin early in life and signs usually progress relentlessly. Syndromes resulting from physical causes, particularly external injury, have a sudden onset and then often stabilize or improve. Signs caused by infectious agents can be acute or chronic, and frequently fluctuate in severity. Immune-mediated diseases often result in fulminant signs that can improve dramatically, particularly with therapy. Progression of metabolic, toxic, and nutritional disorders is variable. Finally, signs due to neoplastic involvement of the nervous system may begin abruptly, but most often are progressive.

Historical data can give clues as to how widespread or focal the disease process is in the nervous system, whether there was evidence of asymmetry, and how severe the signs have been. These aspects of pathogenesis of diseases can also be helpful in the etiologic diagnosis. (See Neuropathology, Chapter 4.)

D. PROCEDURE FOR THE NEUROLOGIC EXAMINATION

The primary aim of a neurologic examination is to confirm whether or not a neurologic abnormality exists. Because omission of parts is the most common mistake made during the neurologic examination, the order in which the examination is performed becomes important. I give here a precise practical format that is logical in sequence, easy to remember with practice, and emphasizes the need for an anatomic diagnosis (where is the lesion?) to be made before an etiologic diagnosis (what caused it?) is made. The rationale for the sequence of this examination is: firstly, it starts at the head and proceeds caudally to the tail; secondly, it is used for patients of all sizes and species, and whether the patient is ambulatory or recumbent; thirdly, it considers the anatomic location of lesions as the examination proceeds. Even if parts of the examination must be omitted because of the nature of the patient, suspicion of fracture, or financial constraints, the sequence ought to be followed through mentally. Frequently, the presence of a neurologic lesion(s) cannot be deducted until the end of a thorough neurologic examination. The following is an outline of the neurologic examination for large animal practitioners.

Different authors use different approaches to the neurologic examination. Some of these other approaches are given in the bibliography.

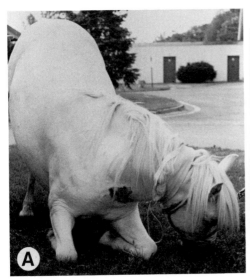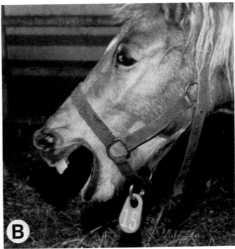

Figure 2–1. Signs of abnormal behavior in horses indicative of cerebral dysfunction may be as dramatic as adoption of abnormal postures and head pressing (A), or may be as subtle as continual yawning (B).

1. Head

a. Behavior

Question the owner about the patient's behavior and normal response patterns. Age, breed, and gender may influence behavior. Sometimes, auditory and tactile stimulation will elicit seizure activity. Partial seizures in neonatal animals may be seen as "chewing gum fits," facial twitching, or periods of tachypnea. Bizarre and inappropriate behavior, such as head pressing, compulsive wandering, circling, changes in voice and appetite, licking objects, and aggressiveness, usually is easy to recognize (Fig. 2–1A). Other subtle behavioral abnormalities, such as continual yawning (Fig. 2–1B), can be regarded as signs of cerebral disease. An animal with a cerebral lesion that compulsively circles tends to circle toward the side of the lesion.

b. Mental Status

An assessment of mental status is made based on the patient's level of awareness or consciousness. The animal's level of responsiveness to its internal and external environment is effected by the ascending reticular activating system (ARAS) in the brainstem, and by the cerebral hemispheres. These can be affected by stimuli received by the sensory nervous system. Coma is a state of complete unresponsiveness to noxious stimuli. The deepest comas usually are related to brainstem, particularly midbrain, lesions. Semicoma is a state of partial responsiveness to stimuli. Other, less profound, levels of loss of awareness are variously described as stupor, obtundation, somnolence, deliriousness, lethargy, and depression. Large animals that are recumbent because of spinal cord disease usually are bright and alert unless they are anorectic, dehydrated, exhausted, or unduly frightened.

c. Head Posture and Coordination

All normal animals maintain the head in a certain posture and maneuver it quickly and smoothly to perform acts such as prehension of food. Lesions involving the vestibular system often cause a mild head tilt that is characterized by the poll deviating laterally while the caudal neck and the muzzle remain on the median plane (Fig. 2–2A). In comparison, a horse with a cerebral lesion that continually turns in circles often has the head and neck deviated to one side. In this case, the poll is not rotated about the muzzle and the muzzle deviates from the median plane (Fig. 2–2B). The presence of a head tilt should be evaluated for only when the muzzle and neck are held as close to the median plane as possible. A severe vestibular lesion can result in a significant head tilt and head and neck turn—usually both toward the side of the lesion. Animals with bilateral (peripheral) vestibular disease frequently show wide swinging movements of the head and neck.

A musculoskeletal disorder must be considered if there is any asymmetry or deviated head and neck posture. Additionally, congenitally blind horses may have abnormal head posture, including a true head tilt along with jerky head movements, and corresponding eyeball deviations. Such a syndrome may be equivalent to amblyopia in children. In addition, congenital, asymmetric strabismus in horses has been associated with a head tilt with no other evidence of vestibular involvement, and abnormal head posture can be seen in Appaloosa horses with night blindness.

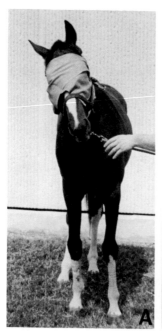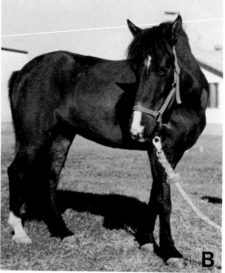

Figure 2–2. The difference between a right head tilt (A) and a right head and neck turn (B) is important. A head tilt most often is indicative of asymmetric vestibular disease, which has been accentuated by blindfolding the horse in A. A head turn usually is associated with asymmetric forebrain disease, such as cerebral abscesses, which the pony in B is suffering from. Most often, the lesion is on the side towards which the head is tilted or turned.

The cerebellum modulates movement of the head and limbs. With cerebellar disease, the fine control of head positioning is often lost, resulting in awkward jerky movements. Even at rest, the lack of control is often seen as bobbing movements of the head, which can be exaggerated by increasing voluntary effort. The resulting fine jerky movements of the head are called intention tremor. Such animals will overshoot when positioning their head, when moving to eat, for example. Newborn foals normally hold their head flexed slightly on the neck (Fig. 2–3) and move it in a jerky manner, especially in response to visual or tactile stimuli.

Animals with neck pain may hold their neck in a fixed position and be reluctant to move the head and neck. Also, diseases causing neck weakness may result in an animal carrying its head lower to the ground. Examples of this include diffuse neuromuscular weakness, which is seen with botulism, and extensive cervical spinal cord lower motor neuron (gray matter) lesions, which are seen in equine protozoal myeloencephalitis. Finally, an extended neck posture may indicate a severe cerebral disorder, such as polioencephalomalacia of ruminants (when it is referred to as "star-gazing"), and diseases causing increased muscle tone, such as tetanus.

d. Cranial Nerves

Abnormalities found in the cranial nerve (CN) examination help in localizing a lesion near or within the brainstem. One should start with the nerve most rostral and proceed caudally, assessing the function of each cranial nerve. In practice it is convenient to evaluate parts of the head and face as outlined on the neurologic examination forms (Figs. 2–19 to 2–20). Thus the evaluation moves from the eyes, face, jaws, and mouth to the pharynx and larynx. When the examination is complete, deficiencies can be related to specific cranial nerves.

I, Olfactory Nerve. Normal function usually is equated with the patient's ability to smell the hand of the examiner or its feed. However, because such

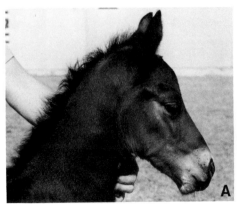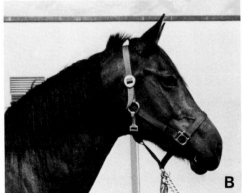

Figure 2–3. The normal head posture of a neonatal foal (A) is quite different from that of an adult horse (B), the head being held flexed more upon the neck in a foal. Additionally, note the different shape of the forehead of a normal newborn thoroughbred foal that does not have hydrocephalus (A).

stimuli can irritate the nasal mucosa, this test evaluates the sensory branch of the trigeminal (V) nerve, as well as cranial nerve I.

II, Optic Nerve. An owner may report that a patient appears to be blind. However, a depressed animal, or one with loss of balance (vestibular disease), may stumble over objects without being blind.

The visual pathway is tested by the menace, blink, or eye preservation response. A threatening gesture of the hand towards the eye elicits immediate closure of the eyelids; the head may be jerked away. In large animals 80 to 90% crossing of optic nerve fibers occurs at the chiasm (Herran et al., 1978). However, for practical purposes, vision in one eye is perceived in the visual cortex of the opposite (contralateral) cerebral hemisphere. The incoming (afferent) pathway for the menace response is the ipsilateral eye and optic nerve, optic chiasm, and contralateral optic tract, lateral geniculate nucleus (thalamus), optic radiation, and occipital visual cortex (Fig. 2–4). The outgoing (efferent) pathway of the menace response is from this contralateral visual cortex to the ipsilateral facial nucleus effecting closure of the eyelids. It is because of this efferent pathway that it can be assumed the visual input reaches the visual cortex. Some stoic, depressed, or even excited animals may not respond to a menace with closure of the eyelids, or they may keep the eyelids closed. A true visual deficiency may be detected while the animal moves about its environment, when objects are placed in front of it, or when nonaromatic objects are dropped noiselessly in its visual field. Partial, unilateral blindness (hemianopia) can be difficult to detect and it may take repeated efforts, such as blindfolding each eye in turn, to determine this.

An ophthalmologic examination should be included in the neurologic evaluation. Lesions of the eye and optic nerve result in ipsilateral blindness. Lesions of the optic tracts and lateral geniculate nucleus cause contralateral blindness.

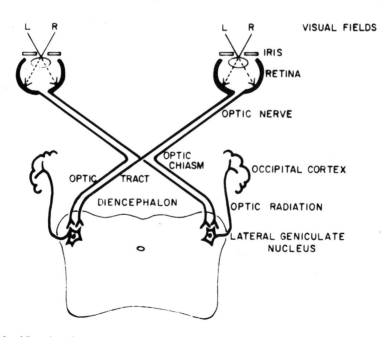

Figure 2–4. Visual pathway.

Space occupying lesions of the brain frequently produce blindness. Animals with various diffuse cerebellar diseases have been observed to have bilaterally deficient menace responses. These animals are not blind, do not have facial paralysis which would explain the menace deficit, and they pull their head away from the menacing gesture, thus demonstrating degrees of amblyopia. It has been assumed that the pathway for the menace response passes from the contralateral occipital cortex, through the ipsilateral cerebellum, and then to the facial nucleus. It is more likely that the cerebellum exerts both stimulatory and inhibitory influences on many cerebral functions, including visual responses (McCormick et al., 1984). Cerebellar disease interferes with these modulating influences, thereby effecting an altered menace response. Foals and calves appear to be able to see by a few hours of age, but do not blink at a menacing gesture until several days of age. They do blink in response to bright light and pull their heads away from a menacing gesture, often in a jerky manner.

III, Oculomotor Nerve. The diameter of the pupillary aperture is controlled by the constrictor muscles of the pupil, which are innervated by the parasympathetic fibers in the oculomotor nerve, and by the dilator muscles of the pupil, which are innervated by the sympathetic fibers from the cranial cervical ganglion (Figs. 2–5, 2–6, 2–7). These autonomic innervations originate from higher centers in the brainstem, and change pupil diameter in response to light (oculomotor nerve), and fear and excitement (sympathetic).

The first observation is the size and symmetry of the pupillary apertures, considering the amount of ambient light and the emotional status of the patient. The response of the pupils to light directed into each eye—the pupillary light responses—can be noted after observing the eyeballs for any lesions that may interfere with the response of the pupil, such as iritis, iris atrophy, or adhesions. The normal response to light directed into one eye is constriction of both pupils;

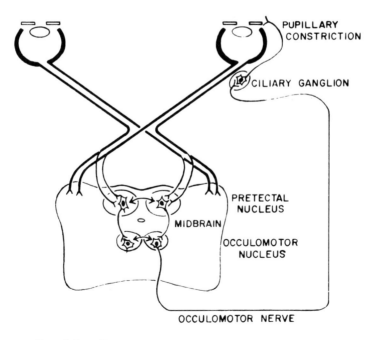

Figure 2–5. Pupillary light reflex.

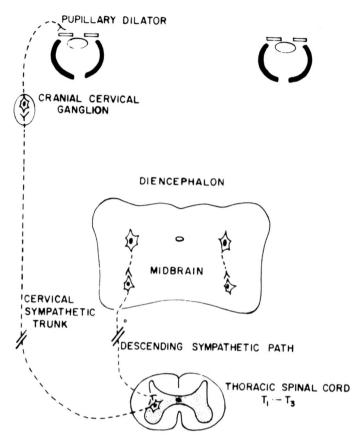

Figure 2–6. Sympathetic pupillary pathway.

this is referred to as a direct response in the same (ipsilateral) eye in which one shines the light and a consensual response in the other (contralateral) eye. The incoming (afferent) pathway for this reflex is similar to that for the menace response to the level of the thalamus. The pathway goes through the optic nerve and optic chiasm (where crossing occurs), through the optic tracts laterally and dorsally to the thalamus, then passes ventrally into the midbrain. Crossover and interconnections occur at this site so that axons pass to the parasympathetic oculomotor nuclei in the midbrain on both sides. The motor (efferent) pathway is from these nuclei (via the oculomotor nerves), to the ciliary ganglia behind the eyeball, and to the constrictor muscles of the pupils (Fig. 2–5).

Because consensual pupillary light responses are awkward to perform alone in large animals, the swinging-light test is a useful alternative. Starting from a distance of approximately 18 in., the light is shone alternately into each eye and the more powerful, direct pupillary light response in an eye is observed as the light reaches it. Most unilateral, afferent pathway lesions in the eyeball, optic nerve, chiasm, or tract to the level of the midbrain, will allow an ipsilateral dilation of the pupil to occur when light reaches the affected eye. This test takes specific advantage of the fact that the ipsilateral pupillary light response is more powerful than the contralateral (consensual) response.

These pupillary light reflexes are within the brainstem and thus are not

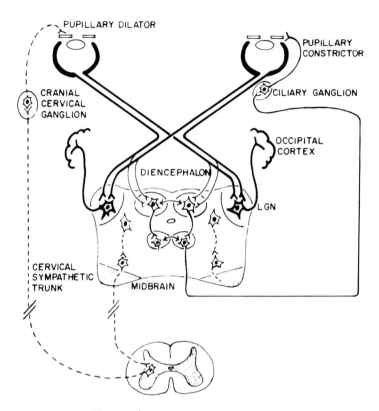

Figure 2–7. Visual and pupillary pathways.

affected by lesions involving the visual cerebral cortex. A widely dilated (mydriatic) pupil in an eye that has normal vision suggests an oculomotor nerve lesion; the pupil being unresponsive to light directed into either eye. The pupil in the contralateral eye, with normal oculomotor function, responds to light directed into both the ipsilateral (direct response) and contralateral (consensual response) eye. The oculomotor nerves are subject to damage from diffuse cerebral swelling and space-occupying lesions in the forebrain. Both can cause pressure to be exerted onto the brainstem. With asymmetric swelling of the cerebral tissue, greater pressure may be applied to one oculomotor nerve. This results in unequal pupils (anisocoria), which is usually evident as ipsilateral pupillary dilation. A severe brainstem contusion can produce various pupillary abnormalities in association with coma or semicoma, and these can change rapidly in the first few hours following injury. Progressive, bilateral, pupillary dilation following cranial injury warrants a grave prognosis.

Nuclei within the brain that control sympathetic motor function are located in the hypothalamus, midbrain, pons, and medulla. First order neuronal fibers descend through the midbrain, medulla, and cervical spinal cord to synapse on cell bodies in the lateral intermediate gray columns in the thoracolumbar spinal cord. The preganglionic, second-order, sympathetic cell bodies supplying the head are situated in this position in the cranial thoracic segments (T_1-T_3). Axons leave these segments of the spinal cord, traverse the thorax, ascend the neck in the cervical sympathetic trunk adjacent to the vagus nerve, and pass to the cranial cervical ganglion that lies under the cranial part of the atlas. In the horse, this ganglion is on the caudodorsal wall of the medial compartment of the guttural pouch. Postganglionic, third-order, sympathetic fibers leave the cranial cervical ganglion to innervate the glands, smooth muscle, and blood vessels of the eyeball, head, and cranial cervical area (Fig. 2–6).

Damage to the sympathetic supply of the eyeball results in Horner's syndrome, which is seen as a slight ptosis of the upper lid, a miosis (constriction) of the pupil, and a slight protrusion of the nictitating membrane. Vision and the pupillary light response are unaffected. In the horse, lesions involving the sympathetic supply to the head result in these ophthalmic signs, as well as additional signs consisting of dilation of facial blood vessels, hyperemia of nasal and conjunctival mucous membranes, and increased temperature and sweating of the face. Sweating is most prominent at the base of the ear and is present over the neck, down to about the level of the atlas with postganglionic lesions, and to the level of the axis with preganglionic lesions (Usenik, 1957). These signs have been seen with various lesions of the sympathetic pathways in the guttural pouches, in the area of the cervical vagosympathetic trunk, and at the thoracic inlet.

Cattle that have lost the sympathetic supply to the head show Horner's syndrome in the eye, dilated blood vessels over the pinna, and lack of sweat production on the muzzle. Only eye signs have been detected with Horner's syndrome in sheep and goats.

Horner's syndrome can be expected to occur with large lesions involving the descending sympathetic pathways in the brainstem and cervical spinal cord. With such lesions in horses, there also will be excessive sweating over the whole affected side of the body because all the sympathetic pathways leaving the spinal cord have lost their central (upper motor neuron) connections.

III, Oculomotor Nerve; IV, Trochlear Nerve, VI, Abducens Nerve. In addition to innervation of the pupillary constrictor muscles, the oculomotor nerve also innervates the extraocular muscles, along with the trochlear and abducens nerves. These muscles and nerves are tested by observing normal position of the eyes within the bony orbits (Fig. 2–8) and by observing eye movement. An abnormal position (strabismus) results when these nerves or muscles are damaged.

When evaluating eye position and movement, consideration must be given to the normal response of the eyes to head posture and movement. When the nose of a large animal is elevated (head extended), the eyes tend to maintain a horizontal axis and thus move ventrally in the bony orbits (Fig. 2–9). As the head is moved to one side, the eyes move in a rhythmical manner until head movement stops. There is slow phase movement in the direction opposite the direction of head movement, which is followed by a fast phase in the direction of movement. These eye movements are regarded as normal vestibular nystagmus and result from the connection between balance centers (vestibular nuclei) in the medulla and the nuclei of the cranial nerves controlling eye movement (III, IV, VI). Normal vestibular nystagmus thus requires an intact vestibular system, intact cranial nerves III, IV, and VI, and the connection between all of these (Fig. 2–10).

The forms of strabismus described for paralysis of each of these cranial nerves should be present in all positions of the head. Such examples of true

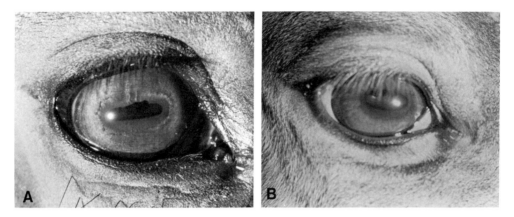

Figure 2–8. The normal posture of the eye of an adult horse is such that the pupillary fissure is almost horizontal (A). In contrast, in a neonatal foal the nasal region of the pupillary fissure is rotated ventrally (B). This apparent ventromedial strabismus slowly disappears so that the eyeball of a weanling foal is like that of an adult.

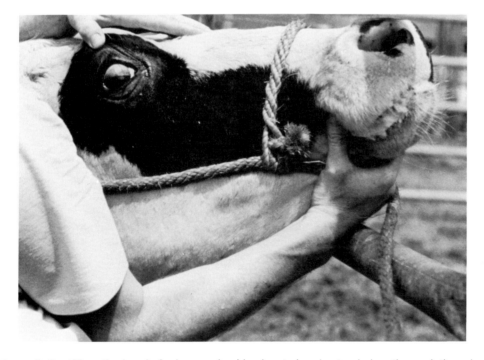

Figure 2–9. When the head of a large animal is elevated and extended on the neck there is a tendency for the eyes to maintain a constant visual axis, which results in a lowering of the globes within their bony orbit: the normal vestibular eyedrop. This is mediated by the vestibular system and its connections with the cranial nerves (III, IV, VI) innervating extraocular muscles (see Fig. 2–10).

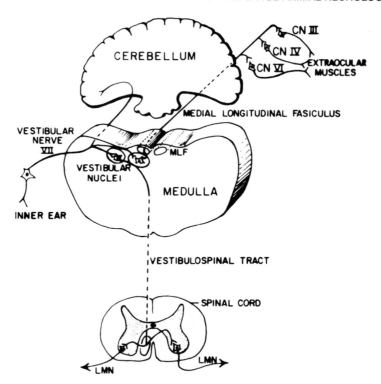

Figure 2–10. Vestibular system.

strabismus are rarely encountered in large animals. Mydriasis is seen with oculomotor nerve disease. A tendency for lateral eyeball deviation has been observed in horses with midbrain (oculomotor) lesions. The dorsomedial, rotational positioning of the eyeball, seen in many diffuse brain diseases in ruminants (especially polioencephalomalacia), may not be a true trochlear paralysis, as the eyeballs can be moved from this position by moving the head. What is most frequently seen in large animals is a deviation of the eyeballs resulting from a disturbance of the vestibular system that alters the normal tonic mechanism controlling eye position. This strabismus is usually ipsilateral to the vestibular lesion. It usually is ventral, but may be medial. The important difference is that the eyeballs can be moved out of this position. Periorbital lesions, particularly trauma and neoplasms, often result in mechanical eye deviations. The eyeball position of newborn foals often is ventromedial, relative to that of adult horses. Also, animals that are congenitally blind may have abnormal eyeball positioning and movement.

By observing the corneal reflex, one can assess sensation from the cornea in the ophthalmic branch of the trigeminal nerve (see below) and the ability to retract the eyeball. The latter is mediated by the retractor oculi muscle innervated by the abducens nerve (VI); however, eyeball retraction in large animals may also require full innervation (III, IV, VI) and function of all extraocular muscles to be effective. Test this reflex by pressing lightly on the closed eyelids while palpating for reflex eyeball retraction, thereby avoiding potential corneal damage.

V, Trigeminal Nerve. This large cranial nerve contains motor nerve fibers that lead to the muscles of mastication in the mandibular branch, as well as sensory nerve fibers from most parts of the head in all three branches—mandibular, maxillary, and ophthalmic.

Loss of motor function of the mandibular nerve bilaterally, results in a dropped jaw and an inability to chew. The tongue may appear protruded because it drops forward in the mouth. Sialosis results because of the lack of jaw movement. After 1 to 2 weeks, atrophy of the temporal and masseter muscles and the distal belly of the digastricus muscle results. Asymmetric lesions cause asymmetric muscle atrophy, and sometimes a slightly deviated lower jaw, without dysphagia. Normal horses frequently have visible asymmetry of the temporalis musculature.

Function of the sensory branches of this cranial nerve is tested reflexly and directly by assessing sensation to the head. Movements of the ear, eyelids, and lower lips, in response to light pricking, are mediated via the sensory branches of the trigeminal nerve and the motor branches of the facial nerve. Thus these reflexes require an intact brainstem and trigeminal and facial nuclei and nerves, but do not require the animal to feel the stimulus. Perception of sensation from the head should be assessed in the distribution of each of the major branches of the trigeminal nerve by observing a behavioral response such as head shaking. In stoic or depressed animals, sensation may be assessed from lightly pricking the internal nares and nasal septum. Lesions of the sensory nucleus of the trigeminal nerve in the lateral medulla oblongata can cause hypalgesia and hyporeflexia of the face, without weakness of the muscles of mastication. This may result in feed impacting in the rostral cheek pouch. It has been observed, especially in horses, that extensive cerebral lesions can produce a contralateral facial hypalgesia without hyporeflexia, which is most evident in the nasal septum. This is due to the involvement of the parietal (sensory) cerebral lobe while sparing the trigeminal nuclei and reflex pathways in the brainstem.

VII, Facial Nerve. This is predominantly a motor nerve innervating the muscles of facial expression, as well as the lacrimal and certain salivary glands. It contains the lower motor neurons for movement of the ears, eyelids, lips, and nostrils, in addition to the motor pathways of the menace, palpebral, and corneal reflexes. Facial paralysis is generally seen as a drooping of the ear, ptosis of the upper eyelid, drooping of the upper lip, and a pulling of the nostrils toward the unaffected side. General inspection for symmetry of facial expression is useful. Some normal horses do appear to have asymmetric external nares and a subtle deviation of the nostrils to one side. Very close inspection is required, especially in food animals, to detect a partial facial paresis. Comparison of tone in the ears, eyelids, and lips on each side may help to detect facial weakness. Occasionally a small amount of food may remain in the cheeks on the affected side. This must not be confused with the dysphagia, which results from sensory and/or motor trigeminal paralysis. Because of lack of muscle tone, saliva may drool from the commissure of the lips with facial paralysis. If only weakness of the lips and a deviated nasal philtrum without a drooped ear and ptosis occur, probably only the buccal branches along the side of the face are involved. As with other cranial nerves, a diagnosis of central, as compared to peripheral nerve involvement can be made by identifiying involvement of adjacent structures in the medulla oblongata. Signs such as depression, weakness, and a head tilt would result. With lesions of the inner (and middle) ear, which cause vestibular signs, there often is accompanying facial nerve paralysis because the facial nerve is only separated from the tympanic cavity by a thin membrane. Lack of involvement of other central pathways is used to differentiate signs of peripheral facial and vestibular nerve disease from involvement of their nuclei and pathways in the medulla oblongata.

With various focal thalamic and cerebral lesions in horses, the facial muscles may be hypertonic and hyperreflexic, resulting in spontaneous and reflexive grimacing of the face. This is due to the involvement of the higher motor centers controlling facial movement (upper motor neuron) that normally calm the facial nucleus and the facial reflexes. Importantly, the facial reflexes are intact, and may be hyperactive. Irritative lesions, such as peracute encephalitis, meningitis, and facial neuritis, can cause facial grimacing also.

VIII, Vestibulocochlear Nerve. The cochlear (auditory) division of this nerve transmits impulses involved with hearing. Bilateral middle ear disease causes deafness, but unilateral hearing loss would be difficult to detect.

The vestibular division of cranial nerve VIII supplies the major input to the vestibular system, thereby controlling balance. Fibers from the inner ear pass through the internal acoustic meatus in the petrosal bone and penetrate the lateral medulla oblongata to terminate in the vestibular nuclei. A few fibers pass to small areas on the cerebellum that are part of the vestibular system. The vestibular system receives input from many higher centers and from the cerebellum; it functions by controlling orientation of the head, body, limbs, and eyes in space (Fig. 2–10). Signs of vestibular disease can be seen with lesions involving any part of the vestibular system. The eyeballs are checked for normal vestibular nystagmus when the head is moved from side to side. The presence of nystagmus with the head in a normal position (spontaneous) and with the head held still in various abnormal positions (positional) indicates a disorder of the vestibular system. In peripheral vestibular system disorders the nystagmus (fast phase) is directed away from the side of the lesion and away from the direction of the head tilt. It usually is horizontal, although it may be rotary or arc-shaped. Only in one horse with peracute signs of bilateral vestibular neuritis, histologically consistent with neuritis of the cauda equina/polyneuritis equi, has transient, dorsally directed nystagmus been observed with peripheral (in this case bilateral) vestibular disorders. With lesions involving the central components of the vestibular system in the medulla oblongata, spontaneous and positional nystagmus may be horizontal, vertical, or rotary and also may change direction with changes in head posture. Such lesions frequently affect adjacent structures, such as the proprioceptive and motor pathways for voluntary limb movement, and the reticular formation, resulting in ataxia, tetraparesis, and depression, respectively. Particularly with acute peripheral vestibular disease, signs often improve within several days because of accommodation, which is probably mediated by other inputs to the vestibular system, including proprioceptive modalities and vision. By blindfolding an animal that has accommodated to a vestibular disease, signs frequently become exacerbated immediately. Conversely, blindness interferes with recovery from vestibular disease.

IX, Glossopharyngeal Nerve; X, Vagus Nerve; XI, Accessory Nerve. A major function of these cranial nerves is achieved through innervation of the pharynx and larynx with both sensory and motor fibers. This is tested by listening for normal laryngeal sounds, observing normal swallowing of food and water, assessing the swallowing reflex by passage of a gastric tube, and finally by inspection of the larynx and pharynx manually, or with an endoscope if necessary. The major centers for control of the pharnyx and larynx via these three cranial nerves are the nucleus ambiguus and nucleus solitarius in the caudal medulla oblongata. The most important clinical signs of deficit are related to paralysis of the pharynx and larynx. The severity of signs depends on whether there is unilateral or bilateral involvement. In pharyngeal paralysis usually food and water can be seen at the nostrils in horses, and at the nostrils and mouth in ruminants. During exercise, unilateral paralysis of the larynx results in an abnormal respiratory noise (roaring) in horses, but usually is subclinical in sedentary animals. Stertorous breathing may be detected with diseases that cause bilateral pharyngeal or laryngeal paralysis.

In the horse, the laryngeal adductor response, or slap test, should be performed (Greet et al., 1980). The skin just caudal to the dorsal part of the scapula is slapped gently with a hand during expiration while the larynx is observed with an endoscope. The contralateral dorsal and lateral laryngeal musculature, over the muscular process of the arytenoid cartilage, can also be palpated with the fingers while the withers are slapped. The normal response to a slap on the withers is brief adduction of the contralateral arytenoid cartilage. This has been detected in cooperative foals as early as 2 weeks of age. Usually this

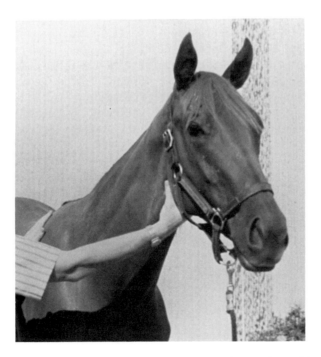

Figure 2–11. Laryngeal adductor response testing (slap test) is performed by slapping a hand on the withers and observing, with an endoscope, adduction of the contralateral arytenoid cartilage. A repeatable form of the test can be performed by palpating for movement of the contralateral, dorsolateral laryngeal musculature with one hand while slapping the withers during expiration with the other hand.

response can be felt externally as a slight tap or muscular contractions under the fingers (Fig. 2–11). The afferent pathway is through the segmental dorsal thoracic nerves, cranially to the (probably contralateral) cervical spinal cord white matter, and to the contralateral vagal nucleus in the medulla oblongata. The efferent pathway is through the vagus nerve, to the cranial thorax, then back up the neck in the recurrent laryngeal nerve to the larynx. The reflex can be interrupted at any of these sites.

Lesions in the nucleus ambiguus and in the swallowing center of the medulla oblongata usually affect adjacent structures, causing depression, ataxia, weakness, and signs of other cranial nerve involvement. Many severe, diffuse brain diseases can result in dysphagia without lesions in the medulla oblongata. This again is the result of interference with the voluntary, higher motor control of swallowing. Because of their close association with the guttural pouch, these three cranial nerves can become involved with guttural pouch diseases. Dysphagia is seen with diseases affecting pharyngeal muscles and the diffuse neuromuscular paralysis of botulism.

XI, Accessory Nerve. This nerve is motor to at least the trapezius and cranial part of the sternocephalicus muscles. Loss of function is difficult to detect, in horses at least, without an electromyographic study. Some cases of cervical scoliosis, associated with lesions such as listeriosis and equine protozoal myeloencephalitis, may involve the accessory nuclei.

XII, Hypoglossal Nerve. This last cranial nerve has its cell bodies in the hypoglossal nucleus of the caudal medulla oblongata. It is the motor nerve to muscle of the tongue. Thus, the tongue must be inspected for symmetry, normal movement, and evidence of atrophy. Normally, there is a strong resistance to withdrawing the tongue from the mouth. A unilateral lesion of the nucleus or nerve results in unilateral atrophy of the tongue, with weak retraction; however, the tongue usually will not remain protruding from the mouth. Bilateral involvement interferes with prehension and swallowing, the tongue usually protrudes, and the animal is not able to withdraw it back into the mouth. Horses that play with their tongue are referred to as tongue-chewers or tongue-suckers and appear to have poor tone in this organ.

In large animals (especially horses) with severe cerebral lesions resulting in depression, but without focal brainstem involvement, the tongue may remain protruded and be slow to return to its normal position when pulled out of the mouth. This is the result of a lesion in the higher motor centers or upper motor neuron, which controls hypoglossal function. The voluntary control pathways for function of the tongue are interfered with, causing weakness without involving the hypoglossal nuclei or nerves.

2. Gait and Posture

After completing an examination of the head, the examiner then evaluates gait and posture of the animal to give a general assessment of brainstem, spinal cord, and peripheral nerve and muscle function.

The two observations to be made when evaluating gait and posture are firstly, which limbs are abnormal, and secondly, is there evidence of lameness, suggesting a musculoskeletal gait abnormality? The essential components of neurologic gait abnormality are weakness and ataxia, the latter often having characteristics of hypometria and hypermetria. Each limb must be evaluated for evidence of these conditions. This is done while the animal is standing still, walking, trotting, turning tightly (pivoting), and backing up. To detect subtle asymmetry in the length of stride one should walk parallel to, or behind the animal, matching step for step. If possible, the gait should also be evaluated while the animal is walking up and down a slope, walking with the head and neck held extended, while blind-folded, and while running free in a field. Often subtle signs are not seen at normal gaits, but are seen as consistent mistakes while the animal performs more involved gait maneuvers. Essentially, these maneuvers comprise the postural reaction tests for large animals. Thus, input to the upper motor centers is altered through changes in many modalities, including the visual horizon, vestibular stimulation, and neck and limb proprioception, that are synthesized into refined motor system signals. Subtle neurologic abnormalities, which may be compensated for under conditions of normal gait, are exaggerated during these maneuvers.

Weakness. Weakness or paresis often is evident when an animal drags its limbs, has worn hooves, or has a low arc to the swing phase of the stride. When an animal bears weight on a weak limb, the limb often trembles and the animal may even collapse on that limb because of lack of support. While circling, walking on a slope, and walking with the head elevated, an animal frequently will stumble on a weak limb and knuckle over at the fetlock.

Pulling the mane and then pulling the tail while the animal is walking forward helps determine weakness. A weak horse is easily pulled to the side (Fig. 2–12). Also, while the animal circles, the examiner can pull on the lead rope and tail simultaneously to assess resistance (strength) (Fig. 2–13). Ease in pulling the patient to the side occurs because of weakness, which is the result

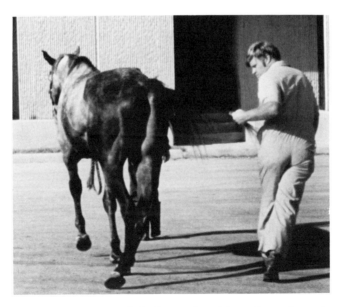

Figure 2–12. Weakness in the pelvic limbs is usually evident when a horse is not able to resist a moderate tail pull while walking. Such a weak animal will easily be pulled to the side and put off stride.

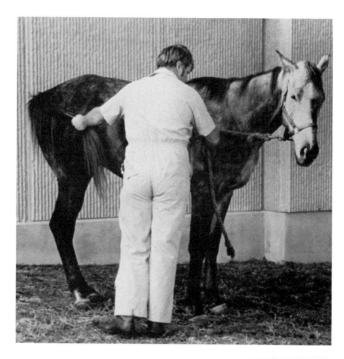

Figure 2–13. Pulling a patient to the side by holding the lead rope or halter and the tail evaluates strength. Making a horse turn in circles while doing this reveals evidence of weakness because any normal adult horse can pull an examiner around and not simply pivot on a foot or be pulled to the side.

of descending upper motor pathway involvement or because of lesions that involve ventral horn gray matter level with the limb or peripheral nerves or muscle (lower motor neuron lesions). With the latter, weakness is often profound and it is easy to pull such a patient to the side while it is standing still and while walking. In contrast, a weak animal with a lesion of the upper motor pathways usually can fix the limb in extension, reflexly, when pulled to one side; thus it resists the pull and appears strong. In this situation, the examiner is simply initiating an extensor reflex (which is intact), whereas while moving, the patient does not have the voluntary motor effort necessary to resist the pull.

With severe weakness in all four limbs, but no ataxia and spasticity, neuromuscular disease must be considered. Profound weakness in only one limb is suggestive of a peripheral nerve or muscle (lower motor neuron) lesion in that limb. Weakness occurs with descending motor pathway (upper motor neuron) lesions in the brainstem and spinal cord, and is present in the limb(s) on the same side, and caudal to, the lesion. A patient with peracute peripheral vestibular syndrome may appear weak in the limbs on the same side as the lesion. This is because of the tendency to fall in that direction, and the increased tone in the contralateral limbs.

Ataxia. Ataxia is an unconscious, general proprioceptive (GP) deficit causing poor coordination when moving the limbs and body. It is seen as a swaying from side to side of the pelvis, trunk, and sometimes the whole body. It may also appear as a weaving of the affected limb during the swing phase. This often results in abducted or adducted foot placement, crossing of the limbs, or

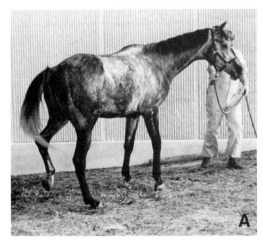 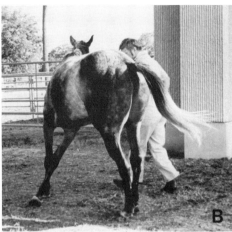

Figure 2–14. An ataxic animal often will demonstrate circumduction and some excessive flexion or hypermetria with resultant wide placement of the pelvic limbs (A), as well as twisting of the body and awkward cross-over placement of thoracic limbs (B) when being turned tightly.

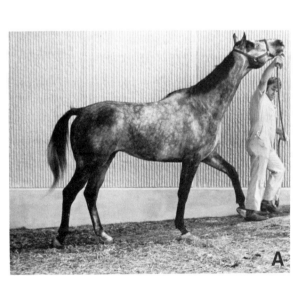 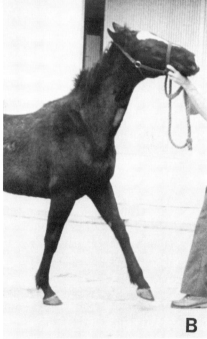

Figure 2–15. Walking a horse in a zig-zag up a slope, with the head elevated, is essentially a postural reaction test. Such a maneuver can exaggerate subtle gait abnormalities, particularly hypermetric ataxia as shown in the thoracic limbs of a horse with cervical vertebral malformation (A). In some cases hypometria becomes more apparent, as in a horse with neck trauma of long duration (B).

stepping on the opposite foot—especially while the animal is circling or turning tightly (Fig. 2–14). Any animal that is significantly ataxic, for any reason, tends to pace when walking. Circumduction of the outside limbs when turning and circling is also considered a proprioceptive deficiency. Walking an animal on a slope, with the head elevated, often exaggerates ataxia, particularly in the pelvic limbs. This maneuver frequently allows expression of a hypermetric or hypometric component of ataxia in the thoracic limbs (Fig. 2–15). When a weak and ataxic animal is turned sharply in circles, it leaves the affected limb in one place while pivoting around it. This may also occur when backing up. Blindfolding does not appear to exacerbate weakness and ataxia that is caused by spinal cord disease. However, the gait abnormality seen with vestibular or cerebellar diseases frequently worsens with blindfolding. An ataxic gait may be most pronounced when an animal is moving freely—in a paddock, or at trot or canter—especially when attempting to stop. This is when the limbs may be wildly adducted or abducted. Proprioceptive deficits are caused by lesions affecting the GP sensory pathways, which relay information on limb and body position to the cerebellum (cerebellar, or unconscious proprioception), and to the thalamus and cerebral cortex (conscious proprioception). Often it is difficult to differentiate weakness from ataxia.

Knuckling the flexed foot while the animal stands on the dorsum of the pastern, to determine how long the animal leaves the foot in this state before returning it to a normal position, is the test for conscious proprioception in dogs and cats. This can be attempted in large animals, but has not been very helpful. Depressed patients, especially calves, often allow the foot to rest on the dorsum for prolonged periods. Horses need to have almost total paralysis of the limb, or a nociceptive (pain) deficit in the limb, before they allow such testing. Other tests, such as crossing the limbs or placing one limb on a sack and slowly sliding the sack to the side, have been tried to test conscious proprioception. I prefer to suddenly stop the patient on numerous occasions, particularly while it is turning in a tight circle, to observe how long the patient adopts and holds an abnormal stance. This tests for deficiencies in conscious proprioception.

Hypermetria. Hypermetria is used to describe a lack of direction and increased range of movement, and is seen as an overreaching of the limbs with excessive joint movement (Fig. 2–15A). Hypermetria without paresis is characteristic of spinocerebellar and cerebellar disease.

Hypometria. Hypometria is seen as stiff or spastic movement of the limbs with little flexion of the joints, particularly the carpal and tarsal joints. This generally is indicative of increased extensor tone, and of a lesion affecting the descending motor, or ascending spinocerebellar pathways to that limb. A hypometric gait, particularly in the thoracic limbs, is seen best when the animal is backed up or when it is maneuvered on a slope with the head held elevated (Fig. 2–15B). The thoracic limbs may move almost without flexing and resemble a marching tin soldier. The short-strided, staggery gait seen with vestibular disease may be considered hypometria.

Dysmetria. Dysmetria is a term that incorporates both hypermetria and hypometria. Animals with severe cerebellar lesions may have a high stepping gait, but have limited movement of the distal limb joints, especially in thoracic limbs. This is best termed dysmetria.

Grading the Gait Abnormalities. The degree of weakness, ataxia, hypo-

Table 2–1.   Types of Gait Abnormalities with Various Nervous and Musculoskeletal Lesions

Site of Lesion	Ataxia	Paresis	Hypermetria	Hypometria
Brainstem or spinal cord white matter [UMN and GP]	+ +*	+ +	+ +	+ +
Vestibular system	+ +			+ +
Cerebellum	+ + +		+ + +	+ +
Ventral gray matter or motor nerves [LMN]		+ + +		
Peripheral nerves; mixed sensory and motor	+ + +	+ + +		+
Musculoskeletal system		+ +		+ +

*Sometimes present (+); often present (+ +); usually present (+ + +).

metria, and hypermetria should be graded for each limb (see Table 2–1). Generally, with focal, particularly compressive, lesions in the cervical spinal cord or brainstem, neurologic signs are one grade more severe in the pelvic limbs than in the thoracic limbs. Thus, with a mild, focal, cervical spinal cord lesion there may be a mild abnormality in the pelvic limbs with no signs in the thoracic limbs. The anatomic diagnosis in such cases may be a thoracolumbar, cervical, or diffuse spinal cord lesion. A moderate or severe abnormality in the pelvic limbs, and none in the thoracic limbs, is consistent with a thoracolumbar spinal cord lesion. With a mild, and a severe change in the thoracic and the pelvic limb gaits respectively, one must consider a severe thoracolumbar lesion plus a mild cervical lesion, or a diffuse spinal cord disease. Lesions involving the brachial intumescence (C_6-T_2), with involvement of the gray matter supplying the thoracic limbs, and diffuse spinal cord lesions may both result in a severe gait abnormality in the thoracic limbs and the pelvic limbs. A severely abnormal gait in the thoracic limbs, with normal pelvic limbs, indicates lower motor neuron involvement of the thoracic limbs; a lesion is most likely present in the ventral gray columns at C_6-T_2, or thoracic limb peripheral nerves or muscle.

Gait alterations can occur in all four limbs, with lesions affecting the white matter in the caudal brainstem, when head signs, such as cranial nerve deficits, are used to define the site of the lesion. Subacute to chronic lesions affecting the cerebrum cause no substantial change in gait. However, postural reactions, such as hopping, are abnormal and sometimes the gait is slowly initiated on the thoracic limb contralateral to the side of a cerebral lesion.

Recumbent Patient. Every effort should be made to help a recumbent patient stand and walk, unless there is suspicion of bone fracture. Heavy animals, in particular, should be moved early in the course of recumbency to avoid secondary problems like decubital sores, decreased blood supply to limbs, and dehydration, which make evaluation difficult.

3. Neck and Forelimbs

If a gait alteration was detected in the thoracic limbs and there were no signs of brain involvement, then this part of the examination can confirm involvement of the spinal cord, peripheral nerves (C_1-T_2), or thoracic limb muscles; it should also localize the lesion within these segments.

Observation and palpation of the neck and forelimbs will detect gross skeletal defects, asymmetry in the neck, and muscle atrophy. These signs may be associated with neurologic disease and thus be localizing findings. The neck should be manipulated to assess normal range of movement. Reluctance to flex the neck or pain being evident during flexion of the neck requires careful assessment before any conclusions are drawn. Cervical vertebral arthrosis, involvement of cervical nerve roots, and marked cervical spinal cord disease can cause scoliosis and even torticollis. Involvement of the peripheral pre- and postganglionic sympathetic neurons in the horse result in localized sweating; this can be an extremely helpful localizing sign. Horner's syndrome will result if the cervical sympathetic trunk is damaged. In the horse, dermatomal patterns of sweating on the neck and cranial shoulder occur with involvement of the C_3-C_8 branches of the sympathetic fibers. These arise segmentally from the vertebral nerve that follows the vertebral artery up the neck after the vertebral nerve has left the stellate ganglion near the thoracic inlet.

When the skin of the lateral neck of a horse (just above the jugular groove between the level of the atlas to the shoulder) is tapped lightly with a probe, the cutaneous colli muscle contracts, which causes skin flicking. The sternocephalicus and brachiocephalicus muscles often contract also, causing the shoulder to be pulled cranially and even the head to be flexed laterally. This response tends to be less obvious in other species. In horses, there also is flicking of the ear rostrally, blinking of the eyelids, and contracture of the labial muscles (smile) when the test is performed. Originally introduced by Rooney (1973), these are termed the local cervical and cervicofacial responses, respectively. The precise anatomic pathways are not known, although they must involve several cervical segments and the facial nucleus in the medulla. Cervical lesions that involve gray and white matter can cause depressed or absent cervical responses.

Sensory perception from the neck and forelimbs must be assessed. This can be difficult to evaluate accurately in stoic animals (Fig. 2–16). Perception of a noxious stimulus is noted by observing the animal's cerebral (behavioral) response while observing the local cervical responses and continuing the skin pricking over the shoulders and down the limbs (see Fig. 16–1, Problem 11).

As with any cutaneous sensory test, a two-step technique is recommended (Bailey et al., 1987). This is accomplished by initially tenting and grasping a fold of skin between the jaws of heavy duty hemostats or needle holders. After pausing to allow the patient to settle, a second, slow, skin pinch is applied to determine superficial sensation. There may be reflex withdrawal of the part with or without a cerebral response, such as vocalization or moving the whole body away from the stimulus.

Pushing against the shoulders to force the animal to first resist and then to take a step laterally, is the sway reaction for the thoracic limb. It is performed while the animal is standing still and while it is walking forward. One forelimb can be held up while the patient is forced to hop on the other. This is considered a modified postural reaction test (see below). Weakness is evident by a lack of resistance to lateral shoulder pressure. Weakness and ataxia may cause tripping and stumbling on the forelimbs when taking lateral steps.

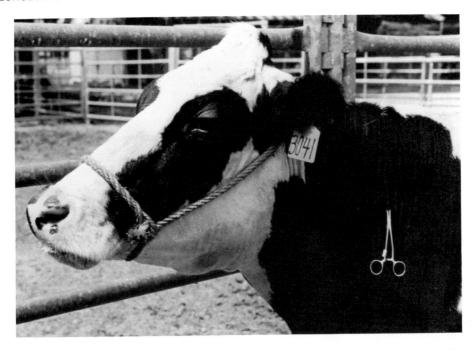

Figure 2–16. Sensory testing can be difficult to interpret accurately, as demonstrated by the lack of response to the hemostats applied to the neck of this normal cow. Such apparent stoicism is frequently found in large animals, particularly cattle and horses. A two-step cutaneous pinch technique is recommended to test superficial sensation (see text).

By pulling laterally on both the tail and the halter simultaneously, an assessment of the resistance (strength) on each side of the body is made (Fig. 2–13). This is analogous to hemiwalking in smaller patients. The patient's voluntary strength is assessed by making the patient turn in circles while the lead rope and tail are pulled firmly to each side in turn. An adult horse should be able to pull the examiner and should not pivot on a limb or be pulled to the side. Pinching and pressing down with the fingers on the withers of a normal animal causes some arching (lordosis), and then resistance to the downward motion. An animal that is weak in the thoracic limbs may not be able to resist this pressure by fixing its vertebral column; it will arch its back more than normally and even buckle in the thoracic limbs.

In smaller patients, other postural reactions can be performed. These primarily help detect signs of subtle proprioceptive and motor pathway lesions when the gait is normal. Wheelbarrowing the patient to make it walk on just the thoracic limbs, hopping it to the left and to the right on each individual thoracic (and pelvic) limb (Fig. 2–17A), and hemistanding and hemiwalking the animal by making it stand and then walk sideways on both left, then both right limbs, are three useful postural reactions to perform. Even in large, adult animals, particularly horses, it is possible to perform a modified hopping response test with the thoracic limbs (Fig. 2–17B). This is done by lifting each thoracic limb in turn while using the shoulder to make the horse hop sideways on the other thoracic limb. This test can help the clinician decide if there are subtle neurologic abnormalities in the horse's thoracic limb control. Brainstem

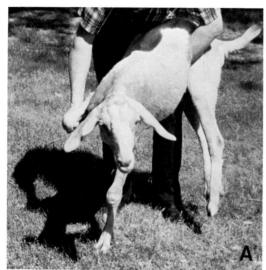

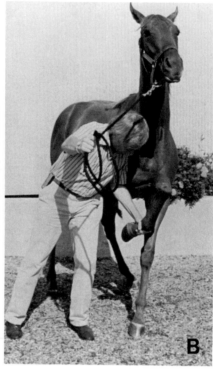

Figure 2–17. Hopping is a simple postural reaction test that allows expression of subtle neurologic abnormalities, especially proprioceptive and motor deficiencies, which may not be evident on gait evaluation. With all smaller patients (A), the pelvic limbs and one thoracic limb are raised off the ground and the patient is forced to hop sideways towards the side of the limb that is on the ground. This is repeated for each of the four limbs.

With adult horses (B), the maneuver is modified by leaving the pelvic limbs on the ground and using a shoulder to coax the horse to hop sideways on each thoracic limb in turn.

and spinal cord lesions appear to result in postural reaction deficits on the same side as the lesion, whereas cerebral lesions produce contralateral abnormalities.

If a large, adult animal has significant gait abnormality and it is feasible to cast it, then this should be done to assess the spinal reflexes. If the animal is ambulating well, it may be assumed that the spinal reflexes are intact. These reflexes can be studied in all smaller patients.

Recumbent Patient. A patient that has recently become recumbent, but uses the thoracic limbs well in an attempt to get up, most likely has a lesion caudal to T_2. If such an animal cannot attain a dog-sitting posture, the lesion is likely to be in the cervical spinal cord. If only the head, but not the neck, can be raised off the ground, there probably is a severe cranial cervical lesion. With a severe caudal cervical lesion, the head and neck usually can be raised off the ground, although thoracic limb effort decreases and the animal usually is unable to maintain sternal recumbency. Assessments of limb function must not be done while a heavy animal is lying on the limb being tested. Muscular tone can be determined by manipulating each limb. A flaccid limb, with no motor activity, is typical of a lower motor neuron lesion to that limb, but in heavy recumbent animals there can be poor tone and little observable voluntary effort in a limb that has been lain upon. A severe upper motor neuron lesion to the thoracic limbs (cranial to C_6) causes decreased, or absent, voluntary effort, but there will be normal, or more likely, increased, muscle tone in the limbs. This is because there is a release of the lower motor neuron that is reflexly maintaining normal muscle tone from the calming influences of the descending upper motor neuron pathways. Interestingly, such a spastic paralysis also can be seen with lesions between C_6 and T_2 if little or no gray matter is affected. A Schiff-Sherrington phenomenon of short duration, with excessive extensor tone in the presence of good voluntary activity and normal reflexes in the thoracic limbs, has been seen rarely in horses, and usually follows a cranial thoracic vertebral fracture (Chiapetta et al., 1985).

Finally, spinal reflexes are tested in the thoracic limbs. The flexor reflex in the thoracic limb involves stimulation of the skin of the distal limb with needle holders and observing for flexion of the fetlock, knee, elbow, and shoulder (Fig. 2–18A). This reflex arc involves sensory fibers in the median and ulnar nerves, spinal cord segments C_6 to T_2, and motor fibers in the axillary, musculocutaneous, median, and ulnar nerves. Lesions cranial to C_6 may release this reflex from the calming effect of the upper motor neuron pathways and cause an exaggerated reflex with rapid flexion of the limb; the limb may remain

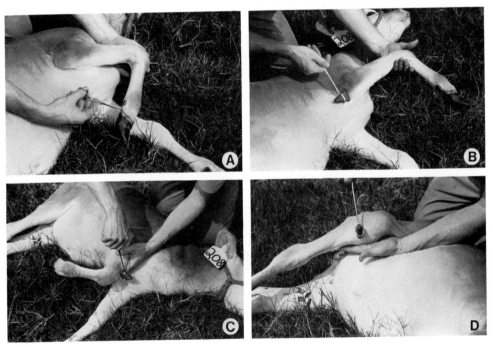

Figure 2–18. Normal spinal reflexes that can be performed reliably in all smaller animals, and most larger normal animals, are the flexor reflex (A), triceps reflex (B), extensor carpi reflex (C), and patellar reflex (D). Neonates show a prominent and normal crossed extensor reflex of the limb contralateral to the one being tested (A). This would be regarded as evidence of a lesion in the descending motor pathways (upper motor neurons) in an adult, and does disappear in neonates within a few weeks of normal ambulation. In larger animals a heavy pipe or orthopedic hammer (rather than rubber neurologic hammer as shown) is required to test the extensor reflexes (B, C, D).

flexed for some time. Such lesions also may result in a crossed extensor reflex, with synchronous extension of the limb untested. This usually occurs only with severe and chronic upper motor neuron lesions. Thus, an animal affected by such a lesion may demonstrate considerable reflex movement following stimuli, but usually will have little voluntary motor activity in the limbs being tested. A spinal reflex can be intact without the animal perceiving the stimulus. Cerebral responses associated with perception include changes in facial expression, head movement, or phonation. Conscious perception of the stimulus will be intact only as long as the afferent fibers in the median and ulnar nerves, the dorsal gray columns at C_6-T_2, and the ascending sensory pathways in the cervical spinal cord and brainstem are intact.

The biceps reflex is performed by placing two or three fingers firmly on the biceps and brachialis muscles (which are on the cranial aspect of the elbow joint), ballotting them with a plexor, and feeling for contraction of those muscles while observing for flexion of the elbow. In adult horses and cattle, the muscle bellies themselves can be percussed with a neurologic hammer or similar plexor. This reflex has its afferent and efferent pathways in the musculocutaneous nerve and involves spinal cord segments C_7 and C_8. It is difficult to evoke, except in small patients.

To perform the triceps reflex the relaxed limb is held slightly flexed and the distal portion of the long head of the triceps and its tendon of insertion is ballotted with a rubber neurology hammer (smaller patients) or a heavy, metal plexor (larger patients) while observing and palpating for contraction of the triceps muscle, which causes extension of the elbow (Fig. 2–18B). The triceps reflex involves the radial nerve for its afferent and efferent pathways and spinal cord segments C_7 to T_1. The triceps reflexes, although present, can be difficult to demonstrate in heavy, adult, recumbent patients.

The musculotendinous portion of the extensor carpi radialis muscle can be ballotted to produce extension of the knee when the relaxed limb is held in a partially flexed position (Fig. 2–18C). This extensor carpi radialis reflex involves afferent and efferent fibers also in the radial nerve but the reflex may not always be present in normal animals.

All these reflexes usually are active in normal neonates and there is a prominent crossed extensor reflex present (Fig. 2–18A), which slowly subsides through the first weeks of life.

By this stage of the examination the clinician should have a clear idea of the presence and location of lesions in the brain, spinal cord (cranial to T_2), and the peripheral nerves and muscles of the thoracic limbs. The more peripheral the lesion, the better defined the sensory and motor deficits. Syndromes resulting from lesions involving the thoracic limb peripheral nerves, such as the suprascapular and radial nerves, involve characteristic abnormalities of gait, paralysis of specific muscles with resulting muscle atrophy, specific reflex loss, and sensory deficits (see Fig. 16–1, Problem 11).

4. Trunk and Hindlimbs

If the examination of the head, gait, and posture, or neck and thoracic limbs reveals evidence of a lesion, then an attempt should be made to explain any further signs found during examination of the trunk and hindlimbs that could have been caused by the lesion. If there are only signs in the trunk and hind-limbs, then the lesion(s) must either be between T_2 and S_2, or in the trunk and pelvic limb nerves or muscles. This part of the examination helps localize the lesion more precisely. However, the examiner must remember that with a subtle (grade 1 +) neurologic gait abnormality in the pelvic limbs, the lesion may be anywhere between the midsacral spinal cord and the rostral brainstem.

The trunk and hindlimbs must be observed and palpated for malformation and asymmetry. Lesions affecting thoracolumbar gray matter cause muscle atrophy, which is a helpful localizing finding. With asymmetric myelopathies scoliosis of the thoracolumbar vertebral column often occurs, initially with the concave side opposite the lesion.

Sweating in the horse is a helpful localizing sign. Ipsilateral sweating caudal to the lesion signals involvement of the descending sympathetic tracts in the spinal cord. Lesions involving specific pre- or postganglionic peripheral sympathetic fibers (second or third order neurons) cause patches of sweating at the level of the lesion.

Gentle pricking of the skin over the trunk, particularly the lateral aspects of the body wall, causes a contraction of the cutaneous trunci muscle, which is seen as a flicking of the skin over the trunk. The sensory stimulus travels to the spinal cord in thoracolumbar spinal nerves at the level of the site of stimulation. Transmission is then cranial in the spinal cord to C_8-T_1, where the lower motor neuron cell bodies of the lateral thoracic nerve are stimulated causing contraction of the cutaneous trunci muscle. Lesions anywhere along this pathway may cause suppression of the response, which is easiest to detect with an asymmetric lesion.

An assessment of sensory perception from the trunk and hindlimbs must be made. This appears as a cerebral response while observing the local response and continuing the skin pricking over the rump and down the limbs (see Fig. 16–1, Problem 11). Degrees of hypalgesia and analgesia have been detected caudal to the sites of thoracolumbar spinal cord lesions, but only when they are severe.

The sway reaction for the pelvic limbs involves pushing against the pelvis and pulling on the tail with the patient standing still and while walking (Fig. 2–12); this allows one to feel the resistance given by the animal and to observe the resulting limb movement. An animal that is weak in the pelvic limbs will be easily pulled and pushed laterally, especially while walking (see above for differences between upper motor pathway involvement and lower motor neuron involvement). Proprioceptive deficits can be observed as overabduction and crossing of the limbs when a step is taken to the side. In younger and smaller patients, pelvic limb hopping, wheelbarrowing, and hemistanding and hemiwalking are useful postural reactions to perform. These yield information on the overall integrity of the proprioceptive and motor pathways (to and from higher centers), the cerebellar control of these pathways, and the lower motor neurons of the pelvic limbs. With subacute to chronic lesions involving one cerebral hemisphere only, such as a hematoma or abscess, there often is an abnormal hopping response in the contralateral limbs. This is seen as a slow onset of movement with stumbling. There will be no observable gait change; however, the animal may be slow to bring the limb back to midline when turning away from that side. With lesions involving the proprioceptive and motor pathways to the pelvic limbs in the brainstem and spinal cord cranial to L_3, there is a slow hopping response in the ipsilateral pelvic limb. Lower motor neuron lesions in one pelvic limb result in poor tone, paresis, and often an extremely slow or absent hopping response in that limb.

Pinching and pressing down on the thoracolumbar or sacral paravertebral muscles with the fingers causes a normal animal to extend slightly, then fix, the thoracolumbar vertebral column. It also resists the ventral motion and usually does not flex the thoracic or pelvic limbs. A weak animal usually is not able to resist the pressure by fixing the vertebral column and thus it over-extends the back and begins to buckle in the pelvic limbs.

Recumbent Patient. The pelvic limb spinal reflexes can be evaluated in all animals that can be restrained in lateral recumbency, and in all recumbent animals. In addition, the amount of voluntary effort and muscle tone present in the pelvic limbs is assessed in recumbent patients. As described for the thoracic limbs, this can be done while watching the animal attempt to get up, or by observing its struggle in response to stimuli while lying in lateral recumbency. Consideration must be given to possibly exacerbating a fracture.

The patellar reflex and the flexor reflex are the two most clinically important spinal cord reflexes involving the pelvic limbs. The patellar reflex is performed by supporting the limb in a partly flexed position, tapping the intermediate patellar ligament with a neurologic hammer or a heavy metal plexor, and observing for a reflex contraction of the quadriceps muscle. This results in extension of the stifle (Fig. 2–18D). The sensory and motor fibers for this reflex are in the femoral nerve; the spinal cord segments involved are primarily L_4 and L_5. The flexor reflex is performed by pinching the skin of the distal limb with needle holders and observing for flexion of the limb. The afferent and efferent pathways for this reflex are in the sciatic nerve and involve spinal cord segments L_5 to S_3.

Although two other reflexes can be elicited in most neonatal animals, they frequently are not clearly reproducible in adult patients. Firstly, the gastrocnemius reflex is performed by ballotting the gastrocnemius tendon and observing and palpating for contraction of the gastrocnemius muscle, which is accompanied by extension of the hock. This reflex involves the tibial branch of the sciatic nerve and spinal cord segments L_5 to S_3. Secondly, the cranial tibial reflex causes contraction of the cranial tibial muscle with hock flexion occurring when the muscle is ballotted and the relaxed limb is held partially extended. Limb movement may be interpreted falsely as a positive, neurologic, reflex muscle contraction when both these reflexes are tested.

Skin sensation of the pelvic limbs should be assessed independently from reflex activity. The femoral nerve is sensory to the skin of the medial thigh region, the peroneal nerve to the dorsal tarsus and metatarsus, and the tibial nerve to the plantar surface of the metatarsus. As for the thoracic limbs, lesions of the peripheral nerves to the pelvic limbs, such as the femoral and peroneal nerves, result in specific motor deficits; however, the precise sensory deficits can be difficult to define (Fig. 16–2, Problem 12).

The patellar reflex is hyperactive in newborn foals, calves, and kids (and probably all large animal neonates); the cranial tibial, and gastrocnemius tendon reflexes are easily performed in healthy, cooperative newborn patients. As with the forelimbs, these patients have normal, strong, crossed extensor reflexes. In addition, an extensor thrust reflex is obtained, in very young foals at least, by rapidly overextending the toe while the limb is already partially extended. This results in forceful extension of the limb, and possibly represents a golgi tendon organ reflex.

At this stage of the neurologic evaluation the clinician has a clear idea of the probable site of any brain or spinal cord lesion that causes abnormal gait or recumbency.

5. Tail and Anus

Tail tone can be assessed prior to testing the perineal reflex. A completely flaccid tail, with no voluntary movement, is indicative of a lesion of sacrococcygeal spinal cord segments, nerves, or muscles. Decreased movement of the tail can be detected with lesions cranial to the coccygeal segment, but usually the spinal cord lesion must be severe for the weakness to be apparent. Some horses are considered natural tail-wringers and flick their tails vertically and laterally while moving.

Torticollis of the coccygeal vertebrae ("wry-tail") should alert the examiner to the possibility of the presence of other midline malformations, but it may, particularly in cattle, be iatrogenic.

The perineal reflex is elicited by lightly pricking the skin of the perineum and observing reflex contraction of the anal sphincter and clamping down of the tail. The sensory fibers are contained within the perineal branches of the pudendal nerve (S_1-S_3). Contraction of the anal sphincter is mediated by the caudal rectal branch of the pudendal nerve, and tail flexion is mediated by the sacral and coccygeal segments and nerves $(S_1-Co.)$. An animal with a flaccid tail and anus, due to a lower motor neuron lesion, will not have an anal (or tail) reflex. However, it may still have normal sensation from the anus and tail provided that the sensory nerves and spinal cord and brainstem white matter nociceptive pathways are intact. Thus, as with all other reflex testing, sensory perception of the stimulus must be evaluated separately from segmental reflex action.

The spinal cord ends at the level of the first or second sacral vertebra in large animals. Therefore, focal lesions of the last lumbar, and of the sacral and coccygeal vertebrae may involve the cauda equina, and thus the spinal nerve lower motor neurons from many sacrococcygeal spinal cord segments. Depending on the level, this causes varying degrees of hypalgesia, hyporeflexia, hypotonia, and ultimately muscle atrophy of the tail, anus, perineum, hips, and caudal thighs. A rectal examination may detect a space-occupying lesion, and fracture or luxation of the lumbar, sacral or coccygeal vertebrae. In addition, assessment should be made of urinary bladder volume, and the tone of the bladder wall and rectum. Adult animals, especially male horses, that are recumbent for any reason, often do not urinate; thus, they usually have a distended bladder that eventually spills over. Manipulating such an animal to help it stand, or violent attempts by the animal itself to stand, can result in rupture of a bladder wall that is already weakened by pressure necrosis.

PATIENT ID
HISTORY

LARGE ANIMAL NEONATAL NEUROLOGICAL EXAMINATION

Physical Examination: _____

Temperature: _____
Pulse: _____
Respirations: _____

EVALUATION OF THE HEAD
BEHAVIOR:
  Affinity for the mare: _____
  Flopping: _____ Shivering: _____
  Flegmen: _____ Odontoprisis: _____ Salivation: _____ Snapping: _____
MENTAL STATUS: _____
HEAD POSTURE AND COORDINATION: _____
CRANIAL NERVES: _____

	RIGHT	LEFT
Ophthalmic Examination:	_____	_____
Vision (II):	_____	_____
Menace (II-VII, Cerebellum):	_____	_____
Pupil Size (II, III, Symp.):	_____	_____
Pupil Symmetry (II, III, Symp.):	_____	_____
PLR (II, III):	_____	_____
Blink to Bright Light (II, VII):	_____	_____
Strabismus (III, IV, VI, VIII):	_____	_____
Nystagmus, vestibular (III, IV, VI, VIII):	_____	_____
Nystagmus, spontaneous (III, IV, VI, VIII):	_____	_____
Corneal Reflex (V, VII):	_____	_____
Ear, Eye, & Lip (V, VII):	_____	_____
Muscle Mass & Jaw Tone (V):	_____	_____
Smile (V, VII):	_____	_____
Swallow (IX, X):	_____	_____
Voice (IX, X):	_____	_____
Tongue (XIII):	_____	_____
Endoscopy:	_____	_____
Slap Test:	_____	_____

FORELIMBS AND NECK

	RIGHT	LEFT
Cervical-local:	_____	_____
Cervical-face:	_____	_____
Muscle Mass:	_____	_____
Sweating:	_____	_____
Triceps Reflex:	_____	_____
Biceps Reflex:	_____	_____
Ex. Ca. Ra. Reflex:	_____	_____
Flexor Reflex:	_____	_____
Crossed Extensor Reflex:	_____	_____
Babinski Sign:	_____	_____
Extensor Strength:	_____	_____
Proprioception:	_____	_____
Recumbent Extensor Thrust:	_____	_____

REARLIMBS, TAIL AND ANUS

	RIGHT	LEFT
Panniculus:	_____	_____
Muscle Mass:	_____	_____
Sweating:	_____	_____
Patellar Reflex:	_____	_____
Cr. Tibial Reflex:	_____	_____
Gastrocnemius Reflex:	_____	_____
Flexor Reflex:	_____	_____
Crossed Extensor Reflex:	_____	_____
Babinski Sign:	_____	_____
Extensor Strength:	_____	_____
Proprioception:	_____	_____
Recumbent Extensor Thrust:	_____	_____
Tail:	_____	_____
Anus:	_____	_____

PASSIVE TONE: FLEXOR VERSUS EXTENSOR STRENGTH
Forelimb: Heel to elbow, acromion, mid-scapular spine, dorsal scapula. _____
Hindlimb: Minimum distance between Tibial Tuberosity and Third Metatarsus. _____

Neck Movement: _____
Trunk Movement: _____

LIMB POSITION AND PASTERN AXIS:

Normal ≅ 50°   Toe on Ground × 50°   Toe off Ground ≅ 30°   Toe 1 cm. off Ground < 30°   Fetlock on Ground   Contracted > 50°

EVALUATION OF GAIT AND STRENGTH: _____

Lesion site(s): _____
Possible etiology: _____
Plan: _____

Signature _____   Date _____

Figure 2–19. Neonatal examination form.

PATIENT ID

NEUROLOGIC EXAMINATION OF LARGE ANIMALS	
OUTPAITENT:	STALL NO.:
DATE:	TIME:
CLINICIAN:	CHARGES:
STUDENT:	ACCOUNT:
HISTORY:	
PHYSICAL EXAMINATION:	

NEUROLOGIC EXAMINATION

HEAD:
- Behavior:
- Mental Status:
- Head Posture:
- Head Coordination:

Craniel Nerves:

	LEFT	RIGHT
EYES		
Ophthalmic Examination:		
Vision; II:		
Menace; II-VII, Cerebellum:		
Pupils, PLR; II-III:		
Horners; Symp:		
Strabismus; III, IV, VI, VIII:		
FACE		
Sensation; Vs, cerebrum:		
Muscle mass, jaw tone; Vm:		
Ear, eye, nose, lip reflex; V-VII:		
Expression; VII:		
Sweating, Symp:		
VESTIBULAR—EAR		
Eye drop:		
Nystagmus; resting:		
positional:		
vestibular:		
Hearing:		
Special vestibular:		
TONGUE		
Tone, mass, fasciculations; XII, cerebrum:		
PHARYNX, LARYNX		
Voice; IX, X:		
Swallow; IX, X:		
Endoscopy:		
Slap test:		

	LEFT		RIGHT	
	FORE	HIND	FORE	HIND
GAIT: Paresis:				
Ataxia:				
Spasticity:				
Dysmetria:				
Total deficit:				
Other:				

NECK & FORELIMBS	LEFT	RIGHT	TRUNK & HINDLIMBS:	LEFT	RIGHT	TAIL & ANUS:	LEFT	RIGHT
Hoofwear:			Hoofwear:			Strength:		
Posture:			Posture:			Muscle Mass:		
Strength:			Strength:			Tone:		
Muscle Mass:			Muscle Mass:			Reflexes:		
Tone:			Tone:			Sensation:		
Reflexes:			Reflexes:			Rectal:		
Sensation:			Sensation:					
Sweating:			Sweating:					

ASSESSMENT

SITE OF LESION(S): General (circle): cerebrum, brainstem, peripheral cranial nerves, cerebellum, spinal cord, peripheral nerves, muscles, skeleton

Specific:

CAUSE OF LESION(S):

PLAN
- DX:
- RX:
- EX:

SIGNATURE: _____ DATE: / /

Figure 2–20. Adult examination form.

An animal that is ambulatory and has nonobstructive distention of the bladder with urinary incontinence probably has a lesion that affects the sacral spinal cord segments or the pelvic nerves. In such cases there usually will be excess feces in the rectum; this will not cause overt constipation unless there is a dense, diffuse, sacral, lower motor neuron lesion.

Paraplegic large patients frequently contuse their perineum and tail while dog-sitting and while attempting to stand. Also, tail ropes and various forms of sling support frequently damage these areas. An assessment of the neurologic function must be made as soon as possible because perineal and tail contusion results in edema, quickly followed by hypotonia, hyporeflexia, and hypalgesia.

Finally, the results of the neurologic examination should be documented and not left to memory. Examples of forms used for documenting the neurologic examination of neonatal and adult large animal patients are given in Figures 2–19 and 2–20.

E. WHERE AND WHAT IS THE LESION?

After completing the neurologic examination, the clinician should be able to accurately localize any lesion(s) within one or more of the following general areas: cerebrum, brainstem, cerebellum, cranial nerves, spinal cord, peripheral nerves, and muscles. In particular, the syndrome being evaluated will fall into one or more of the major problems discussed in Part II. After localizing the lesion, consideration can be given to the possible mechanisms that cause disease.

F. INITIAL PLAN

Following consideration of anatomic and etiologic diagnoses, an initial plan must be devised. This will include use of ancillary aids to help rule in and rule out certain disease processes, a therapeutic plan, and a plan for client education, including economic advice, herd health management, and prognostic considerations.

BIBLIOGRAPHY

Adams R, Mayhew IG. Neurologic diseases. Vet Clin North Am [Equine Pract] *1*:209–234, 1985.
Barlow R. Neurological disorders of cattle and sheep. In Practice [Suppl Vet Rec] *5*:77–84, 1983.
Brewer BD. Neurologic diseases of sheep and goats. Vet Clin North Am [Large Anim Pract] *5*:677–700, 1983.
deLahunta A. *Veterinary Neuroanatomy and Clinical Neurology.* 2nd Ed. Philadelphia: WB Saunders, 1983, pp. 389–406.
Hofmeyr CFB. Evaluation of neurological examination of sheep. J S Afr Vet Assoc *49*:45–48, 1978.
Oliver JE, Hoerlein BF, Mayhew IG. *Veterinary Neurology.* Philadelphia: WB Saunders, 1987, pp. 7–56.
Palmer AC. *Introduction to Animal Neurology.* 2nd Ed. Oxford: Blackwell Scientific Publications, 1976, pp 91–113.
Wells GAH. Locomotor disorders of the pig. In Practice [Suppl Vet Rec] *6*:43–53, 1984.

REFERENCES

Bailey CS, Kitchell RL. Cutaneous sensory testing in the dog. J Vet Int Med 1987; *1*:128-135.

Chiapetta JR, Baker JC, Feeney DA. Vertebral fracture, extension hypertonia of thoracic limbs, and paralysis of pelvic limbs (Schiff-Sherrington syndrome) in an Arabian foal. J Am Vet Med Assoc 1985; *186*:387–388.

Greet TRC, Jeffcott LB, Whitewell KE, et al. The slap test for laryngeal adductory function in horses with suspected spinal cord damage. Equine Vet J 1980; *12*:127–131.

Herran MA, Martin JE, Joyce JR. Quantitative study of the decussating optic axons in the pony, cow, sheep and pig. Am J Vet Res 1978; *39*:1137–1139.

McCormick DA, Thompson RF. Cerebellum: essential involvement in the classically conditioned eyelid response. Science 1984; *223*:296.

Rooney JR. Two cervical reflexes in the horse. J Am Vet Med Assoc 1973;*162*:117–118.

Usenik EA. Sympathetic innervation of the head and neck of the horse; neuropharmacological studies of sweating in the horse. PhD Thesis, University of Minnesota, 1957.

CHAPTER 3

Ancillary Diagnostic Aids

ROUTINE CLINICOPATHOLOGICAL TESTS

A routine hemogram can assist in the diagnosis of some infectious and inflammatory diseases, lymphosarcoma, and trauma with blood loss.

Routine blood chemistry tests assist in defining many metabolic diseases affecting the nervous system, particularly liver disease, hypocalcemia, hypomagnesemia, hypokalemia, and hypoglycemia. Special serum enzyme assays and organ biopsies may be performed to confirm liver and muscle disease. These are covered under the specific diseases listed in Part II.

Specific serum antibody titers, particularly when assayed on acute and convalescent sera, are helpful in diagnosing infectious diseases such as equine viral encephalitides, equine infectious anemia, equine herpesvirus-1, pseudorabies, and bovine leukemia virus infection. Blood and tissue toxins and nutrient concentrations can assist in diagnosing intoxications and nutritional disorders.

CEREBROSPINAL FLUID ANALYSIS

The collection and analysis of cerebrospinal fluid (CSF) from large animals has been described and simplified (deLahunta, 1983), (Mayhew, 1975, 1981), and techniques for analysis also have been published (Mayhew, 1981), (Mayhew et al., 1980). Sites of CSF collection from the horse are given in Figures 3–1, 3–2, and 3–3. The collection sites for other large animal species can be extrapolated directly from the horse. In foals, calves, sheep, goats, and piglets it is advantageous to use a 1.5 in., 20 g disposable hypodermic needle with a plastic hub for all atlanto-occipital CSF collections. These needles are atraumatic and cause less patient reaction; more importantly, CSF appears in the hub of the needle immediately after it enters the subarachnoid space. A sample can be obtained and the needle withdrawn much more rapidly than if a stiletted needle is used; in a nonanesthetized patient this is clinically important. The results of CSF analysis can reflect diseases in the brain and spinal cord just as a hemogram detects many systemic diseases. Thus, CSF analysis is one of the most helpful aids in determining the cause of CNS lesions.

Normal CSF is clear and colorless, with a refractive index of 1.3347 to 1.3350; in addition it contains no erythrocytes and usually less than 6 small mononuclear cells per μl. Protein content is between 50 and 100 mg/dl in the

49

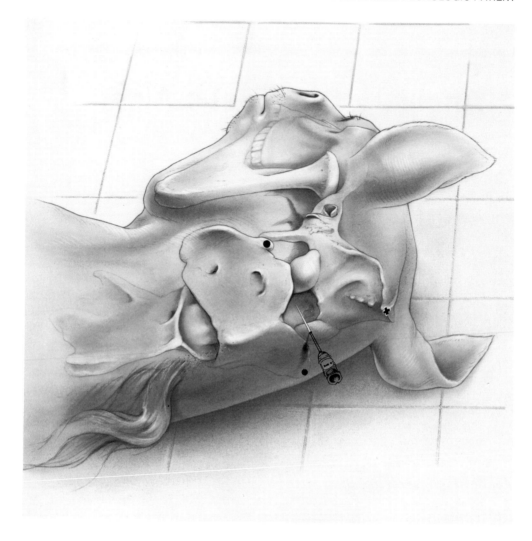

Figure 3–1. Atlanto-occipital cerebrospinal fluid collection from the recumbent horse. Spinal needle in position with stilette removed. Palpable landmarks are the cranial borders of the atlas (●---●), and the external occipital protuberance (+) on the dorsal midline. (From Mayhew, IG. Collection of cerebrospinal fluid from the horse. Cornell Vet 1975; 65:500–511, with permission.)

horse (absolute range 10 to 120 mg/dl), and can be higher (up to 180 mg/dl) in neonatal foals. Ruminants and swine usually have CSF with a protein content of less than 75 mg/dl. Neonates may have slightly xanthrochromic CSF.

In most CNS malformations the CSF will be normal. If a malformation of the calvarium or vertebral column causes damage to underlying nervous tissue, the CSF may reflect compression with evidence of subtle hemorrhage.

Infectious diseases can result in CSF pleocytosis and elevation of protein content. The cell type present varies considerably, although generally, there are neutrophils with bacterial diseases and small mononuclear cells with viral diseases. Fungal and protozoal diseases usually cause mixed cell responses. Protozoal, and particularly helminth parasite infestations, may produce an

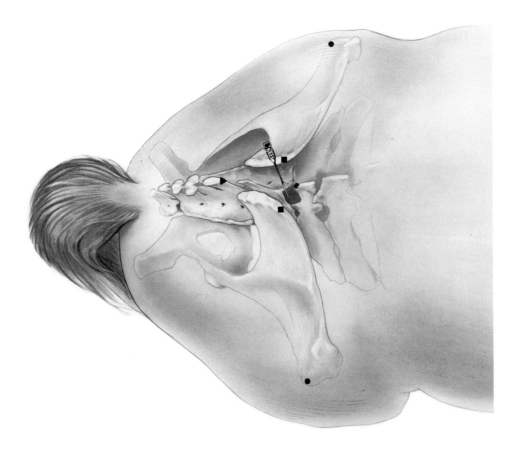

Figure 3–2.   Lumbosacral cerebrospinal fluid collection from the standing horse. Spinal needle in position with stilette removed. Palpable landmarks are the caudal borders of each tuber coxae (●---●), the caudal edge of the spine of L_6 (+), the cranial edge of the second sacral spine (▶), and the cranial edge of each tuber sacrale (■---■). (From Mayhew, IG. Collection of cerebrospinal fluid from the horse. Cornell Vet 1975; 65:500–511, with permission.)

eosinophilic response in the CSF, as well as hemorrhage. In most chronic inflammatory states, and in diseases in which there is much CNS tissue necrosis, the CSF can contain many large mononuclear cells or macrophages.

    With traumatic injury to the CNS, there is often some hemorrhage into the CSF with resulting yellow discoloration. This xanthochromia remains after red cells have been centrifuged off. Trauma also results in leakage of red cells and some protein into the CSF, particularly if meningeal vessels are damaged. Neutrophils, not showing toxic changes followed by macrophages, usually will appear in the CSF as a result of hemorrhage.

    In most toxic, nutritional, and metabolic neurologic diseases, the results of routine CSF analyses are normal. However, for those diseases in which there can be considerable tissue destruction, such as lead poisoning and polioen-

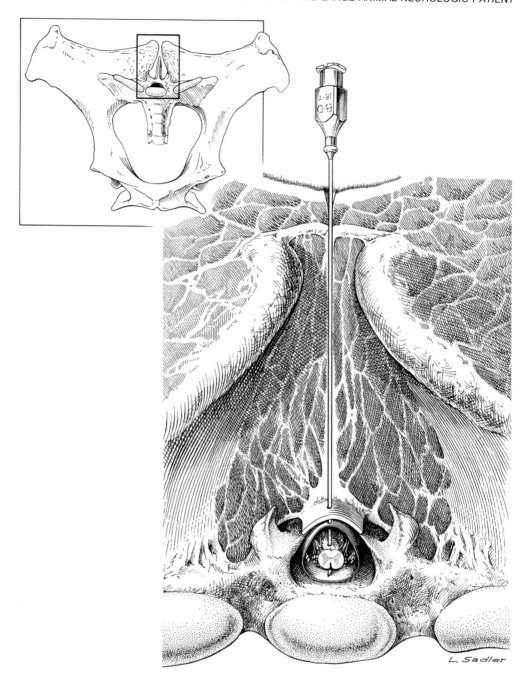

Figure 3–3.   Lumbosacral spinal fluid collection from the horse. Transverse dissection through lumbosacral articulations, cranial view. Spinal needle passes through the skin, thoracolumbar fascia adjacent to the interspinous ligaments, interarcuate ligament, dorsal dura mater and arachnoid, dorsal subarachnoid space; and conus medullaris. Needle point is in the ventral subarachnoid space. Cranial view of pelvis, sacrum, and area of dissection (inset). (From Mayhew, IG. Collection of cerebrospinal fluid from the horse. Cornell Vet 1975; 65:500–511, with permission.)

cephalomalacia in ruminants, and moldy corn-associated leukoencephaloma-lacia in horses, there may be some protein leakage and a mononuclear cell response in the CSF.

Typically, there is leakage of protein and some xanthochromia without any significant pleocytosis in many vascular diseases. If the hemorrhage is large, then neutrophils and macrophages also may be seen.

Degenerative diseases do not typically cause any changes in CSF, and most frequently the CSF analysis is normal.

Neoplasms can act like other space-occupying lesions, such as abscesses and hematomas, and increase CSF pressure. The most frequent CSF change in patients with neoplasia is a slight elevation in protein content. Rarely are there atypical lymphocytes in CSF from cattle with CNS lymphosarcoma. Sometimes there is evidence of mild injury, xanthochromia, and a few macrophages.

Any process that is contained within the parenchyma of the CNS, without contact with the subarachnoid space, is unlikely to cause leakage of pigments or protein, or exfoliation of cells into the CSF.

ELECTRODIAGNOSTIC TESTING

Electroencephalography, electromyography, and nerve stimulation and conduction testing contribute to a complete neurological evaluation. The techniques used in large animals are the same as those used in small animal neurology (Oliver et al., 1987). Considerable experience in using these ancillary aids is required to be able to interpret electroencephalograms and nerve conduction studies in large animals, because findings in normal animals are not yet well defined (Mysinger et al., 1985), (Strain et al., 1986). This fact, and the expense of the equipment, make these procedures somewhat prohibitive to most large animal clinicians. However, visual-evoked and auditory brainstem response testing, as well as spinal and somatosensory-evoked potential testing definitely will be more widely used in large animal neurology in the near future (Wilson et al., 1982), (Wilson et al., 1986), (Rolf et al., 1987).

Needle electromyography to detect abnormal electrical activity present in muscle that has been denervated and in several myopathies can be just as helpful in localizing lower motor neuron lesions in large animals as it is in small animals (Oliver et al., 1987). The equipment is moderately priced and interested clinicians should contact a neurologist at a referral clinic or Veterinary College.

NEURORADIOLOGY

Radiography of the calvarium and vertebral column is indispensable for identifying bony malformations, fractures, and osteomyelitis (Oliver et al., 1987), (Rantanen et al., 1981), (Whitewell et al., 1987).

The techniques of positive contrast myelography have been described in the horse (Beech, 1979), (Nyland et al., 1980), (May et al., 1986), (Rantanen et al., 1981). These procedures are useful for defining spinal cord compression and swelling of the spinal cord. Some experience is required to be able to obtain satisfactory studies. Complications do occur, and the procedures can be prolonged and distressful to the patient. Consequently, it is suggested that these procedures be done only by an experienced radiographer who has the correct equipment, and only when the clinician is prepared to attempt whatever surgical and medical therapy is indicated, including euthanasia if it is necessary at the end of the procedure. I do not condone performing positive contrast myelography on unanesthetized large animal patients.

THERMOGRAPHY

Infrared, electronic thermography is a completely noninvasive method of determining skin temperature (Purohit et al., 1980). Thermography is well suited for horses because of their short, even, haircoat and because radiography of the thoracolumbar vertebral column, which is so useful in smaller patients, does not usually contribute to a patient's neurologic work-up.

Superficial temperature primarily depends on cutaneous blood flow. Because many neurologic disorders can be associated with local alterations in blood flow, this diagnostic modality can help localize neuromuscular lesions. In this manner, exercise-exacerbated focal, thoracolumbar myopathies, with associated pelvic limb gait abnormalities, have been corroborated by focal and asymmetric thermographic patterns before and after exercise. Also, neurologic and disuse muscle atrophy have been associated with a lower overlying superficial temperature, when compared with the normal, opposite side.

Because loss of sympathetic innervation in the horse causes demarcated cutaneous vasodilation and hyperhidrosis, thermography can be of great assistance in localizing any lesion affecting the sympathetic nervous system— particularly those involving peripheral nerves that contain sympathetic fibers. For example, the well known facial hyperthermia of Horner's syndrome in the horse produces a characteristic, abnormal thermographic pattern (Purohit et al., 1980).

REFERENCES

Beech J. Metrizamide myelography in the horse. J Am Vet Rad Soc 1979; *20*:2–322.

de Lahunta A. *Veterinary Neuroanatomy and Clinical Neurology.* 2nd Ed. Philadelphia: WB Saunders, 1983.

May SA, Wyn-Jones G, Church S, et al. Iopamidol myelography in the horse. Equine Vet J 1986; *18I*:199–202.

Mayhew IG. Cerebrospinal fluid. In: Howard JL, ed. *Current Veterinary Therapy, Food Animal Practice.* Philadelphia: WB Saunders, 1981. pp 1078–1080.

Mayhew IG. Collection of cerebrospinal fluid from the horse. Cornell Vet 1975; *65*:500.

Mayhew IG, Beal CR. Techniques of analysis of cerebrospinal fluid. Vet Clin North Am [Small Anim Pract] 1980; *10*:155–176.

Mysinger PW, Redding RW, Vaughan JT, et al. Electroencephalographic patterns of clinically normal, sedated, and tranquilized newborn foals and adult horses. Am J Vet Res 1985; *46*:36–41.

Nyland TG, Blythe LL, Pool RR, et al.: Metrizamide myelography in the horse: Clinical, radiographic and pathologic changes. Am J Vet Res 1980; *41*:204–211.

Oliver JE, Hoerlein BF, Mayhew IG. *Veterinary Neurology.* Philadelphia: WB Saunders, 1987.

Purohit RC, McCoy MD. Thermography in the diagnosis of inflammatory processes in the horse. Am J Vet Res 1980; *41*:1167–1174.

Purohit RC, McCoy MD, Bergfield WA. Thermographic diagnosis of Horner's syndrome in the horse. Am J Vet Res 1980; *41*:1180–1182.

Rantanen NW, Gavin PR, Barbee DD, et al. Ataxia and paresis in horses, Part II. Radiographic and myelographic examination of the cervical vertebral column. Comp Cont Ed Pract Vet 1981; *3*:S161–S171.

Rolf SL, Reed SM, Melnick W, et al. Auditory brain stem response testing in anesthetized horses. Am J Vet 1987; *48*:910–914.

Strain GW, Olcott BM, Braun WF. Electroencephalogram and evoked potentials in naturally occurring scrapie in sheep. Am J Vet Res 1986; *47*:828–836.

Whitwell KE, Dyson S. Interpreting radiographs: equine cervical vertebrae. Equine Vet J 1987; *19*:8–14.

Wilson RD, Witzel DA, Verlander JM: Somatosensory-evoked response of Angora goats in suspected haloxon-delayed neurotoxicity. Am J Vet Res 1982; *43*:2224–2226.

Wilson RD, Beerwinkle KR: Somatosensory-evoked potential induced by stimulation of the caudal tibial nerve in awake and barbiturate anesthetized sheep. Am J Vet Res 1986; *47*:46–49.

CHAPTER 4

Pathologic Responses of the Nervous System

This section reviews the gross and cellular reactions of nervous tissue in disease states and covers the general clinicopathologic characteristics of the various mechanisms of neurologic disease. The aim of this section is not to review veterinary neuropathology, but to provide a basic understanding of clinically important, neuropathologic principles. The reader is referred to general pathology references for more detailed coverage of most of these aspects of neuropathology (see bibliography).

General reactions seen in the nervous system, and their associated terminology, should be understood. We must be able to communicate with each other about neurologic diseases and understand the pathogenesis of these diseases. Importantly, such an understanding allows us to sensibly investigate a neurologic disorder of unknown cause and to understand, evaluate, and clinically interpret pathology reports on animals dying of neurologic diseases.

A. GROSS CHANGES VISIBLE IN NERVOUS TISSUE

(i) Finding the Lesion

A complete necropsy, including the removal of the entire brain and spinal cord from a large animal, is arduous. Nervous tissue shows the effects of autolysis rapidly and is extremely susceptible to distortion before it is well fixed. There is nothing more frustrating for a pathologist than scanning numerous histologic sections of "soup." However, because of these facts, and because so much vital information can be gained by a thorough neurologic necropsy, it is worth doing if it is done well. Sometimes an abbreviated necropsy will suffice in obtaining a diagnosis. There is no need to remove the petrosal bones and vestibular nerves from a horse with only tail paralysis. However, this presupposes an accurate neuroanatomic diagnosis. Failing this, a compromised (or no) pathologic diagnosis can be expected. Inadequate specimens for study, such as removal of only the cervical spinal cord from a wobbler with a thoracic lesion, or only the brain from a horse with tetraplegia, or no peripheral nerves and muscles from a horse with monoplegia, all can be expected to frustrate both the clinician and pathologist.

A practical approach to the postmortem examination of a large animal with neurologic disease is to begin at the site suspected of having a lesion (e.g., cervical vertebrae), but continue to harvest more tissues if no gross explanation for the signs is evident. Histopathologically, most compressive lesions of the spinal cord—whether they be caused by previous external injury, a stenotic vertebral canal, osteomyelitis or a tumor—are the result of trauma. Thus, the burden is often on the gross prosector to supply such etiologic information.

Some guidelines for collecting CNS tissues from a large animal are outlined in Figures 4–1 and 4–2. A technique for removal of the brain and spinal cord from the horse can be consulted (Mayhew et al., 1982).

In lieu of the technique outlined in Figure 4–1, which requires facilities

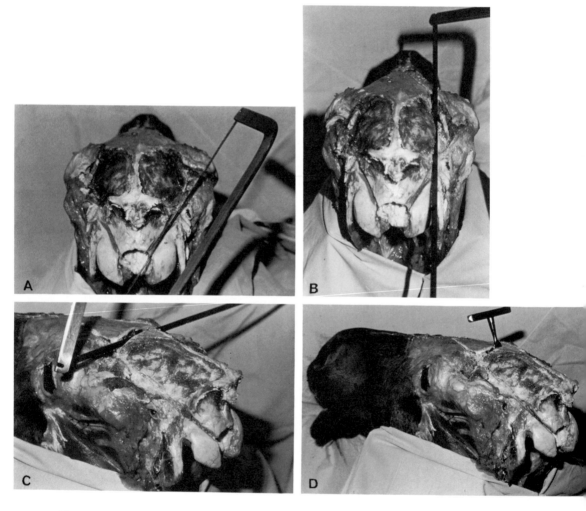

Figure 4–1. Technique for removal of the brain from a large animal. (A) The head of a horse is held in a vise with spiked jaws. Alternatively, it may be held by an assistant or a small wood vise can be applied to the lateral and medial surfaces of the horizontal ramus of one mandibular bone. Soft tissues over the calvarium have been removed and the first bone cut is being made with a hacksaw on a 45° angle from the lateral aspect of the foramen magnum to just above the zygomatic arch. This is repeated on the other side. (B) A longitudinal cut directed medially is then extended from the first cuts, above the coronoid process of the mandible into the lateral part of the frontal sinus. This is repeated on the other side. (C) The final cut is made transversely at a level just caudal to the caudal canthi of the eyes.

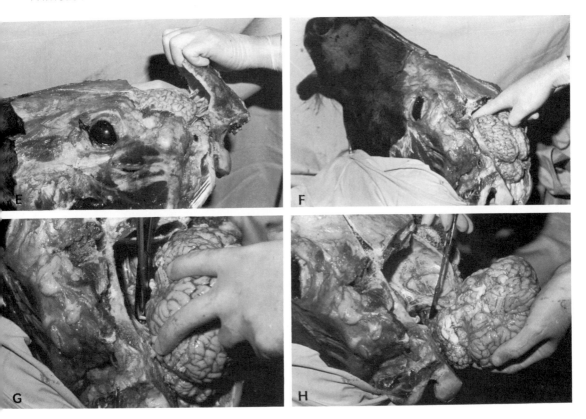

Figure 4–1. (D) The cap of the calvarium then can be pried free using a bone-wedge, screwdriver or chisel wedged into each cut in turn. This is the most difficult stage and some of the bone cuts may need to be deepened. In addition, the occipital crest can be struck from each side with moderate force using a hammer to help free the bony cap. (E) The bone cap then is removed, taking care to cut any attached dura mater and particularly the tentorium cerebelli. (F) Elevating the nose and using the first two fingers allows the frontal lobes to be separated from the olfactory bulbs. (G, H) Careful caudal retraction of the cerebral hemispheres exposes the remaining cranial nerves, which are cut with scissors or a scalpel, until the entire brain is extracted.

and time, there are other, less suitable techniques for brain removal. A midline saw or hatchet cut allows for the removal of the brain halves. However, it is better to make two, transverse saw cuts through the calvarium: one at the level of the external auditory meati, the other at a level halfway between the caudal aspect of the bony orbit and the external auditory meatus. This allows removal of four sections of brain (after the pons is sectioned to remove the central sections) and preserves midline structures.

The spinal cord can be harvested in three sections by performing a dorsal laminectomy or sagittal vertebral cut (cervical, thoracic, thoracolumbosacral), and labeling each for orientation (Fig. 4–2). The dura mater should be carefully split along the dorsal surface and almost complete transverse sections made with a razor blade through the cord, at least at every segment. Alternatively, in wobblers, the cervical vertebrae may be disarticulated and each segment of spinal cord labeled and oriented cranial versus caudal.

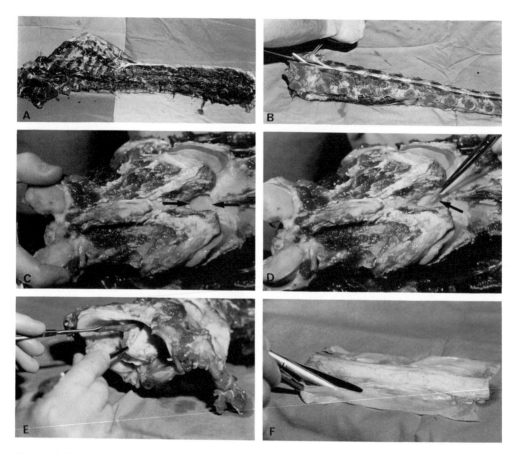

Figure 4–2. Removal of the spinal cord from a horse. (A) The vertebral column with soft tissue and ribs removed can be prepared in three segments: the cervical region, a thoracic region, and a thoracolumbosacral region. At this stage, each of these may be cut and labelled into smaller segments, and immersed in formalin for transport to a pathologist. (B) A dorsal laminectomy (shown) or sagittal vertebral cut can be made with a bandsaw or even a meat saw. The spinal cord, with dura mater intact, then can be removed as the nerve roots are cut. (C) If a cervical compressive lesion is suspected, each cervical vertebra can be disarticulated or sawn off the column. Most cervical spinal cord compressions occur at the level of the intervertebral junctions; thus, particular attention is directed to these sites. Each dorsal intervertebral space (between arrows) is opened by removing the interarcuate ligament to expose the epidural fat. (D) The epidural fat pad is elevated (arrow) and removed before the dura and spinal cord are cut transversely. If there is no epidural fat and if the dura mater is pushed against the vertebral arch or articular processes, then a compressive lesion can be suspected. (E) After each segment of spinal cord is cut free of the remaining cord, it is grasped from the cranial orifice and removed after cutting the respective spinal nerve roots. Shown here is a cranial view of the atlas with the first cervical segment (C_1) being held by the dura mater by forceps and the C_1 nerve roots being cut with a scalpel. (F) The dorsal dura mater is split and each segment or removed portion of spinal cord is identified. A cut is placed in the cranial border of dura mater for orientation prior to fixation.

Removal of the spinal cord from an adult large animal is particularly difficult. Therefore, sectioning the entire, or appropriate part of the vertebral column with enclosed spinal cord, trimming off excess soft tissues, and immersing the sections of vertebral column in a large volume of formaldehyde is an appropriate alternative means of preservation.

A bandsaw may not be available to perform a laminectomy or sagittal vertebral cut to remove the spinal cord, and it may be unsuitable to preserve large sections of vertebral column for the pathologist. A hatchet may then be used to remove the vertebral bodies from the vertebral arches using a ventral approach. The cuts are made in a slightly medial direction, from the angle between the vertebral bodies and the transverse processes in the cervical and lumbar regions, or from the rib remnants in the thoracic region (see Rooney's technique in Mayhew and MacKay, 1982).

(ii) Gross Artifacts

Vertebral and cranial fractures frequently occur postmortem in large animals. This may be the result of falling, electrocution, dragging, or slinging. Surprisingly, considerable hemorrhage may be present around these fracture sites and the histologic appearance can be difficult to interpret. Large, mainly subarachnoid hemorrhages also occur frequently, especially if decapitation is performed immediately after death.

Gross estimates of an excessive volume of CSF are almost impossible to make, and except for a major malformation, evaluation of an apparent, slight increase in the size of ventricles should await measurements after fixation.

Areas of postmortem damage to nervous tissue can appear as a softening (malacia) and discoloration. Saw cuts and sites of tension may be apparent but the spinal cord, in particular, must be removed carefully to avoid a "toothpaste effect." Tension or compression on the spinal cord within its dura easily causes constrictions, areas of softening, discoloration, and dislocation of parts of the cord.

Partial and differential fixation can produce localized changes in texture and color, so comment is best reserved until fixation is complete. This does not preclude initial sectioning of the brain and spinal cord, as this aids in fixation.

(iii) Gross Lesions

Malformations of the CNS usually are apparent on gross inspection; however, associated structures, such as eyeballs, peripheral nerves, and muscles, should be scrutinized.

The outside of the brain and spinal cord should be studied for abnormalities in color, configuration, size, and texture; the brain can then be cut into four to six transverse sections to assist in fixation. Examining these freshly-cut surfaces, especially for symmetry, can help locate areas of malacia, hemorrhage, atrophy, and swelling. If cerebellar disease is suspected, the cerebellum to whole brain weight ratio should be calculated (normal >7%). Parasite tracts and inflammatory lesions can be inconspicuous. A culture taken from the meninges and saving a small portion of brain tissue for viral and bacterial isolation (especially from areas of discoloration), is advisable. In animals suspected of having rabies, the whole head may be submitted for rabies diagnosis. Because this may preclude an accurate diagnosis if the animal does not have rabies, one half of the brain can be submitted fresh and one half submitted in formaldehyde. This requires that appropriate precautions be followed during brain removal.

If care is used in removing the spinal cord, areas of compression and discoloration associated with necrosis, hemorrhage, or inflammation can be detected easily.

Obviously, one cannot section every part of the CNS, so an effort must be made to maintain orientation of the parts. If one suspects the presence of a gross lesion, then examination of newly made cut surfaces of the fixed tissue should provide clarification.

B. GENERAL HISTOLOGIC REACTIONS OF CELLS OF THE NERVOUS SYSTEM

(i) Reactions of Neurons

Artifacts are extremely common in microscopic specimens and usually are the result of fixation, sectioning and staining procedures. Disappearance of neurons is good evidence of a lesion, but can be difficult to detect. Neuronal changes, without associated glial or other cellular reactions, must be interpreted cautiously. Neuronal fiber (axon and myelin sheath) degeneration can be a useful sign of a neuronal defect, even at a site distant from the cell body.

Swelling and shrinkage are two changes frequently seen in neurons and are reasonably reliable findings if they are present in well-preserved tissue. Swelling of the cytoplasm (pale, basophilic) and nucleus often is the earliest observable change in infections, toxicities, and hyperthermia, and it might be reversible. When there are excessive numbers of glia (microglia) surrounding such cells (satellitosis), or there is actual neuronophagia, then the change is irreversible. Shrinkage of a soma often is seen in hyperthermia, hypoxia, and trauma. Shrinkage with eosinophilic homogenization (chromatolysis) of cytoplasm and a shrunken, densely basophilic nucleus is indicative of ischemia or hypoglycemia (ischemic nerve cell change).

Simple atrophy of CNS neurons with axonal loss is part of the aging process, and is present in many abiotrophies (delayed onset, degenerative disorders), and when chronic, trans-synaptic atrophy occurs. Neurofibrils in atrophic axons undergo shrinkage, hyperchromia, and beading.

Injury to neuronal processes can be divided functionally and morphologically into three stages. Neurapraxis is the state of loss of function only; axonotmesis is severance of axons; and neurotmesis is severance of the entire nerve fiber. In the PNS, wallerian degeneration and regeneration occur following interruption of axons. The nerve fiber that is distal to the site of damage disintegrates in 3 to 4 days, and more slowly, the myelin degenerates as ellipsoids and droplets, to be phagocytosed. The end plate, or receptor organ, atrophies and disintegrates, and Schwann cells begin proliferation. The nerve fiber proximal to the site of damage disintegrates minimally, but the cell body shows a reactive change, including central chromatolysis and swelling with margination of the nucleus. Regeneration of several axonal stumps, with budding into proliferated Schwann cells and endoneurial columns, begins early, with further growth at about 1 to 4 mm a day. Individual fiber replacement can be complete, but total quantitative nerve function is not.

In the CNS, wallerian-like degeneration occurs following focal axonal damage, but the regenerative process is markedly curtailed. The mapping of degenerated, distal neuronal fibers following damage is used to help define the site(s) of lesions in the CNS, particularly in the brainstem and spinal cord. Thus, in a pathology report, if degeneration is only described in fibers in ascending (afferent) white matter pathways cranial to C_6, and only in descending (efferent) fibers caudal to C_6, then a focal lesion at C_6 most likely is present. However, if ascending and descending fiber degeneration is present in the T_{10} segment, there must be at least one lesion cranial to T_{10}, and one lesion caudal to T_{10}, or diffuse degeneration of neuronal fibers.

With many metabolic, toxic, and nutritional insults, axons may undergo degenerative changes that often are recognized as swellings. Such swollen axons, or spheroids, can be prominent in particular nuclear regions where neuroaxonal dystrophy is occurring. This process is common in some nutritional diseases and intoxications, and in certain hereditary disorders; it also occurs during aging.

Accumulation of iron- and calcium-containing pigments in neurons (often around neurons and blood vessels), may indicate a previous influx of blood pigments to the area. Such pigmentations occur with aging, along with often spectacular intraneuronal accumulation of lipofuscin—the aging or wear and tear pigment. All these changes can be prominent in the brainstem and basal nuclear regions of aged animals. Accumulation of specific lysosomal products are the hallmark of the inherited lysosomal storage diseases, as well as a few intoxications.

(ii) Reactions of Astrocytes

Astrocytes which occur in the gray and white matter, appear to be a major component of the cytoskeleton framework of the CNS. Their processes, with basal laminae, form part of the blood-brain and blood-CSF barriers, and they appear to act as a guide to migrating neurons during development. They tend to be relatively resistant to noxious stimuli and are associated with reparative processes. For unknown reasons, repair of substantial areas of damaged CNS parenchyma often does not occur, leaving a void that is occupied by CSF-like fluid, which is surrounded by a lamina of astrocyte processes. On the other hand, the common response to CNS damage is astrocyte hyperplasia and hypertrophy with prominence of their processes (fibrillary astrogliosis). Shrinkage and necrosis of astrocytes occurs with the death of other CNS elements during infarction, hemorrhage and pressure. Astrocytes imbibe tissue fluid after it has leaked into extracellular spaces; this is an early finding in various edematous states, such as trauma, infarction, and vascular disorders. Astrocytes do act as phagocytes, but to a lesser degree than microglia and macrophages. Reactive astrocytes often are found at the periphery of subacute and chronic lesions. They often show prominent nuclear enlargement and eosinophilic cytoplasmic swelling and are called gemistocytes.

(iii) Reactions of Oligodendrocytes

The oligodendrocyte cell bodies can show hydropic swelling in many edematous states, although the edematous fluid often is transferred to astrocytes and microglial cells. The oligodendrocyte processes and associated myelin sheaths are susceptible to any noxious stimulus.

Oten the enclosed axons are damaged, but several immune-mediated, infectious, and toxic insults cause a disintegration of myelin sheaths with or without oligodendrocyte loss; therefore, the functionally vital oligodendrocyte-axon relationships are disturbed. This process is demyelination. If such a perturbation occurs prior to the developmental, perinatal process of myelination, it is termed hypomyelination. Some toxic and inherent disorders of oligodendrocytes result in disturbances of the myelin sheath, which are seen as vacuoles or fluid in the white matter (status spongiosus). Many of the disorders that affect myelin alone cause asynchrony of axonal conduction, which is seen clinically as congenital, or delayed onset whole body tremor.

Remyelination of demyelinated CNS axons can occur under various conditions, but is not consistent. Interestingly, remyelination in the CNS is just as likely to be performed by resident and immigrant Schwann cells as by oligodendrocytes.

(iv) Reactions of Microglial Cells

These fixed histiocytes, or tissue macrophages, of the CNS respond quickly to any insult that results in necrosis and tissue debris, which they phagocytose. They thus can hypertrophy into macrophages. During proliferation these histiocytes may form nodules or stars at sites of damage to CNS parenchyma, and may also accumulate in perivascular cuffs along with monocytic and polymorphonucleated inflammatory cells. They are involved with removal of dead neurons (neuronophagia). Focal or diffuse microgliosis often remains for years as the last recognizable change following lesions in the CNS.

With prominent damage to CNS parenchyma, often phagocytic mononuclear cells filled with lipid (myelin) debris accumulate. These are gitter cells and for the most part are believed to arise from an influx of circulating monocytes, as opposed to proliferation of microglial cells.

(v) Reactions of Meningeal, Choroidal, and Ependymal Cells

These cells tend to be relatively unreactive. Invasion by infectious agents, and direct injury, result in an influx of circulating inflammatory and phagocytic cells with some proliferation. Subependymal and subpial gliosis can be prominent in some superficial CNS infections. These cells become flattened when

CSF pressure is increased within the neuraxis. Fibroblasts associated with the meninges are effective in proliferation and migration; they cover any meningeal or submeningeal defects that occur with damage.

(vi) Reactions of Schwann Cells

Proliferated Schwann cells mainly guide and ensheath regrowing axons during the process of wallerian regeneration in the PNS. Thus, following focal or diffuse PNS axon lesions, such proliferation is evident. Schwann cells, like oligodendrocytes, are subject to immune and toxic attack and are sometimes affected by inherent metabolic disorders. This may occur before, or after, normal developmental myelination, causing hypomyelination, or demyelination, respectively. Unlike oligodendrocytes, Schwann cells are extremely efficient at recoating bare PNS axons and repairing lesions.

C. NEUROPATHOLOGIC RESPONSES IN THE VARIOUS MECHANISMS OF DISEASE

Just as each mechanism of disease has its own clinical characteristics (see above chapter on Neurologic Examination), so each has certain morphologic characteristics. One must understand that vascular disorders result in abrupt, localized hypoxia and tissue necrosis, as well as leakage of blood protein and pigments. This is as clinically relevant as understanding that such diseases usually have a sudden onset of signs that remain static or, more frequently, improve with time.

(i) Malformations

Neurologic signs can result from malformations that involve nervous tissue, or involve the tissues surrounding the neuraxis, particularly the cranium and vertebral column. Cranial and vertebral malformations do not always affect the nervous system, but when they do it is affected by trauma and often signs are progressive. Malformations may be congenital, or acquired, and in both cases can have a hereditary, infectious, toxic, traumatic, or even vascular basis. The type of nervous tissue malformation that results often depends more on the time and site of action, rather than the causative factors. Thus, certain infections and toxins may result in the same malformation (e.g., cerebellar hypoplasia or arthrogryposis) when acting at the appropriate developmental stage.

(ii) Infectious, Inflammatory and Immune Disorders

With few exceptions these result in degrees of inflammatory cell infiltrate, at least in the early stages.

a. Viral

Most viral diseases cause nonsuppurative inflammation with lymphocytes, plasma cells, and monocytes, especially in perivascular cuffs. A few fulminant viral infections, particularly those that result in considerable necrosis of CNS tissue, are characterized by neutrophil invasion. Neurotropic viruses, such as rabies and the arboviral encephalitides, destroy neurons so there is neuronal degeneration, satellitosis, and neuronophagia. The rarer slow-viral infections may not induce much of an inflammatory response and are slowly progressive.

b. Bacterial

Suppurative meningitis is most common in neonatal animals, especially those with failure of passive transfer of immunoglobulin. Often there is considerable protein exudate with tissue swelling. Brain abscesses act as space-occupying lesions and cause compression and edema of adjacent tissue. Because of the rigidity of the calvarium these forms of cerebral edema can result in herniation of adjacent parts of the brain. Vertebral osteomyelitis most often causes spinal cord compression rather than myelitis, and septic emboli, at least initially, damage CNS tissue because of ischemic and hemorrhagic infarction.

c. Fungal

Fungal infections of the nervous system are rare. The usual result is a mixed neutrophilic and mononuclear inflammation, and granulomata may form.

d. Protozoa

Encysted protozoal forms may be associated with little cellular reaction. Often there is severe necrosis with hemorrhage and inflammation comprised of lymphocytes and macrophages, sometimes neutrophils, eosinophils, and multinucleated giant cells.

e. Helminth and Arthropod Parasites

Penetration of the CNS by fly larvae (myiasis) and roundworms (nematodiasis) usually is accidental; however, invasion by some nematodes and tapeworm cysts (coneurosis) is part of the respective life cycle. In the natural host, minimal damage may result. Usually, however, massive tissue destruction, hemorrhage, protein exudate, and an influx of neutrophils and macrophages, with variable numbers of eosinophils, and giant cells, occurs. Such parasites can arrive in the CNS through natural foramina or via the blood supply. Subsequent, usually random migrations, can be tortuous, and may simply separate the tissues without causing much inflammation. Also, parasites can leave the CNS after creating devastation.

f. Immune Mediated

Type I, anaphylactic immune reponses in the CNS are rare, partly because the CNS is well-isolated from the immune system. Cytotoxic, autoimmune, type II reactions, directed against natural or altered antigens (such as myelin), occur in the CNS and PNS causing nonsuppurative encephalitis or neuritis. Antigen-antibody complex, type III-mediated vasculitis occurs in the CNS in some diseases and, like other forms of vasculitis, CNS damage results more from infarction than inflammation. The latter can be neutrophilic, lymphocytic, or mixed.

(iii) Physical Disorders

Concussion, with loss of function, is only the mildest effect of CNS trauma, whereas contusion and laceration causes morphologic lesions with degrees of cell death, hemorrhage, edema, and neutrophil and macrophage infiltration. Microglial, then astrocytic activation, proliferation and hypertrophy occur in adjacent viable tissue. The site of major tissue damage may not be directly related to the site of traumatic impact on the calvarium or vertebral column. Parenchymal and subarachnoid bleeding is common, but subdural and epidural hematoma formation is less frequent in domestic animals than in man. Hematomas, like cerebral abscesses and other space-occupying lesions, create local pressure and edema that can cause herniation of parts of the brain. Destroyed tissue is removed by activated microglia, but if it is more extensive, by infiltrating monocytic macrophages; this results in pools of lipid-laden macrophages (gitter cells). Such large lesions may heal to form an astrogial scar or a fluid-filled cavity. Secondary neuronal fiber degeneration will occur along fiber tracts that are separated from their cell bodies by the injury.

Heat, cold, chemicals, and ionizing irradiation can cause immediate cell death with massive vascular breakdown and tissue infarction. Some delayed effects, particularly on maintenance of myelin, may be noted with irradiation.

Hypertension, perhaps on a compartmental basis, may play a role in the vascular accidents associated with the so-called neonatal maladjustment syndrome of foals.

(iv) Toxic Diseases

Some toxins, such as cyanide, interfere with oxygen transport. Water and salt intoxications directly alter osmolality of cells by interrupting many metabolic functions, and by swelling or shrinking cells. Lesions, if present, usually are symmetrical, often diffuse, and usually end with tissue necrosis. Some plant (e.g., yellow star thistle) and microbial (e.g., *Clostridium perfringens* type D) toxins produce extremely selective and focal lesions, suggesting that they are mediated by selective neurotransmitter disruption or, more likely, by selective vascular derangements.

(v) Nutritional Diseases

Starvation, and disorders associated with vitamins A and D and calcium and phosphorus intake, can be associated with vertebral fractures. Depending on the animal species, thiamin deficiency can cause cerebrocortical neuronal necrosis, hemorrhagic necrosis of white matter, and axonal degeneration. Lesions of cell death tend to be symmetrical with nutritional diseases.

(vi) Metabolic Diseases

Many metabolic disorders, such as hypocalcemia, hypomagnesemia, and ketoacidosis alter nervous tissue function (especially electrical transmission) when there are no morphologic lesions. Some cause degeneration of neurons, and ultimately necrosis, often in selective areas of the CNS. These include hypoglycemia, hypoxia, and hepatoencephalopathy. The latter can produce a striking hypertrophy of astrocytes. Most are characterized by a lack of inflammation.

Inherited, neuronal, metabolic disorders often are expressed as abiotrophies with selective neuroaxonal degeneration, or as lysosomal storage disease with accumulation of metabolic products in macrophages and neurons. Other metabolic disorders result in hypomyelination or demyelination.

(vii) Vascular Lesions

Interruption of the blood supply results in hemorrhagic or ischemic infarction and tissue necrosis, with neutrophilic and then monocytic phagocytosis of debris. Emboli and thrombi may be septic, parasitic, or fibrocartilaginous. More generalized infarction may occur with cardiopulmonary deficiencies, disseminated clotting defects, and septicemia.

(viii) Degenerative Processes

Many of these diseases, which involve morphologic degeneration of CNS tissue, are familial or hereditary and may be considered metabolic disorders (see above). Of the remaining, most are of unknown origin, although hereditary, toxic, metabolic, nutritional, and viral factors often are suspected.

(ix) Neoplastic Diseases

With the exception of neurofibroma and lymphosarcoma in cattle, neoplasms involving nervous tissue are rare in domestic large animals.

Neoplasms replace or compress nervous tissue, and both forms often cause adjacent edema because of local vascular perturbations. As a result of the space-occupying effect and the associated edema, brain herniations occur with brain neoplasms just as they occur with cerebral abscesses and hematomata. These include herniations of the cingulate gyrus under the falx cerebri, the occipital lobes under the tentorium cerebelli, and the cerebellar vermis through the foramen magnum. All these tissue movements cause compression of other parts of the brain. Primary CNS tumors are extremely rare in large animals, but can arise from meningeal, ependymal, choroidal, glial, or endothelial cell lines. Neuronal cell line neoplasms are even less frequent; however, a proliferation of primitive neuroepithelial cells from the hind brain sometimes occurs in young calves, and is a medulloblastoma. Ganglion and Schwann cell neoplasms occur in the PNS. Neoplasms involving the skull and vertebrae, as well as metastatic neoplasms, usually compress nervous tissue; the effects are identical to those of external injury. Lymphosarcoma probably is the most common metastatic neoplasm involving the brain in large animals, although probably it should be considered a primary tumor when it is in the epidural space and when it encompasses the peripheral nerves of cattle.

(x) Idiopathic Disorders

In many clinical neurologic syndromes, no consistent gross or light microscopic findings exist. This includes "shivering" and self-mutilation syndrome. In some cases, a thorough search for lesions is not undertaken for various reasons. Other problems, such as roaring and stringhalt, may be associated with consistent neuropathologic lesions, but the etiology still is unknown.

BIBLIOGRAPHY

Davis RL, Robertson DM, eds. *Textbook of Neuropathology.* Baltimore: Williams and Wilkins, 1985.

Hume Adams J, Corsellis JAN, Duchen LW, eds. *Greenfield's Neuropathology.* 4th Ed. New York: Wiley-Medical, 1984.

Innes JRM, Saunders LZ. *Comparative Neuropathology.* New York: Academic Press, 1962.

Jones TC, Hunt RD. *Veterinary Pathology.* 5th Ed., Philadelphia: Lea & Febiger, 1983. Ch 27, pp 1637–1728.

Mayhew IG, MacKay RJ. The nervous system. In: Mansmann RA, McAllister ES, Pratt PW, eds. *Equine Medicine and Surgery.* 3rd Ed., Vol 2, Santa Barbara: American Veterinary Publications, 1982. Ch. 21, pp 1159–1252.

Sullivan ND. The nervous system. In: Jubb KVF, Kennedy PC, Palmer N, eds. *Pathology of Domestic Animals.* 3rd Ed., Vol 1, Orlando: Academic Press, 1985. Ch. 3, pp 201–338.

PART II

PROBLEMS IN LARGE ANIMAL NEUROLOGIC PATIENTS

CHAPTER 5

Problem 1:
Disorders of Behavior and Personality [Including Diffuse CNS Disorders]*

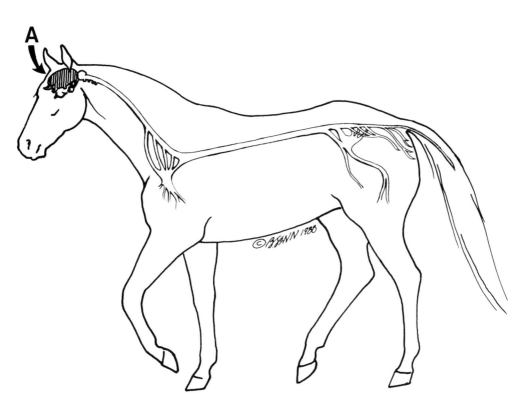

Location of lesions resulting in disorders of behavior and personality: focal and diffuse forebrain (A).

Normal behavior is extremely variable between species, breeds, and individuals. Thus, if after a neurologic examination, the only finding is a subtle change in expected behavior, the examiner must be cautious when assuming that a morbid lesion in the forebrain accounts for the signs.

Subtle alterations in behavior, resulting from organic brain disorders, in-

---

*See also Problem 13, for unusual behavior.

clude continual yawning that can be prominent in hepatoencephalopathy, a tendency to drift to one side that often is present with asymmetric lesions, and a lack of recognition of familiar animals, people, and objects, which often is the earliest expression of cerebral disease in foals. More severe signs are compulsive walking, circling, head pressing, biting at animate and inanimate objects, leaving food in the mouth, and adopting bizarre postures. Such signs usually are referable to lesions in the frontal and temporal lobes, internal capsule, limbic system, thalamus and basal nuclei, or to diffuse brain disease.

Usually, local and diffuse lesions affecting the forebrain only result in combinations of behavioral changes (Problem 1), seizures (Problem 2), blindness (Problem 3), and depression (Problem 4). Little or no alteration in gait occurs, at least in the subacute to chronic stage.

With no other neurologic signs, it is dificult to be sure whether subtle behavioral syndromes are psychologic or neurologic in origin. Examples of these include licking, head shaking, tail-wringing, aggressiveness, and refusing to take jumps. Some of these syndromes are discussed in Problem 13, although for a more detailed evaluation of equine behavioral (psychologic) aberrations, the reader is directed to Crowell-Davis and Houpt (1986) and Kiley-Worthington and Wood-Gush (1987).

Categories of Disease and Differential Diagnosis
*NOTE: Only diseases marked * are discussed in this section.*

   I. Congenital and Familial
       *1. Hydrocephalus
       *2. Hydranencephaly
       *3. Lysosomal Storage Diseases
       *4. Citrullinemia
       *5. Miscellaneous Forebrain Malformations
        6. Maple Syrup Urine Disease of Calves (Problem 8A)
        7. Hypomyelinogenesis (Problem 8B)
        8. Neuraxial Edema (Problem 8B)
        9. Shaker Calf Syndrome (Problem 8B)
       10. Congenital Swayback (Problem 10)
  II. Physical
       *1. Head Trauma (Problem 4)
       *2. Dehorning Injuries
        3. Intracarotid Injection (Problem 2)
        4. Heat Stroke (Problem 4)
 III. Infectious, Inflammatory, Immune
       *1. Equine Togaviral Encephalomyelitides
       *2. Malignant Catarrhal Fever
       *3. Rabies
       *4. Enteroviral Encephalomyelitis of Pigs
       *5. Hemagglutinating Encephalomyelitis Virus
       *6. Pseudorabies (Problem 13)
       *7. Porcine Paramyxovirus (Blue Eyes)
       *8. Scrapie (Problem 9 and 13)
       *9. Chronic Wasting Disease of Captive Deer

    *10. Bovine Spongiform Encephalopathy
    *11. Equine Infectious Anemia Ependymitis—Meningitis
    *12. Sporadic Bovine Encephalomyelitis
    *13. Thromboembolic Meningoencephalitis
    *14. Bacterial Meningitis and Meningoventriculitis
    *15. Brain Abscess
    *16. Mycotic Encephalitis
    *17. Verminous Encephalitis (Problem 10)
    *18. Parasitic Thromboembolism (Problem 10)
    *19. Miscellaneous Diffuse Meningoencephalomyelitides
    20. Basillar Empyema—Pituitary Abscess (Problem 6)
    21. Equine Protozoal Myeloencephalitis (Problem 10)
    22. Infectious Bovine Rhinotracheitis (Problem 13)
    23. Louping Ill (Problem 9)
    24. Visna/Maedi (Problem 10)
    25. Caprine Arthritis—Encephalomyelitis (Problem 10)
IV. Metabolic
    *1. Hypoglycemia
    *2. Hypocalcemia (also Problems 2 and 8)
    *3. Hypomagnesemia (also Problems 2 and 8)
    *4. Anesthetic Hypoxia—Anoxia (Problem 3)
    *5. Hepatic Encephalopathy
    *6. Miscellaneous
V. Toxic
    *1. Lead
    *2. Salt and Water
    *3. Urea—Ammonia
    *4. Cyanide
    *5. Locoweed, and Darling Pea
    *6. *Kochia scoparia* (Mexican fireweed)
    *7. Miscellaneous Plants
    *8. Moldy Corn
    *9. Focal Symmetrical Encephalomalacia, Edema Disease
    10. Organophosphates, Chlorinated Hydrocarbons, and Strychnine
        (Problem 2)
    11. Organomercury (Problems 9 and 10)
VI. Nutritional
    *1. Thiamine Responsive Polioencephalomalacia of Ruminants
    *2. Vitamin E Deficiency—Mullberry Heart Disease of Swine
    *3. Vitamin A Deficiency (see Hydrocephalus I.1 above)
VII. Neoplastic (Problem 2)
VIII. Idiopathic
    *1. Neonatal Maladjustment Syndrome of Foals
    2. Grove Poisoning (Problem 2)
    3. Nervous Coccidiosis (Problem 2)

  I. Congenital and Familial
    1. Hydrocephalus

This is sometimes a rare inherited trait in cattle, or an isolated occurrence in all species (Bester et al., 1976), (Foreman et al., 1983) (Fig. 5–1). Vitamin A deficiency in calves can result in altered bone growth and a deformed calvarium, particularly involving the temporal bone, which obstructs CSF flow and results in hydrocephalus (Divers et al., 1986).

2. **Hydranencephaly**

This may be more common than hydrocephalus is in large animals, particularly in calves; it is frequently associated with bovine viral diarrhea virus, Akabane virus, and other in utero viral infections (Konno et al., 1982a,b), (MacLachlan et al., 1983). Cerebellar signs and arthrogryposis predominate the clinical syndromes, but depression and blindness ("dummies") may be evident because of hydranencephaly. (See Problems 9 and 10.)

3. **Lysosomal Storage Disorders**

These rare diseases result from an inborn error or acquired defect in a metabolic enzyme pathway, often reflected by accumulation of substrates and by-products in all cells of the body, particularly in the nervous system (Jolly et al., 1977). Some examples are:

a. *GM$_1$–Gangliosidosis in Freisian Calves* (Donnelly et al., 1977). Depression and ataxia are seen at birth, and death occurs in 6 to 8 months. This is an autosomal recessive disease.

b. *GM$_2$–Gangliosidosis in Yorkshire Swine* (Kosanke et al., 1978). This disease causes hypermetria and weakness within 3 months of birth. Recumbency occurs in 4 to 6 months.

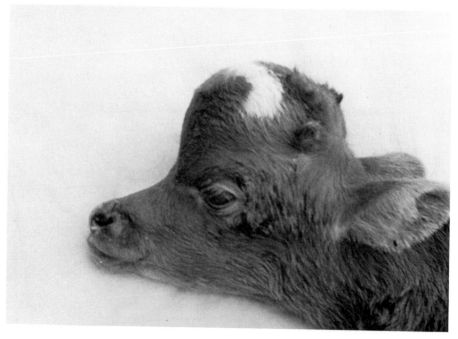

Figure 5–1. Newborn hydrocephalic calf, with profound malformation of the calvarium and ventromedial eye deviation, which is presumed to be due to the deformed bony orbit.

   c. *α–Mannosidosis in Aberdeen Angus and Murray Gray Cattle.*
      Aggressiveness, cerebellar ataxia, and ill thrift are seen (Leipold
      et al., 1979). Progressive signs begin at birth or several months
      of age. This disease is mimicked by *Swainsona* sp and locoweed
      plant intoxications (Huxtable et al., 1982), (Molyneux, et al.,
      1982).
   d. *β–Mannosidosis in Anglo-Nubian Goats.* The affected animal is
      recumbent at birth, with profound cerebellar signs evident (Healy
      et al., 1981), (Kumar, et al., 1986).
   e. *Ovine* (Mayhew et al., 1985), *Caprine* (Luttgen et al., 1982) *and*
      Bovine Ceroid-Lipofuscinosis (Harper et al., 1988). At 9 to 12
      months of age, affected South Hampshire lambs show blindness,
      head nodding, jaw chomping, facial twitching, weight loss, and
      depression (Fig. 5–2). They succumb to the disease by 30 months
      of age. Kid goats with the disease show evidence of cerebellar
      involvment (see Problem 9). Affected Devon cattle demonstrate
      blindness by 14 months of age and may become weak. They
      usually die from misadventure by 3 to 4 years of age.
   f. *Generalized Glycogenosis in Beef Shorthorn and Brahman Cat-*
      tle. Although glycogen is deposited in central and peripheral
      neurons, signs generally include ill thrift, respiratory difficulty,
      and muscle weakness (Cook et al., 1982).

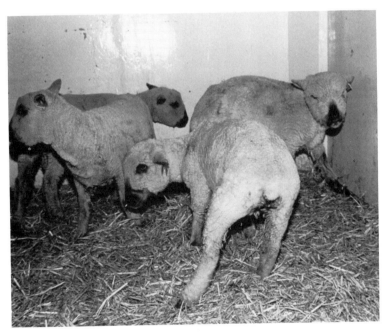

Figure 5–2. Ovine ceroid lipofuscinosis (OCL) in a group of 18- to 22-month-old South Hampshire sheep homozygous for OCL. As with many inherited "storage diseases," the sheep demonstrate weight loss. The neurologic syndrome representing progressive cerebral (and retinal) disease consists of being unaware of the environment, wandering in circles, adopting abnormal postures, head pressing, blindness, and periodic episodes of face, head, neck, and thoracic limb tremor, which are interpreted as mild diffuse seizure episodes.

4. Citrullinemia

This is a fatal, neurologic disorder affecting Holstein-Fresian Calves 1 to 4 days of age. Affected calves are normal at birth, but develop acute depression, blindness, head pressing, aimless walking, tremor, seizures, and opisthotonus; they usually die within several hours. Diffuse cerebrospinal edema, with some neuronal degeneration, is present on histologic examination of the brain and is associated with elevated plasma citrulline concentrations (<1000 mmol/L; normal 66 ± 19 mM/L, N = 6) without elevated argininosuccinic acid concentrations. It is suggested that this disease is inherited argininosuccinate synthetase deficiency (Harper et al., 1986).

5. Miscellaneous Forebrain Malformation

Many congenital and inherited brain malformations occur that involve the forebrain. These are best described in calves (Cho et al., 1977). Depression, behavioral changes, blindness, and failure to thrive frequently occur. Great variability in the severity of the clinical syndrome may accompany the same morphologic defect, such as agenesis of the corpus callosum. The latter anomaly occurred along with polymicrogyria in 23 of 345 (7%) Murray Gray dominant X Aberdeen Angus calves over a period of 6 years (Read, 1983).

Holoprosencephaly, with undivided, hypoplastic cerebral hemispheres and associated flattened skull may be common in Border Leicester lambs (Roth et al., 1987).

II. Physical

1. Trauma

Patients may have dementia following head injuries. This usually is transient, but may last a few weeks in mild cases, and up to several months in severe cases. Management of head injuries is discussed under Problem 4.

2. Dehorning Injury.

Signalment. Young ruminants.

History. A few hours to several weeks following hot iron dehorning, young ruminants, especially kids, may circle, become depressed and blind, and have seizures or die (Nation et al., 1985), (Wright et al., 1983), (Dickson, 1984).

Examination. Pyrexia may be present, and the animal usually is anorectic. Diffuse or localizing cerebral signs occur, although sudden death most often is reported. Signs include acute or progressive depression, blindness, circling, opisthotonus, seizures, recumbency, and death.

Assessment. This condition is rare in calves, but occurs particularly in young kids. Overzealous use of a hot iron, or even caustic dehorning paste may cause coagulative necrosis of the parieto-occipital lobes, with or without secondary infection (Fig. 5–3).

Treatment. Glucocorticosteroids, other anti-inflammatory agents and antibiotics, along with debridement and topical therapy are indicated. Tetanus prophylaxis should be undertaken; however, with prominent signs the outlook is bad.

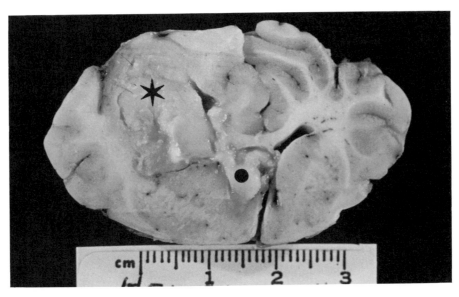

Figure 5–3. Dehorning injury. Excessive heat from a hot iron used for dehorning has caused profound coagulative necrosis in the frontoparietal cortex of one cerebral hemisphere (star) in this goat kid. Some of the necrotic debris is displaced into the lateral ventricle (filled circle). (Courtesy of A. de Lahunta.)

III. Infectious, Inflammatory, Immune

1. **Equine Togaviral Encephalomyelitides**

These diseases are common in particular areas and countries.

The viruses associated with this disease complex include Eastern, Western, Venezuelan, Semiliki Forest, St. Louis, Japanese B, Murray Valley, louping ill, and Russian spring-summer encephalitis (togaviruses), Borna disease, and Near-East equine encephalomyelitis. Clinical signs, which vary in severity with each virus, usually are referable to diffuse cerebral disease, but sometimes, such as with louping ill in horses, signs of spinal cord disease predominate. Borna disease is a rare encephalomyelitis, which is caused by an unclassified virus that mainly affects horses, but may infect sheep, cattle, goats, and rabbits. The disease occurs in Europe and ticks, presumably, spread the virus. Signs include blindness, teeth-grinding, hyperexcitability, seizures, and ataxia. The role of Snowshoe Hare virus (Lynch et al., 1985), Main Drain virus (Emmons et al., 1983) and Powassan virus (Little et al., 1985) in the clinical syndrome of viral-type encephalomyelitis in North American horses is unclear. The remainder of this section refers particularly to the alphaviruses: Eastern, Western, and Venezuelan encephalomyelitis (EEE, WEE, VEE), which predominate in the Americas.

Signalment. Horses of any age, breed, and sex. The diseases are not common in suckling foals under 3 months of age.

History. There is a progressive, but often abrupt onset of depression and fever, then peracute to acute diffuse brain signs. Usually the disease follows vector mosquito (or tick) movement. In the southeastern part of the United States, the disease may occur year-round.

Physical Examination. Fever, prodromal malaise, colic, and anorexia may be evident.

Neurologic Examination. Dementia, head pressing, ataxia, blindness, circling, and seizures usually are evident (Fig. 5–4). Signs of spinal cord or brainstem involvement rarely may occur first.

Virus Ecology. Birds are reservoir hosts for these viruses, and horses (and human beings) are infected by mosquitoes (transfer hosts). The transfer seasons depend on (migratory) bird life and vector seasons, and may be year-round in the southeastern part of the United States with EEE.

Assessment. These viruses are neurotropic and directly cause neuronal necrosis throughout the entire CNS, particularly in the cerebrum. In the fulminant syndrome, which usually occurs with EEE, a prominent neutrophilic infiltrate results from tissue necrosis. This slowly is replaced by a more nonsuppurative inflammation if the horse survives. Frequently with EEE, massive necrosis and softening (malacia) occurs, and blood vessels are disrupted, resulting in diffuse, patchy hemorrhage, which is seen as congestion and dark staining of the freshly cut brain. In addition, the resulting brain

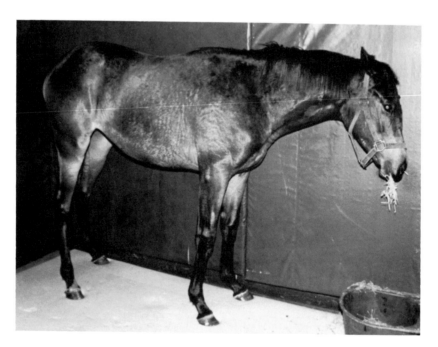

Figure 5–4. Eastern Equine Encephalomyelitis (EEE). This horse was febrile and rapidly developed depression, a tendency to wander and stumble into objects, and would leave food hanging from the mouth although swallowing was not impaired. Analysis of cerebrospinal fluid revealed a prominent neutrophilic pleocytosis with xanthochromia. These signs of diffuse cerebral disease, typical of togaviral encephalitis, progressed to seizures and coma. The horse was euthanized and EEE was confirmed at the postmortem examination.

swelling causes occipital and cerebellar herniations under the tentorium cerebelli and occipital bone, respectively, compressing vital brainstem structures. These movements of brain tissue are associated with terminal events, including dilated pupils (cranial nerve III), irregular breathing patterns, cardiac arrhythmias, and death.

"Brain-heart" Syndrome. The cardiac irregularities detected in fulminant EEE have been related to conduction defects on electrocardiograms, release of heart specific muscle enzymes (serum hydroxybutyric dehydrogenase activity), and severe, multifocal cardiac ischemic lesions. Brain-heart syndrome (King et al., 1982) can be caused by many profound intracranial events and appears to be mediated via the upper motor neurons of the autonomic nervous system, to the blood supply, and to the neural control of the myocardium.

Diagnostic Aids. Rising acute and convalescent serum HI titers, or a high terminal titer for a specific strain can be used in a clinical diagnosis. The use of IgM specific enzyme immunoassays may help in the ante mortem diagnosis of EEE (Scott, et al., 1986). Viral isolation from brain tissue usually is possible but it is difficult to isolate the virus from cerebrospinal fluid. Analysis of CSF shows leukocytosis, which is often initially neurotrophilic (especially with EEE), as well as increased protein content and xanthochromia. Occasionally, a prominent CSF eosinophilic pleocytosis is detected with EEE. The CSF changes are less prominent with WEE, and probably with VEE also.

Therapy. This primarily entails intense nursing care, including intravenous fluid therapy and forced feeding. Glucocorticoids (dexamethasone, 0.1–0.25 mg/kg IV, QID) may be tried in the peracute phase for a short term; 10% DMSO (1 g/kg daily IV) also appears to have been useful.

Prognosis. The outlook for survival is poor for EEE and for VEE; it is fair to bad for WEE. Survival may leave residual signs such as a "dummy syndrome." Horses suspected of having EEE that have survived had some previous exposure to EEE vaccine, but with insufficient protection. They appeared to have a modified disease course, initially with a slow progression of signs, and sometimes with only evidence of spinal cord and brainstem disease.

Control. Mosquito control and immunization have significantly reduced the incidence of these diseases. However, outbreaks still are frequent in the southern United States because of the short duration of vaccine immunity (4 to 6 months) and the long vector season. Thus, horses must be vaccinated at least in the early spring and again in summer. Foals may become tolerant to EEE if they are repeatedly vaccinated at a young age (J. Wilson and P. Gibbs, pers. comm.). Thus, initial vaccination should occur at 3 to 4 months of age and then twice yearly.

2. **Malignant Catarrhal Fever (MCF).**

Signalment. Usually adult cattle are affected. It is rare under 6 months of age.

History. Usually this is a sporadic disease. There have been outbreaks of acute diarrhea, rhinitis, ophthalmitis, and dermatitis with terminal encephalitis (James et al., 1975). Recovery is rare.

Physical Examination. Panophthalmitis, purulent nasal and ocular discharges, exudative dermatitis, and lymphadenopathy may be present.

Neurologic Examination. There is depression, blindness, wandering, seizures, and recumbency. Neurologic signs occur 3 to 10 days after systemic signs.

Assessment. Terminal encephalitis occurs in this multisystem disease which is caused by a herpesvirus. Cattle usually are in contact with sheep, and sometimes deer, when the disease occurs (Pierson et al., 1974). The disease appears to be distinct from wildebeest-associated MCF in Africa, but has been transmitted experimentally from affected cattle and deer to calves (Horner et al., 1975), (Selman et al., 1978).

Diagnostic Aids. Urinalysis may reveal proteinuria because of nephrosis. Skin and lymph node biopsy may show a necrotizing fibrinoid vasculitis, which characterizes the lesions present in all organs, including the brain and meninges.

Plan. Treatment is palliative. The disease is usually fatal, although it is sporadic. Separating cattle from sheep and deer is a sensible preventative precaution.

3. Rabies

This is a rare disease, but it is significant because of public health concerns.

Signalment. Any age, breed, and sex of warm-blooded animals.

History. The patient may have been bitten by a racoon, skunk, fox, or bat several months prior to the onset of signs. Once the signs start, the untreated clinical course is less than 14 days, but usually less than 5 days, and the animal dies (Joyce, et al., 1981). Modified, live, virus (MLV), vaccine-induced rabies in cats, dogs, and horses has occurred.

Physical Examination. There is nothing diagnostic; usually bite wounds are healed. Fever may occur independently from seizure activity (Joyce et al., 1981), (Reid, 1985).

Neurologic Examination. In the cerebral, or furious form, aggressive behavior, photophobia, hydrophobia, hyperesthesia, straining, and convulsions (Fig. 5–5) occur. In the brainstem, or dumb form, depression and dementia with ataxia, excessive drooling, and pharyngeal paralysis occur. The spinal cord, or paralytic form, is characterized by progressive, ascending paralysis. Self-mutilation, often directed to one part of the body, may be associated with any form, particularly the latter (Fig. 5–5). The ascending spinal cord form, progressing to brainstem involvement, has been seen in the vaccine-associated form in horses (West, 1985).

Although the clinical signs vary, a few generalizations are worthy of mention. The rabies virus passes along neurons within the nervous system. Initially, there may be hyperactivity of affected neurons with signs such as hyperesthesia, tremor, straining, and

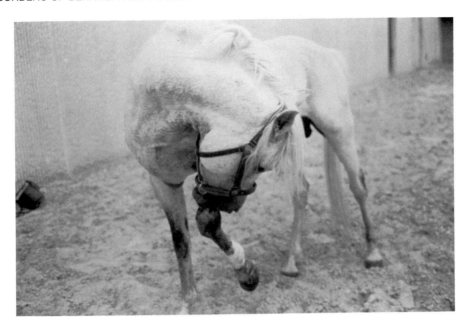

Figure 5–5. Rabies. Bizzare behavior—biting the forelimbs as well as inanimate objects and humans—characterized this particular case of equine rabies.

salivation. Ultimately the neurons die and signs such as flaccid paralysis, dysphagia, and anesthesia then can be expected. The disease is progressive, but the course may be prolonged by anti-inflammatory therapy. If the patient does not succumb with brainstem involvement, ultimately the virus reaches the forebrain causing altered behavior, such as vocalization and aggressiveness, seizures, coma, and death.

Frequently occuring signs recorded in large animals dying of rabies (in decreasing order of frequency) include: for cattle, salivation, bellowing, aggressiveness, paresis/paralysis, and straining; for goats, aggressiveness, bleating, and salivation; for sheep, aggressiveness, salivation, and overt sexual activity; and for horses, aggressiveness, paresis/paralysis, hyperesthesia, chewing at inanimate objects, salivation, and seizures (Reid, 1985), (Joyce et al., 1981), (Barnard, 1979), (West, 1985), (Pepin et al., 1984).

Assessment. This is a rare but fatal viral infection of warm-blooded animals in most countries. It is unusual because of mandatory vaccination laws for dogs in the Western world; however, it is still present in wildlife, so occasional domestic large animals may succumb to the disease. Because it is transmissible to man and is fatal, great precautions must be taken by the veterinarian who examines a patient suspected of being rabid.

Generally, the virus does not evoke a prominent cellular reaction, and the associated nonsuppurative myeloencephalitis can be mild in large animals. When the patient dies spontaneously, often the virus is recoverable from brain and salivary gland tissue, and characteristic eosinophilic intracytoplasmic Negri bodies are present in neurons. If an animal is euthanized early in the course of disease, particularly if only signs of spinal cord disease are present, virus and Negri bodies may not be detectable in brain tissue and can be confined to the spinal cord alone (Meyer et al., 1986). Thus, premature euthanasia may not be prudent.

Diagnostic Aids. If rabies is suspected, caution should be used in performing further diagnostic work; however, the animal should be treated for any other possibly treatable disease. The animal may be evaluated for 10 days and if it dies, the head or ½ fresh and ½ formalin-fixed brain and fresh salivary gland, are sent to a veterinary diagnostic laboratory equipped to handle rabies virus-infected tissue. Fluorescent antibody testing for rabies may be done there, as well as mouse inoculation studies.

Therapy. There is no treatment. Anti-inflammatory therapy for other diseases may delay progression of signs.

Prevention. Inactivated diploid vaccines* now are licensed for use in sheep, cattle, and horses, and appear to be quite protective (Blancou et al., 1984). Thus, a currently vaccinated animal that is bitten by a rabid animal, probably will not die of rabies.

However, the usefulness of vaccinating large animals against rabies is complicated by several factors. Because of public health concerns, it is recommended that any animal bitten by another animal known to be rabid should be destroyed. An animal, partially protected by vaccination, that is bitten by a rabid animal may have a modified course of disease, may shed the wild rabies virus, and may survive. Thus, a definitive diagnosis is obviated. Also, vaccinating livestock may create a false sense of security concerning rabies, that is detrimental. Efforts to vaccinate all dogs and cats, destroy feral dogs and cats, and control association of racoons, skunks, and foxes with livestock, must be maintained. Finally, vaccination does involve an expense, and the chance of a rare vaccine reaction still exists.

Thus, the decision and responsibility taken for vaccinating large animals against rabies rests with field veterinarians. Consideration should be given to the pros and cons concerning vaccination, including the above points, before undertaking a rabies vaccination program.

All rabies vaccines must be given in the muscles of the thigh.

4. **Enteroviral Encephalitis of Pigs (Porcine Polioencephalomyelitis, Teschen Disease)**

Signalment. All ages of pigs may be involved in an initial outbreak. Suckling-weanling piglets usually are affected in an endemic area. See Table 5–1 for a comparison of the viral encephalitides of swine (Brown, 1981).

---

*IMRAB-1®; Pitman-Moore, Inc,; Washington Crossing, NJ.—sheep (1 ml), cattle (2 ml), horses (2 ml) at 3 mos, then annually (sheep triennially).
RABGUARD®; Norden Laboratories, Inc.; Lincoln, NE.—sheep, cattle, horses, 1 ml at 3 mos, then annually.

Table 5–1. *Syndromes Associated with Various Encephalomyelitis (EM) Viral Infections of Swine*

Disease	Group Often Affected	Morbidity %	Mortality %	Fever*	Vomiting–Diarrhea	Nervous Signs**
Enteroviral EM (European-type)	all	50	<100	+	±	+ + + +
Enteroviral EM (USA-type)	nursing-weanling	<30	<100	±	–	+ +
Hemagglutinating EM	nursing	<100	<100	±	+	+ + +
	growing	low	low	–	±	+
Pseudorabies	nursing-weanling	<100	<100	+	+	+ + +
	adult	low	low	±	±	+ +
Paramyxovirus	nursing	low	high	+	±	+ +
Rabies	all	low	100	±	–	+ + + +
Hog cholera	all	<100	<100	+	+	+
African Swine Fever	all	<100	<100	+	+	+

*Present (+); absent (–); sometimes present (±).
** + to + + + + indicates increasing likelihood and severity of neurologic signs.
Adapted from Brown, 1981.

History. There is a peracute or subacute (most common in North America) onset of paresis or paralysis, convulsions, and death. Usually the morbidity rate is high. Signs of generalized systemic illness may occur.

Neurologic Examination. Signs of diffuse, spinal cord gray matter disease, such as weakness, reflex loss, and analgesia, may be masked by acute, diffuse, brain involvement, which produces depression, seizures, and recumbency.

Assessment. There are several strains of this enterovirus of swine, including Talfan disease, Teschen disease, enzootic paresis of swine, and poliomyelitis suum. These are neurotropic enteroviruses having a predilection for spinal cord ventral gray columns. Also there is a polioencephalitis with diffuse brain involvement.

Diagnosis. CSF and EMG studies should be useful in diagnosis but do not appear to be recorded in the literature. Necropsy examination with typical histologic lesions and virus isolation, which is difficult, are the best diagnostic aids. Hemagglutinating encephalomyelitis virus infection, pseudorabies, rabies, hog cholera, and African swine fever, are clinically and pathologically similar (see Table 5–1).

Therapy. None, isolate affected litters.

Prognosis. Older pigs may show prominent ataxia and improve with time, but the disease is fatal in suckling piglets.

5. Hemagglutinating Encephalomyelitis Virus (see Table 5–1)

This corona virus usually causes chronic "vomiting and wasting disease" in piglets. Encephalitis with depression, hyperesthesia, ataxia, tremor, convulsions, and death sometimes occurs; this acute form is "Ontario disease." There is no treatment. It is diagnosed using serologic testing and virus isolation (Mengeling, 1981).

6. **Pseudorabies (also see Table 5–1 and Problem 14)**

Signs of diffuse brain disease occur with this herpesvirus in piglets (Lee et al., 1979). These include blindness, seizures, wandering, recumbency, and death. A high morbidity and mortality rate, which is often associated with severe pruritus in other species, frequently occurs (Benfield, et al., 1986). The disease appears to be rare or nonexistent in horses (Crandell, 1981). A pseudorabies monoclonal antibody* is now available to reduce death during outbreaks of the disease in pigs.

7. **Porcine Paramyxovirus (Blue Eyes) (See Table 5–1)**

This newly reported, diffuse, nonsuppurative encephalitis of piglets 2 to 15 days old is characterized by depression, ataxia, weakness, and tremor, with seizures and blindness sometimes prominent (Stephan et al., 1988) Panophthalmitis with corneal opacity (blue eyes) is a conspicuous finding. Gastrointestinal signs and reproductive failure also occur.

8. **Scrapie (also Problems 9 and 14)**

This disease of sheep and goats is predominantly characterized by cerebellar ataxia (Problem 9) and pruritus (Problem 14), but later in the disease severe depression, dementia, and blindness may occur.

9. **Chronic Wasting Disease of Captive Deer**

Signalment. Captive Mule Deer and Elk, 2.5 to 4 years of age.

Syndrome. Chronic wasting, listlessness, behavioral changes, and gastrointestinal signs occur. Deer become oblivious to their surroundings and stand with head lowered, ears drooping, and a fixed stare. They then revert to normal awareness. Excessive salivation, teeth grinding, dysphagia, regurgitation, and a depraved appetite sometimes are seen. A scrapie-like, slow-viral agent may cause this disease (Williams et al., 1980).

Assessment. Status spongiosis and astrogliosis occur, as in Scrapie (see Problem 9).

Outcome. The disease is fatal; there is no treatment.

10. **Bovine Spongiform Encephalopathy**

Signalment. Only Holstein-Friesian, British Dairy Cattle, 3 to 6 years of age, have been reported with this disease (Wells et al., 1987).

Clinical Syndrome. Usually an insidious onset of apprehensiveness and hyperesthesia occurs, which progresses to belligerency, hypermetric ataxia, and finally frenzy and falling down. This all occurs within 6 months.

Diagnosis. No definitive diagnosis can be made antemortem. Initially, the possibility of rabies must not be overlooked. One affected Friesian bull demonstrated weight loss, ataxia, and facial twitching—with no behavioral abnormalities (Gilmour et al., 1988).

Assessment. There is a classic neuronal spongiform change in many brainstem gray matter areas. A mild gliosis and sparse mononuclear infiltrate occurs; scrapie-like filamentous particles have been detected in affected brains (Wells et al., 1987). It is possible that this disease is bovine scrapie (Wells, 1988, pers com.).

Outcome. The disease is fatal.

*Molecular Genetics Inc.; Minnetonka, Minn.

Significance. As with other spongiform encephalopathies (which are presumably contagious), including scrapie and chronic wasting disease of deer, the public health ramifications and its relationship to Kuru and Creutzfeldt-Jakob disease in man are not clearly understood.

11. **Equine Infectious Anemia (EIA) Ependymitis-Meningitis**

A granulomatous ependymitis, choroiditis, meningitis, and encephalomyelitis with lymphoreticular proliferation can occur subsequent to chronic EIA infection. The anemia and weight loss may be minimal. Occasionally, signs of ataxia and weakness may refer only to spinal cord involvement, but usually chronic behavioral changes, leading to dementia and blindness, occur (Held et al., 1983).

12. **Sporadic Bovine Encephalomyelitis (Buss Disease)**

Signalment. All ages are affected, but usually it involves weanling to yearling cattle (Harshfield, 1970).

History. An isolated case of respiratory diseases or arthritis may occur, and occasionally an outbreak occurs. Progressive depression and recumbency usually ensue in calves.

Physical Examination. Evidence of polyserositis, such as pleuritis, arthritis, and fever, are evidence of systemic involvement.

Neurologic Examination. Mild, diffuse, cerebral signs usually are seen in adults, and severe signs of recumbency, blindness, opisthotonus, and coma occur in weanlings.

Assessment. Diffuse nonsuppurative meningoencephalitis, caused by *Chlamydia pecoris,* is evident. Primarily, the disease is a polyserositis. Elementary bodies may be demonstrated in glial cells and mononuclear inflammatory cells.

Ancillary Aids. A moderate mononuclear pleocytosis with elevated protein may be present in the CSF. Thoracocentesis, arthrocentesis, and abdomenocentesis may confirm a polyserositis. There is a serum complement fixation test for antibodies.

Plan. Chlamydia are sensitive to tetracycline and tylosin and these drugs should be considered. Nursing care is mandatory for survival. The morbidity varies from 5 to 60%, with mortality up to 50%. The mortality rate is highest in growing cattle.

13. **Thromboembolic Meningoencephalitis (TEM)**

Signalment. This disease is seen primarily in feedlot cattle of any age, but usually occurs in the weanling to young adult stage (Beeman, 1985).

History. There is an acute onset of anorexia, staggering, and coma. Death may occur from 2 hours to several days later.

Physical Examination. Fever up to 108° F. Other forms of the disease, such as polyarthritis and respiratory disease, may be present in the patient or in pen-mates.

Neurologic Examination. Separation from the rest of the cattle, with depression and apparent blindness, often are the earliest signs. Paralysis, coma, tonic-clonic seizures, opisthotonus, and partial paralysis of multiple cranial nerves may be present. The main differential diagnoses of encephalopathy in feedlot cattle are, TEM, polioencephalomalacia, lead poisoning, and water intoxication (Little et al., 1969).

Assessment. This disease is a thromboembolic, suppurative meningoencephalitis of cattle produced by *Hemophilus somnus.* Bacteremia results in thrombosis of the small vessels of the brain, which is likely to initiate disseminated coagulopathy (Little, 1986). The same organism can cause outbreaks of pneumonitis and septicemia. Usually there is low morbidity and high mortality with the neurologic form of *H. somnus* infection.

Diagnostic Aids. CSF analysis reveals many neutrophils and increased protein with xanthochromia.

Therapy. Antibiotics that can be used include tetracyclines, sulfonamides, penicillin, chloramphenicol, and ampicillin. Electrolyte- and glucose-containing fluids given orally and anticonvulsants, such as phenobarbital or chloral hydrate, may be necessary (see Problem 2).

Prognosis. With the patient still ambulatory, the outlook is fair to good with intensive therapy. Few cattle survive after becoming recumbent. With a herd problem the diagnosis should be confirmed by necropsy. Effective vaccines now are available, and they appear to be useful at reducing the incidence and severity of the neurologic disease. However, with a low morbidity the economic value of a vaccination program must be considered.

14. Bacterial Meningitis and Meningoventriculitis

This disease is common, especially in neonatal foals, calves, and lambs.

Signalment. This is rare in adults (Rumbaugh, 1977), but common in neonatal large animals.

History. Primary complaints include hyperesthesia, stiff neck, depression, seizures, and blindness. Sometimes there is a history of another illness, such as enteritis. In addition, there may be information relating to a wound near the calvarium or vertebrae (especially in adults), infections of sinuses and inner ears, omphalophlebitis, lack of colostral intake, and prematurity.

Physical Examination. This disease can result in fever (103° to 106° F), but often this is absent in neonates. Depression, anorexia, tactile hyperesthesia over the entire body, neck pain, extended neck posture, omphalophlebitis, polyarthritis (especially in pigs), and ophthalmitis are common in large animals.

Neurologic Examination. Ataxia, often with spasticity and mild paresis, may be seen in all four limbs. Spinal reflexes are normal to hyperactive. Hyperesthesia and neck pain may be detected. Head signs frequently are seen in foals, calves, lambs, and piglets, and they include depression, wandering, star-gazing, abnormal vocalization ("barking"), and seizures. Young pigs with *Streptococcus suis* septicemia frequently have vestibular signs because of otitis media (Problem 6).

Assessment. Meningitis may be caused by bacterial, viral, protozoal and fungal infection or by immunologically mediated processes. The former cause is the most common and important in large animals. Lack of absorption of adequate colostral immunoglobulins (failure of passive transfer—FPT) is the primary predisposing factor (Brewer, et al., 1987a).

Histologic meningoventriculitis often occurs with neonatal septicemia in ungulates, with overt neurologic signs being absent. It is possible that the meningeal tissues become involved by infected monocytes migrating through normal pathways to maintain a surface (CSF) population of macrophages (Cordy, 1984).

Occasionally in animals with septicemia, there may be a showering of emboli to the brain, producing multiple granulomatous foci or microabscesses and resulting in behavior disorders. *Corynebacterium, Pasteurella, Haemophilus, Streptococcus,* and *Actinobacillus* are some bacterial species associated with embolic disease.

Streptococcus spp frequently cause meningitis and polyarthritis in calves, lambs, and piglets. *S. suis* type I (2 to 4-week-old piglets) and type II (10 to 14-week-old piglets) cause septicemia, meningitis, polyarthritis, and otitis interna in swine; *S. pneumoniae* causes meningitis, polyarthritis, and endophthalmitis in calves. Sepsis with coliforms, *Salmonella* spp, and *Pasturella* spp in calves, coliforms, *Salmonella* spp, and *Actinobacillus equuli* in foals, *Corynebacterium* spp, *Pasturella* spp and coliforms in lambs, and *Erysipelothrix rhusiopathiae* in piglets frequently are cultured from animals with meningitis and meningoventriculities (Sullivan, 1985)

Diagnostic Aids. A complete blood count may reveal a neutrophilic leukocytosis, but neonates, especially foals, frequently have neutropenia with sepsis. CSF, in bacterial cases, contains increased numbers of neutrophils. Mononuclear cells and increased protein content often are present as well. Glucose content of CSF measured on a urinary reagent strip is negative and is a good field test, although hypoglycemia must be considered as a cause of this. Blood cultures are often positive. A sepsis score based on predisposing factors and clinical parameters is useful in predicting sepsis in critically ill foals (Brewer et al., 1988a), (Brewer et al., 1988b).

Therapy. Four to 6 weeks of antibiotic therapy as determined by culture and sensitivity is indicated in bacterial infections. In meningitis, the blood brain barrier is damaged and most antibiotics may get into the CSF; however, the organisms are often pathogenic and resistant to many antibiotics. Third generation cephalosporins, such as cefotaxime and moxalactam, may be worth using, though they are expensive. Plasma is needed if FPT has occurred (serum $ZnSO_4$ turbidity test results <800 mg/dl in hospital or <400 mg/dl in field).

Prognosis. The prognosis for survival is fair to poor (25%) for bacterial infections when a specific organism is isolated and treated aggressively (Brewer et al., 1987). Chronic CNS and other foci of infection (e.g., osteoarthritis) may be recurrrent and difficult to control. Essentially the prognosis is guarded, particularly if no immunoglobulin transfer has occurred.

15. Brain Abscess

Signalment. Mostly in mature cattle and horses.

History. Brain abscesses may follow a pyogenic disease elsewhere in the body, such as polyarthritis, omphalophlebitis, traumatic reticuloperitonitis, and pododermatitis. In horses, a history of strangles, with secondary *Streptococcus equi* abscesses forming in the cerebrum, frequently is given (Sweeney et al., 1987), (Allen et al., 1987), (Ford, et al., 1980). Signs of behavioral changes and blindness, which frequently fluctuate, are seen, although vestibular syndromes or tetraparesis may first be evident.

Physical Examination. Evidence of other pyogenic foci may be found. Vital signs usually are normal. Evidence of metastatic *S. equi* abscesses may be present in horses (Sweeney et al., 1987).

Neurologic Examination. Compulsive circling, a head turn, depression, unilateral, bilateral, central or peripheral blindness, and a sluggish or ataxic gait—all of which may fluctuate—most often occur (Sharma, et al., 1975), (Raphel, 1982). Papilledema is not frequently reported in horses (Rumbaugh, 1977), but is seen in cattle with cerebral abscesses (McCormack, 1973), (Sharma, et al., 1975).

Assessment. Signs, for the most part, are due to the space-occupying nature of the abscess, rather than the inflammatory response (Fig. 5–6A). Brain herniations (see Neurologic Examination, Chapter 2) can occur and can be lethal (Fig. 5–6B). The lesions frequently occupy one or both lateral ventricles, and perhaps have a similar genesis to bacterial meningoventriculitis (see above).

Diagnostic Aids. Unless septic foci are present elsewhere in the body, few, if any hematologic indicators of inflammation are evident.

Cerebrospinal fluid is often abnormal with inflammatory cells, frequently of mixed cell type; a slightly elevated protein content is usually present. However, prominent suppurative meningitis may accompany a cerebral abscess (Rumbaugh, 1977).

Cerebral angiography has been used to define a space-occupying mass in a cow (Sharma et al., 1975).

Visual evoked potential and electroencephalographic recordings assisted in localizing a *Corynebacterium pyogenes* cerebral abscess in a steer (Strain et al., 1987).

Computed axial tomography (CT) has been used to define the site of a *Streptococcus equi* cerebral abscess in a horse (Allen et al., 1987).

Therapy. Antimicrobial therapy alone has not been successful in treating cerebral abscesses in large animals. Surgical drainage and appropriate, prolonged, antimicrobial therapy has been successful and is recommended (Sharma et al., 1975). Following measurements taken from CT scan images of a *S. equi* cerebral abscess, successful surgical drainage has been achieved in a yearling filly (Allen et al., 1987).

Prognosis. Without surgical drainage the outlook is bad.

16. Mycotic Encephalitis

On rare occasions fungi produce fatal meningoencephalomye-

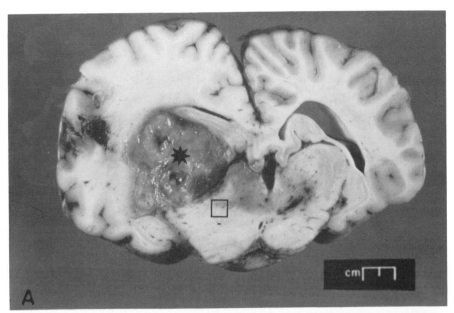

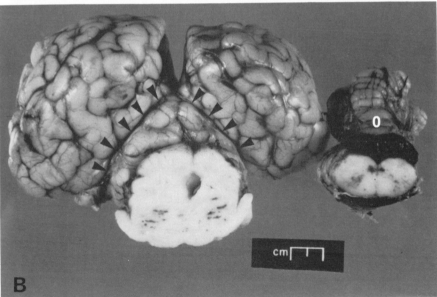

Figure 5–6. Cerebral abscesses in a pony. A transverse section of forebrain through the thalamus is shown in A. B shows the caudal aspect of the occipital lobes with midbrain and pons beneath (left) and the caudal aspect of the cerebellum with medulla oblongata beneath (right).

In the region of the left choroid plexus is a pyogranulomatous mass with abscess formation (star). There is associated swelling of the left cerebrum and protrusion of the left hemisphere to the right side. The left thalamus (open square) is significantly compressed.

Asymmetric swelling of the forebrain has resulted in the herniation of the ventral occipital lobes (arrowheads) under the tentorium cerebelli, compressing the midbrain beneath. Also the cerebellum has been forced caudally so that the caudal tonsil of the cerebellar vermis (white O) was forced through the foramen magnum. Beneath this is a hematoma associated with these severe herniations of brain tissue.

litis in large animals. Amebic encephalitis has been produced experimentally in ruminants, but does not seem to occur naturally in intact large animals.

Terminal *Aspergillus* sp septicemia and meningoencephalitis can follow prolonged antimicrobial and immunosuppressive therapy; local spread of *Aspergillus* gutturomycosis can produce localized meningoencephalitis that causes blindness (Hatziolos et al., 1975).

Cerebral phycomycosis may occur as part of a primary disseminated disease (Austin, 1976), (Juck et al., 1978), or in association with other organisms in cattle and horses (Seamen, 1977).

Neonatal mycotic encephalitis, caused by *Mortierella wolfii,* has occurred in conjunction with mycotic pneumonia and placentitis in cattle (Neilan et al., 1982).

Cryptococcal meningitis has occurred in large animals, particularly horses, and is associated with a wide variety of clinical signs, including cerebral syndromes. Mixed inflammatory cell, CSF pleocytosis usually should be present, and the presence of cryptococcal organisms in CSF is diagnostically significant. Treatment with drugs, such as amphotericin B, is feasible and has been attempted (Steckal et al., 1982).

17. **Verminous Encephalitis (also Problem 10)**

Signalment. Any aged animal is susceptible.

History. This sporadic disease may occur endemically in certain regions (e.g., Kumri in horses in India because of *Setaria* sp). Usually there is an acute onset of signs with progression (Blunden et al., 1987), though this varies tremendously (Mayhew et al., 1982a).

Neurologic Examination. Signs usually reflect tortuous, usually asymmetric, random migrations (*Stronglyus* sp, *Hypoderma* sp, *Habronema* sp, *Setaria* sp) or diffuse brain or spinal cord involvement (*Setaria* sp, *Micronema [Halicephalobus] deletrix*). Thus, progressive forebrain, brainstem, cerebellar, or spinal cord signs may predominate.

Micronema deletrix does have a predilection for the basillar, pituitary region of the brainstem and has been detected in a pair of sibling foals on the same property, in two successive seasons.

Coenurus cerebralis, the larval stage of *Taenia multiceps* of canidae, frequently forms large cysts in the brains of cattle, and particularly sheep, resulting in asymmetric cerebral syndromes that most often include circling, blindness, head pressing, and depression. The condition is colloquially referred to as "gid" in the UK (Tirgari et al., 1987). The larval stage of *Taenia solium,* a large tapeworm in man, is *Cysticercus cellulosae;* in some countries it occurs commonly in the brains and other tissues of swine (Gonzalez et al., 1987).

Assessment. Tissue destruction, hemorrhage and inflammation, or a space-occupying effect (depending on the parasite), cause clinical signs.

Ancillary Aids. Circulating eosinophilia and CSF eosinophilic or neutrophilic leukocytosis with hemorrhage are helpful ancillary findings, but they may not be present. *Micronema deletrix* may be detected in CSF and urine. Plain and contrast radiography can help diagnose and localize *Coenurus cerebralis* in sheep (Tirgari et al., 1987); computed tomography clearly defines cerebral cysticercosis in pigs (Gonzalez et al., 1987).

Treatment. Appropriate antiparasitic and anti-inflammatory therapy appears to be rewarding; some amazing recoveries from acute syndromes may be expected. Suggested anthelmintic doses include: Ivermectin 200 µg/kg (may take up to 2 weeks to destroy the parasite); fenbendazole 50 mg/kg daily for 1 to 3 days; thiabendazole 440 mg/kg daily for 2 days; diethylcarbamazine 50 mg/kg; and routine doses of organophosphates (Mayhew et al., 1982). Phenylbutazone, flunixin, or dexamethasone at routine anti-inflammatory doses also should be included in the therapy.

Surgical removal of *C. cerebralis* cysts from sheep has resulted in excellent recovery rates (Tirgari et al., 1987), (Skerritt et al., 1984).

18. **Parasitic Thromboembolism (also Problem 10)**

Signalment. Any age, breed, and sex of animal is susceptible, but most cases have been suspected in young adult horses.

History. Acute seizures as well as depression, with violent or passive behavior, usually occurs with recumbency at the onset. Signs may be static or improve with time.

Physical Examination. This usually is unremarkable, although there may be evidence of self-inflicted injury.

Neurologic Examination. Initially, there may be recumbency with seizures. Asymmetric cerebral signs, including circling and wandering towards the side of lesion, blindness, facial hypalgesia, and subtle gait abnormalities opposite the side of the lesion, are expected.

Many cases do not show progression of the signs, as no parasite migration occurs and signs can improve dramatically. However, marked, diffuse, cerebral edema can occur, resulting in herniations and death.

Assessment. Usually *Strongylus vulgaris* thromboarteritis in the great vessels leads to an embolic shower from the carotid arteries to the ipsilateral cerebrum. In horses, the carotid artery supplies the cerebrum and rostral brainstem, whereas the pons, medulla oblongata, and cerebellum receive the majority of arterial blood from the vertebral and basillar arteries.

Diagnosis. A circulating eosinophilia often is not found. CSF pleocytosis with neutrophils, and often eosinophils, and erythrocytes, and xanthochromia, can be expected.

Therapy. Usually it must be assumed that a potentially viable parasite still is present, and anthelmintics and anti-inflammatory therapy should be instituted (see 17 Verminous Encephalitis above).

Prognosis. Without parasite migration, prognosis is fair to good after the acute seizure episode occurs, provided brain swelling can be controlled. If the animal survives, residual signs of depression, seizures, and partial visual dysfunction may result.

19. Miscellaneous Diffuse Meningoencephalomyelitides

Toxoplasma gondii in cattle and sheep, *Sarcocystis* sp-like organisms in sheep (Hartley et al., 1974), (Stubbings et al., 1985), (Morgan et al., 1984) and cattle (Dubey et al., 1987), *Trypanosoma evansi* infection of horses (surra) (Seiler et al., 1981) and bovine cerebral theileriosis ("turning disease") (Valli, 1985), (Giles et al., 1978), all have been associated with clinical neurologic syndromes. Some of these have been referable to focal spinal cord disease (Hartley et al., 1974), (Stubbings et al., 1985) or to focal or diffuse brain involvement (Dubey et al., 1987), (Seiler et al., 1981), (Giles et al., 1978), (Valli, 1985). Degrees of nonsuppurative meningoencephalomyelitis are detected at postmortem examination. Theoretically, treatment with folic acid antagonists, which are used to treat equine protozoal myeloencephalitis (see Problem 11), could be tried.

Encephalitis associated with *Borrelia burgdorferi* infection has been reported in the horse (Burgess et al., 1987) and could well occur in other large animals. *B. burgdorferi* infection was associated with uveitis and arthritis in a pony (Burgess, 1986). The spirochete causes Lyme Disease, a zoonotic, tick-borne infection of man and animals, characterized by a skin rash, polyarthritis, heart disease, and nervous symptoms. The organism is sensitive to tetracyclines and to ampicillin.

Heartwater disease (*Cowdria ruminantium*), cerebral babesiosis (*Babesia* spp), and turning sickness (*Theileria* spp), which occur in the tropics are tick-borne cattle diseases that may present with signs of diffuse brain involvement (Schillhorn van Veen, 1987).

IV. Metabolic Disturbances

1. Hypoglycemia

Hypoglycemia in large animals usually produces signs of abnormal behavior such as confusion and depression (delerium). Sometimes hypoglycemia is associated with seizures (also Problem 2) and may complicate the clinicopathologic workup of a foal with neonatal maladjustment syndrome (Ross et al., 1983). See VIII.1 (below).

2. Hypocalcemia

Hypocalcemia may produce confusion, but it usually produces depression, ataxia, and tetraplegia in ruminants (also Problem 10) and convulsions and tremor in other species (also Problems 2 and 8B).

3. Hypomagnesemia

Hypomagnesemia usually produces tremor and tetany, then weakness (also Problems 2, 8, and 10).

4. Anesthetic Hypoxia—Anoxia

Residual behavior changes may occur following an episode of anoxia or hypoxia, as in anesthetic accidents; however, blindness and depression are the most common residual signs (also Problem 3).

5. Hepatic Encephalopathy

Signalment. Acute hepatic necrosis, often associated with prior administration of an equine-origin biologic, occurs in adult horses, not foals. Hepatotoxicity, associated with ingestion of pyrrolizidine alkaloid-containing plants, occurs in any grazing animal. Cirrhosis generally occurs in adult animals. Particularly in New Zealand ruminants, cirrhosis commonly is associated with ingestion of sporidesmin—produced by the toxigenic pasture fungus *Pithomyces chartarum* (facial eczema)—and can result in hepatoencephalopathy (Thompson et al., 1979). Tyzzer's disease, caused by *Bacillus piliformis,* results in sudden death in foals. Congenital portosystemic shunts are rare in large animals (Keane et al., 1983; Buonanno et al., 1988). Finally, ferrous fumarate appears to have been the compound present in a now discontinued microorganism culture product that caused the death of many foals between 1981 and 1983 in the USA. Fulminant hepatic failure followed administration of 1 or 2 doses of this nutrient supplement to foals (Divers et al., 1983).

History. Periods of ataxia, blindness, aimless wandering, dementia, and seizures are seen frequently. A history of exposure to toxic plants may be evident. In horses, tetanus antitoxin (TAT) or other equine-origin biologics may have been administered 1 to 3 months previously.

Physical Examination. There may be ascites or signs of acute liver failure. Young animals may be emaciated and poorly developed; a degree of anorexia is usually present. Photosensitivity is seen in herbivores. Rectal prolapse has been a presenting complaint in calves.

Neurologic Examination. Dementia or coma, head pressing, and yawning are common signs (Fig. 5–7). Ataxia, seizures, and blindness frequently accompany these signs, and tenesmus can be seen in cattle with hepatoencephalopathy. Bilateral laryngeal paralysis (also Problem 5H), with pronounced inspiratory stridor, has been observed in horses with liver disease. The pathogenesis of this finding remains obscure.

Assessment. Protein, carbohydrate, and fat metabolism, is severely impaired; detoxification, particularly of nitrogenous wastes, is reduced. Factors involved in the encephalopathy may include hypoglycemia, hyperammonemia, decreased branched chain to aromatic amino acid ratio (Gulick et al., 1980), excess short-chain fatty acids, and induction of "false neurotransmitters" in the brain.

Diagnostic Aids. Total serum protein concentration usually is low, often less then 5.0 g/dl. Blood-urea nitrogen (BUN) concentration can be low, often 5 to 10 mg/dl. Sulfobromophthalein sodium (BSP) T½ is prolonged to more than 4 minutes (horses and cattle). Blood ammonia concentration is elevated (normal levels vary depending on the laboratory). Blood glucose concentration may be low. Radiographs of the abdomen may show a small shrunken liver. Liver biopsy reveals hepatitis, cirrhosis, or necrosis.

A portosystemic shunt was confirmed in a 6-month-old Quarter-

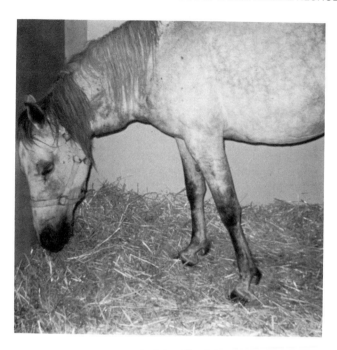

Figure 5–7. Hepatoencephalopathy. Animals with this nonfebrile, metabolic, diffuse encephalopathy frequently show head pressing and depression as shown in this horse with pyrrolizidine alkaloid-induced hepatopathy, as well as blindness and eating/swallowing difficulties.

horse (showing intermittent depression and ill thrift) using quantitative nuclear scintigraphy and intra-operative mesenteric contrast portography (Buonanno et al., 1988).

Therapy. Removal of any hepatotoxins from the environment is essential. Protection from direct sunlight is appropriate. A low protein and high carbohydrate diet, oral neomycin to kill gut bacteria that aid in splitting protein to ammonia, and crystalloid-containing fluids and glucose IV usually are indicated. Glucocorticosteroids probably are not indicated. Tetracyclines can be tried if *Bacillus piliformis* is suspected.

Prognosis. In most cases of profound liver function loss, the prognosis is grave. With intensive support, horses with acute hepatic necrosis have survived. Some horses with active, nonsuppurative hepatitis and mild signs of encephalopathy have recovered with nursing care. By the time significant encephalopathy ensues, with pyrrolizidine toxicity, the liver lesions are permanent and regeneration is essentially impossible.

6. Miscellaneous Metabolic Disturbances

There are several diseases which may secondarily affect acid base balance, electrolyte concentrations, and various organ system functions, resulting in cerebral signs. Terminal renal disease often causes signs of confusion and seizures, and a spongiform encephalopathy may be present (Summers et al., 1985). Ketosis in cattle often produces muscle weakness, tremor, dementia, head pressing, and compulsive licking. Fatty liver syndrome in dairy cows may terminate with hepatoenceophalopathy. Pregnancy toxemia in ewes causes behavioral signs, including wandering and stargazing, as well as depression, blindness, and seizures. Severe alkalosis usually produces seizures (also Problem 2) and severe acidosis usually produces coma (also Problem 4). Shock is discussed in Problem 4.

V. Toxic
   1. Lead
   Signalment. Any age animal, although calves most commonly are affected because of their tendency to lick and chew objects. Horses rarely, if ever, show any cerebral signs other than depression, although ataxia and recumbency may occur at high levels of intoxication (Dollahite et al., 1978). They show signs of cranial neuropathy, particularly laryngeal and pharyngeal paralysis (Problem 5).

   History. There may have been contact with lead-based paint, linoleum, caulking compounds, batteries, old machinery oil, or heavy industrial pollution of forages. Seizures, hysteria, hyperactivity, and tremor occur with acute lead poisoning. Diarrhea, or constipation may be evident in chronic lead poisoning. Blindness, aimless walking, head pressing, and bellowing are common complaints in cattle.

   Physical Examination. Often nothing is remarkable but sometimes lead-based paint is on the hair coat. Bloat and tenesmus, with diarrhea or constipation, frequently are present in ruminants. Roaring and dysphagia, associated with pharyngeal and largyngeal paralysis, are the most common signs in horses.

   Neurologic Examination. The animal may be ataxic and generally weak. It may be irritable and convulse during examinations. Amaurosis, wandering, head pressing, opisthotonus, odontoprisis, and bellowing often are seen in cattle (Fig. 5–8). Usually, just dysphagia and roaring are seen in horses, and those are probably the result of peripheral neuropathy (also problems 5F and 5H).

   Assessment. Lead interferes with normal heme synthesis, resulting in erythrocytes with decreased oxygen-carrying capacity. Signs are caused by an ischemic effect on cerebral cells; cerebral edema may develop. The primary effect is on neurons, but vascular endothelium and peripheral nerves also are affected.

   Diagnostic Aids. In large animals the hemogram usually reveals no anemia, but nucleated erythrocytes are occasionally present. Elevated (>200 mg/dl) delta-amino levulinic acid concentrations can be detected in urine, but this is an inconsistent finding. Blood lead concentrations may or may not be elevated (>0.6 ppm is diagnostic of poisoning), but urinary lead excretion following ethylenediaminetetraacetic acid (EDTA) chelation therapy is more helpful. A distinction must be made between exposure to lead, with resulting elevated blood lead concentrations, and lead poisoning (Osweiler et al., 1978). Free erythrocyte porphyrin estimations appear to be closely correlated with blood lead concentrations, and inversely correlated with time since last lead exposure (Osweiler et al., 1978).

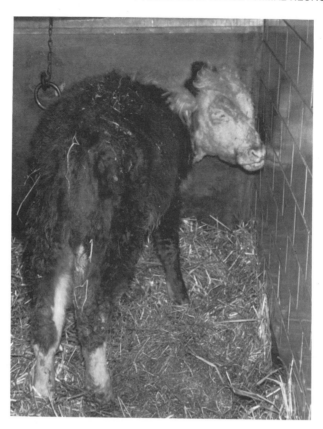

Figure 5–8. Lead poisoning. The major differential diagnosis for this calf with lead poisoning confirmed at postmortem examination included thiamin-responsive polioencephalomalacia and water intoxication. The profoundly depressed calf is showing compulsive circling and head pressing. It was blind and had dorsomedial strabismus. Continuous bellowing and tenesmus, along with constipation or diarrhea (if present), are consistent with lead poisoning.

Therapy. Removal from access to lead may be all that is required to halt an outbreak; slow reversal of signs can occur (Osweiler et al., 1978). Calcium disodium EDTA chelation therapy over several days is indicated. One regimen is 50 to 100 mg/kg, slowly IV, SID, or BID, for 2 days, repeated in several days as necessary.

Prognosis. It is fair, provided aggressive chelation treatment is initiated early in the course of the syndrome; otherwise it is bad.

2. **Salt and Water**

Signalment. Feeder pigs, range cattle, feeder calves, and lambs.

History. Often access to water is restricted (because of drought or frozen water supply); usually this is followed by free water access. High NaCl in the diet (pigs) and high ambient temperatures can be contributing factors.

Physical Examination. Colic, a fluid-filled rumen, diarrhea, cardiac arrhythmias, and hemoglobinuria may be seen in calves (Kirkbride, 1967). Fever has also been reported (Scarratt et al., 1985).

Neurologic Examination. Ataxia, lethargy, then severe depression, aimless wandering, head pressing, blindness, and seizures ("walking backward fits" in pigs) occur. Loss of squeal is characteristic in pigs. These signs are followed by recumbency and coma.

Assessment. The basic lesion is a laminary cerebrocortical necrosis with brain edema. Eosinophils are characteristically seen in this lesion in pigs, presumably attracted by the cellular necrosis. The pathophysiology probably involves hyposmolality and hyponatremia in water intoxication, and hyperosmolality and hypernatremia in salt poisoning (Fountain et al., 1975), (Scarratt et al., 1985), (Padovan, 1980). Sudden shifts in osmolality produce rapid alterations in intracellular water and a subsequent metabolic blockade.

Diagnostic Aids. High (>320 mOsmol/kg) or low (<210 mOsmol/kg) serum osmolality, and high (>160 mEq/L) or low (<105 mEq/L) serum sodium concentration, with concomitant changes in CSF osmolality and CSF sodium concentration, as well as the presence of hemoglobinuria and hemoglobinemia, all are helpful findings.

Treatment. Low doses of furosemide (0.5 mg/kg), along with IV normal saline, is indicated if hyponatremic water intoxication has occurred. A regimen of small but frequent amounts of water per os and IV D5W is a reasonable treatment for hypernatremia. Mannitol, 0.25 g/kg IV may be worth trying in water intoxication, but it should not be used in salt poisoning/hypernatremia. Therapeutic alterations in serum osmolality should be made slowly. If the serum osmolar status is not known, then conservative therapy is indicated (Scarratt et al., 1985), (Kirkbride et al., 1967).

Prognosis. Spontaneous recovery occurs, thus conservative management often is wise. Individual mortality is approximately 50%. One prevents recurrence by correcting management errors.

3. Urea—Ammonia

Signalment. Cattle of all ages, and occasionally horses are affected.

History. A new batch of urea-containing cattle feed may have been fed to the animal. Cattle, calves, and horses may have access to cattle feed, or ammonia-treated forages may be used (Kerr et al., 1987). Initial signs often include acute staggering, recumbency, and death.

Physical Examination. Bloat, dyspnea, muscle tremor, and abdominal pain can be present.

Neurologic Examination. Incoordination, blindness, struggling, bellowing, hyperesthesia, seizures, and coma, all may be evident (Kerr et al., 1987). The disease associated with ammoniated forage feeding in cattle is "Bovine Hysteria" or "Bovine Bonkers" (Miksch, 1985).

Assessment. Ruminants can receive up to 3% of urea in their diet as a protein (nitrogen) supplement. Incorrect amounts, failure to slowly build up the amount of urea fed, or accidental access to feed containing urea or ammonia, result in intoxication. Urea is converted to ammonia in the rumen and the liver, and alkalosis and ammonia encephalopathy result.

The syndrome of abnormal behavior associated with feeding ammoniated feedstuffs to cattle may result from the production of nitrogenous intoxicants other than ammonia or urea. One such compound is 4-methylimidazole (Miksch, 1985).

Diagnosis. An elevated blood and CSF ammonia concentration, in the absence of evidence of liver disease, is diagnostic of ammonia or urea intoxication (Kerr et al., 1987).

Treatment. The stomach or rumen should be lavaged and evacuated. Acidifying solutions, such as 5% acetic acid or vinegar, can be given orally at doses between 0.5L (sheep) and 5L (cattle) along with additional water. Sedation may be necessary (Kerr et al., 1987).

Prognosis. The disease is fatal. Preventive measures usually are obvious.

4. Cyanide

Goats and other ruminants that eat plants containing high concentrations of hydrocyanic acid (HCN), such as cherry trees, *Sorghum* sp, grasses *Brassica* crops, and many weeds, can develop cyanide poisoning.

Clinical Syndrome. Dyspnea, excitement or depression, tremor, opisthotonus, convulsions, and sudden death are reported.

Assessment. Bright red blood and mucous membranes, because of histotoxic anoxia, are readily seen.

Diagnostic Aids. A picric acid paper test is available for detecting HCN, and many laboratories can perform semiquantitative assays on blood and feed samples for cyanide content.

Treatment. Systemic sodium nitrite and sodium thiosulfate therapy can be rewarding. This mixture firstly produces methemoglobin from hemoglobin that combines with HCN to produce nontoxic cyanmethemoglobin. Suggested doses for small to large ruminants are 1 to 3 g sodium nitrite and 2.5 to 15 g sodium thiosulfate, in 50 to 200 ml H_2O, given slowly IV (Blood et al., 1979).

5. Locoweed and Darling Pea

History. Adult horses and cattle that have access to these poisonous plants show progressive signs of aggressive behavior, ataxia, and weight loss.

Clinical Syndrome. Poisoning by locoweeds (*Astragalus* and *Oxytropis* spp) in the USA, and by Darling pea (*Swainsona* sp) in Australia can produce a syndrome of dementia, with periods of aggression and hyperesthesia when handled, along with cerebellar ataxia.

Assessment. Alkaloid toxins in these plants induce a lysosomal storage disease (mannosidosis) in affected animals (Alroy et al., 1985). The syndrome of "blind staggers," thought to be the result of chronic selenium intoxication of horses that ingest selenium-accumulating locoweeds, probably is associated with induced mannosidosis, rather than simple selenium toxicity (James et al., 1981).

Treatment. Removing the animal from the plants can result in alleviation of some signs, but behavioral changes may be permanent (James et al., 1981). Reversal of signs, with an apparent permanent cure, has been achieved using combinations of mood elevators (tranylcypromine and protriptyline), and reserpine (Staley, 1978).

6. *Kochia scoparia* **(Mexican fireweed)**

This plant occurs in the Plain States and intoxication has been seen in cattle. Depression, anorexia, nystagmus, head pressing, recumbency, and opisthotonus occur. Multiple organ involvement, including laminar cerebrocortical necrosis also occurs (Dickie et al., 1983).

7. **Miscellaneous Toxic Plants**

Many other plants cause signs of diffuse encephalopathy, with various combinations of signs, including blindness, depression, seizures, and behavioral changes. Some reported examples are: *Helichrysum sp* in South African cattle (Basson et al., 1975); *Halogeton glomeratus* poisoning in range cattle in the western USA (Lincoln et al., 1980); and Nardoo ferns (*Marsilea sp*) in Australian sheep (Pritchard et al., 1978), which probably contain thiaminase.

The therapeutic regimen should include, removal of the offending plant from the environment, gastric lavage, catharsis, diuresis, large doses of thiamin, and nursing care.

8. **Moldy Corn (Leukoencephalomalacia)**

Signalment. Horses of any breed, sex, or age are affected. Outbreaks do occur.

Primary Signs. Dementia, blindness, convulsions, and sudden death.

History. Ingestion of moldy corn over approximately 1 month, with the development of cerebral signs or sudden death is typical; however, the source of the putative mycotoxin can be elusive. Also, the disease has occurred when feeding commercial horse rations (Wilson et al., 1985).

Physical Examination. Usually there are no significant findings, although there may be evidence of liver disease, such as jaundice.

Neurologic Examination. Dementia, drowsiness, blindness, circling, excitability, seizures, and ataxia are found in various combinations. Signs may be asymmetric. There may be brainstem involvement with pharyngeal paralysis and other cranial nerve deficits.

Assessment. Toxins produced by *Fusarium moniliforme* in moldy corn are incriminated. Horses ingesting toxin-containing feed develop liquefactive cerebral necrosis, especially in the subcortical white matter (Fig. 5–9A). Associated inflammation may include plasma cells and eosinophils (Marasas et al., 1976). Associated brain swelling frequently results in herniations and brainstem compression (Fig. 5–9B). Experimentally, attempts at reproducing the disease are not all successful. Toxic hepatopathy can occur and may contribute to the syndrome. That cultures of *Fusarium* can produce the disease is well accepted, but the putative toxin is not identified (Wilson et al., 1971), (Wilson et al., 1985), (Marasas et al., 1976).

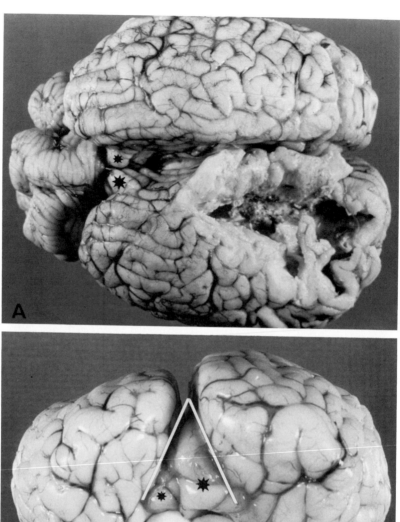

Figure 5–9. Equine leukoencephalomalacia. Shown is a dorsal view of the entire brain (A) and a caudal view of the occipital lobes with the midbrain beneath (B). An outbreak of leukoencephalomalacia occurred in a herd of miniature horses fed a commercial ration; this brain came from a horse found dead. The brain is swollen with flattened gyri, and massive destruction of the right cerebrum is evident (A). Herniation of the swollen occipital lobes (stars), which is worse on the right, has occurred under the tentorium cerebelli. The position of the latter in vivo is indicated by the white bars. The midbrain is compressed by this herniated tissue on the right side, and this can account for sudden death.

Aflatoxicosis in horses with liver and kidney necrosis and associated cerebral edema and necrosis is reported (Angsubhakorn et al., 1981). The relationship this has with moldy corn poisoning is unclear.

Diagnosis. This is based on the history, the neurologic examination findings, and the presence of liver disease. Note that up to 80% of corn samples contain *Fusarium* sp, so this finding alone does not confirm a diagnosis. However, feed containing high numbers of *Fusarium* spores often may be associated with outbreaks of leukoencephalomalacia.

Analysis of CSF taken from affected horses may be normal, or may reveal a pleocytosis that includes neutrophils and elevated protein content (Masri, pers comm, 1987).

Therapy. Removal of the moldy feed and the use of cathartics seems appropriate. Glucocorticosteroids and other drugs, such as dimethyl sulfoxide (DMSO) to reduce brain swelling, may be tried.

Prognosis. If only mildly affected, the animal may be taken off the diet and live with residual or no brain damage. Animals usually die shortly after the onset of the signs (in a few hours to a few days).

9. **Focal Symmetrical Encephalomalacia of Lambs and Kids, and Edema Disease of Swine**

Signalment. Usually feedlot lambs, adult sheep and goats, and growing feeder pigs are affected. Young cattle have been reported to have a similar disease (Buxton, 1981).

History. Outbreaks of "overeating disease" or "pulpy kidney" are the result of *Clostridium perfringens* type D enterotoxemia in ruminants. Edema disease, caused by *Escherichia coli* enterotoxemia, occurs in swine. Changes in the ration being fed is often part of the history (e.g., weaning). An acute onset of head pressing, aimless wandering, opisthotonus, recumbency, and death in several animals usually are the primary clinical signs. This usually occurs in several animals involved in an outbreak of enterotoxemia, or can occur as an isolated event. A chronic, dummy syndrome is described in sheep (Gay et al., 1975) (Fig. 5–10A).

Physical Examination. Diarrhea may be present, especially in sheep. The animal may become recumbent some time prior to presentation. Edema of the forehead in pigs ("edema disease"), along with acute diarrhea, may be detected.

Neurologic Examination. Dementia, head pressing, wandering, opisthotonus, seizures, and coma occur.

Assessment. The pathogenesis probably relates to the effect of *Clostridium perfringens* type D (sheep and goats) and *Escherichia coli* (pigs) exotoxins on blood vessels in the brain and spinal cord, which results in leakage of fluid and brain edema (Kurtz et al., 1976), (Worthington et al., 1975). Areas affected include, the basal nuclei, internal capsule, thalamus, midbrain, vestibular nuclei, and cerebellar white matter (Kurtz et al., 1969) (Fig. 5–10B). Spinal cord gray matter also may be affected. Glycosuria, caused by nephrosis, is commonly present in lambs with "pulpy kidney."

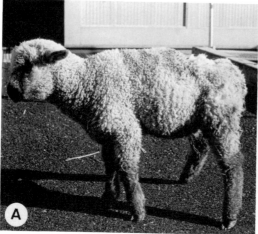

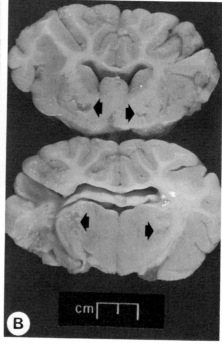

Figure 5–10. Focal symmetrical encephalomalacia (FSE). This lamb, now showing a chronic dummy syndrome (A), survived an outbreak of enterotoxemia presumed to be associated with *Clostridium perfringens* type D, but became depressed, separated from the flock, wandered in circles, and demonstrated opisthotonus (star-gazing). Transverse sections of the fresh forebrain from another case of FSE (B) reveal typical, soft (malacic) areas of necrosis in the internal capsule (top) and lateral thalamus (bottom) indicated by arrows.

Treatment. Diuretics may be of some use in pigs; mannitol is worth trying. Oral antibiotics, such as chlortetracycline or trimethoprim-sulfadiazine should be administered early in the course of the disease. *Clostridum perfringens* type D antiserum is useful in lambs and kids, and the remainder of the at-risk flock should receive a toxoid or antitoxin.

Prognosis. Mortality is high. The farmer should be reminded to make slow dietary changes. Vaccination with *Cl. perfringens* type D toxoid is an important prophylactic measure in ruminants.

VI. Nutritional

1. Thiamin Responsive Polioencephalomalacia of Ruminants

Signalment. This is common in calves 6 to 12 months old (Little et al., 1969), and lambs and kids 2 to 6 months old (Smith, 1979), (Pierson et al., 1975); it is less common in adult ruminants.

History. Outbreaks occur in feedlots, but sometimes while animals are at pasture. Isolated cases occur in adult animals. Usually there is an acute onset of ataxia, tremor, blindness, opisthotonus, convulsions, and recumbency (Rammell et al., 1986).

Physical Examination. Usually this is unremarkable, and the rumen usually remains motile.

Neurologic Examination. Amaurosis, staggering gait, wandering, opisthotonus, and dorsomedial strabismus (eye deviation) are characteristic. Muscle tremor, recumbency with decerebrate posturing, tonic-clonic seizures, and coma eventuate (Little et al., 1969), (Pierson et al., 1975), (Smith, 1979) (Fig. 5–11A).

Assessment. Several rumen organisms have been isolated that produce thiaminase. A high carbohydrate diet (grain, lush forage) promotes proliferation of these organisms in the animal. Thiaminase has been found in pasture swards. Also, it is proposed that some thiamin analogs can be produced in the rumen. Type I thiaminase production by *Bacillus thiaminolyticus* and growth of the organism in rumen liquor are significantly depressed by the presence of thiamin hydrochloride and thiamin propyldisulfide (Thomas, 1986b). This is the basis for oral therapy of subclinical thiamin deficiency and of polioencephalomalacia. Laminar cerebrocortical necrosis results from lack of glycolysis, with resulting brain edema and herniations. Feedlot diets high in sulfates (e.g., gypsum) may promote this disease (Raisbeck, 1982) and competitive, thiamin analogues, such as amprolium, may be factors in the pathogenesis of individual cases and outbreaks. Anthelmintic use has been associated with the onset of clinical signs and may be a triggering factor (Smith, 1979). Subclinical thiaminase production in the bowel has been related to poor weight gain in sheep. From an economic viewpoint, this may be more significant then the overt clinical disease (Thomas, 1986a), (Rammell et al., 1986).

At postmortem examination a swollen, slightly yellow cerebrum usually is evident; cerebral and cerebellar herniations may occur in the acute disease. Autofluorescence of a freshly cut surface of cerebral cortex placed under ultraviolet light is good presumptive evidence of polioencephalomalacia (Markson et al., 1982).

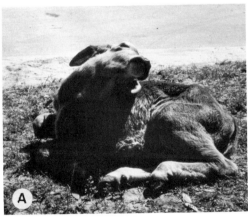 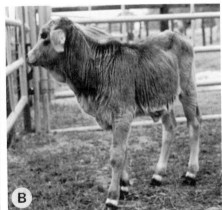

Figure 5–11. Thiamin responsive polioencephalomalacia. This suckling Brahman calf was found recumbent in the field. It could get up but was unaware of its surroundings and wandered around with its head and neck extended. With stimulation it would fall to the ground, convulse, and then sit sternal with its head held back while flopping from side to side (A). It was blind. Several 1-g doses of thiamin were given along with supportive care. In 48 hours the calf was normal (B).

Diagnosis. Blood pyruvate and lactate concentrations may be elevated, and erythrocyte, thiamin-dependent transketolase activity is low (Rammell et al., 1986). Atlanto-occipital CSF analysis usually is abnormal, with a slight mononuclear pleocytosis (5 to 50/μl) and a mild protein elevation (50 to 150 mg/dl) with xanthochromia. The response to vitamin B_1 is a good diagnostic and therapeutic tool.

Therapy. Administer at least 250 to 1000 mg thiamin IV or IM, BID, for 1 to 5 days. Nursing care is important when the animal is recumbent and anorectic.

Prognosis. Usually an excellent response is seen when thiamin is given early in the course of disease (Fig. 5–11A and B). If the animal is not recumbent the prognosis is good. Even recumbent animals can survive, but may be blind and somnolent.

Prevention. Reduce high grain diet and increase roughage if possible. Check sulfate content of diet, and reduce if excessive. Supplementing the diet with thiamin hydrochloride or mononitrate at 10 to 30 mg/kg of feed or 300 mg/head daily is useful as a prophylactic measure if the problem persists in a herd. Increasing the forage allotment to feedlot animals often prevents further cases from developing.

2. Vitamin E Deficiency—Mullberry Heart Disease of Swine

Young swine surviving an episode of vitamin E deficiency-related mullberry heart disease may be depressed, blind, wander in circles, convulse, and show ataxia. Signs result from a microangiopathy and encephalomalacia (Robinson et al., 1985).

VIII. Idiopathic

1. Neonatal Maladjustment Syndrome (NMS) of Foals

A common problem, particularly in thoroughbred breeding regions.

Signalment. Newborn foals, up to 1 week old, usually of the light breeds are affected. The same clinicopathologic syndrome rarely occurs in calves.

History. The newborn foal is normal during the first few minutes to hours of its life (occasionally it is normal for a few days). It then loses affinity for the dam, loses suckling ability, wanders, and convulses.

Physical Examination. Evidence of sepsis, with or without meningitis, and primary respiratory disease can be confounding factors, frequently making the specific diagnosis of uncomplicated NMS difficult (Clement, 1985). Hyperextension of fetlocks, thin supple skin, and soft ears indicate a premature state that can be associated with fading foal syndrome on day 2 to 4 (Vaala, 1986), (Leadon et al., 1986). Other than these signs, physical characteristics of NMS do not exist.

Neurologic Examination. Signs of NMS include combinations of dementia, circling, blindness, loss of suck reflex, seizures, specific cranial nerve deficits, tetraparesis and hyporeflexia (Fig. 5–12). Compared to adult horses, normal neonatal foals have increased extensor tone and hyperreflexia (Adams et al., 1985).

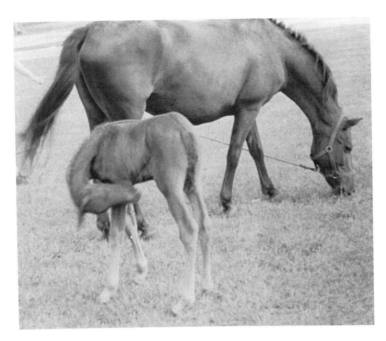

Figure 5–12. Neonatal maladjustment syndrome (NMS). Signs of lack of affinity for the dam and abnormal posturing as shown are frequent signs in NMS. In addition, seizures, depression, blindness, wandering, and abnormal vocalizaiton often are evident—usually after several hours of normal behavior immediately after birth.

Lesions. Combinations of parenchymal and subarachnoid hemorrhages, neuronal necrosis, and edema and malacia in the spinal cord and brain are presumed to be the neuropathologic bases of the syndrome (Haughey et al., 1976), (Mayhew, 1982b), (Palmer et al., 1976), (Palmer et al., 1984).

Frequently there is poor correlation between the presence, site and extent of such lesions and the presence and characteristics of the clinical syndrome (Mayhew, 1982b), (Palmer et al., 1984). Foals that have had numerous uncontrolled seizures or that survive status epilepticus, can have neuronal necrosis in various areas of the brain, including the cerebral cortex, hippocampus, dorsal thalamus, and basal nuclei (Mayhew, 1988). Such changes probably represent the effects of severe seizures and hypoxia (Montgomery et al., 1983).

Assessment. The lesions represent vascular accidents occurring around the time of parturition. Hypertension, hypotension, hypoxia, hypercapnia, acidosis, hypoglycemia, and rapid changes in such parameters, probably result in hypoxic and ischemic damage to vessels and CNS parenchyma. There is, however, poor correlation between the presence and severity of cerebral dysfunction and the presence of unequivocal hypoxic-ischemic brain damage in individual foals dying after demonstrating signs of NMS (Mayhew, 1988).

Spinal cord lesions can be associated with tetraparesis or with a hypotonic ("floppy-foal") syndrome, sometimes with no sign of brain involvement (Adams et al., 1985), (Mayhew, 1982).

Diagnosis. Sepsis should be ruled out, but may coexist with NMS (Brewer et al., 1988a), (Adams et al., 1985). CSF analysis sometimes reveals mild hemorrhage with xanthochromia.

Therapy. Seizures must be controlled with diazepam in 5 to 10 mg doses, pentobarbital to effect or phenobarbital to effect at 5 to 10 mg/kg over 20 min IV then 2.5 to 10 mg/kg, orally TID (also Problem 2). Corticosteroids are not definitively effective and probably are not indicated because of the concern for sepsis. DMSO, 1 gm/kg, 20% in D5W slowly IV may be worth trying, although the effects of DMSO on the foal's defense systems, including neutrophil function, are not known and could be deleterious (Pesanti et al., 1985). Round-the-clock nursing care is absolutely vital to success.

Prognosis. Without sepsis, up to 80% can survive, and the quality of survival is generally considered good. Some mares have given birth to foals having NMS over consecutive years.

REFERENCES

Allen JR, Barbee DD, Boulton CR, et al. Brain abscess in a horse: diagnosis by computed tomography and successful surgical treatment. Equine Vet J 1987; *19*:552–555.

Adams MR, Mayhew IG. Neurologic Diseases. Vet Clin North Am [Eq Pract] 1985; *1*:209–234.

Alroy J, Orgad U, Ucci AA, et al. Swainsonine toxicosis mimics lectin histochemistry of mannosidosis. Vet Pathol 1985; *22*:311–316.

Angsubhakorn S. Poomvises P, Romruen K, et al. Aflatoxicosis in horses. J Am Vet Med Assoc 1981; *178*:274–278.

Austin RJ. Disseminated phycomycosis in a horse: case report. Can Vet J 1976; *17*(3):86–89.

Barnard BJH. Simptome van hondsdolheid by huis-en plaasdiere in Suid-Afrika en Sudwes-Afrika. J S Afr Vet Assoc 1979; *50*:109–111.

Basson PA, Kellerman TS, Albl P, et al. Blindness and encephalopathy caused by *Helichrysum argyrosphaerum* DC (compositae) in sheep and cattle. Onderstepoort J Vet Res 1975; *42*:135–148.

Beeman KB. *Haemophilus somnus* of cattle: an overview. Comp Cont Ed Pract Vet 1985; *7*:S259–S264.

Benfield DA, Libal MC. Pseudorabies in a flock of lambs. Case report. Comp Cont Ed Pract Vet 1986; *8*:F116–F118.

Bester RC, Cimprich RE, Evans LH. Hydrocephalus in an 18-month-old colt. J Am Vet Med Assoc 1976; *168*:1041–1042.

Blancou J, Pépin M, Soulebot JP, Brun A. Vaccination des bovins contre la rage. Cinetique des anticorps, résistance a l'épreuve trois ans aprés vaccination. Ann Rech Vét 1984; *15*(4):543–547.

Blood DC, Henderson JA, Radostits OM. *Veterinary Medicine.* 5th Ed. Philadelphia: Lea & Febiger, 1979. pp 966–968.

Blunden AS, Khalil LF, Webbon PM. *Halicephalobus deletrix* infection in a horse. Equine Vet J 1987; *19*:255–260.

Brewer BD, Koterba AM. Neonatal Septicemia. In Robinson NR, ed. *Current Therapy in Equine Medicine.* Philadelphia: 1987. pp 222–225.

Brewer DB, Koterba AM. The development of a scoring system for the early diagnosis of equine neonatal sepsis. Equine Vet J 1988a; *20*:18–22.

Brewer DB, Koterba AM, Carter R, et al. Comparison of an empirically developed sepsis score with a computer generated and weighted scoring system for the identification of sepsis in the equine neonate. Equine Vet J 1988b; *20*:23–24.

Brown TT. Enteroviral Encephalomyelitis of Pigs. In: Howard JL, ed. *Current Veterinary Therapy: food animal practice.* Philadelphia: WB Saunders, 1981. pp 607–609.

Buonanno AM, Carlson GP, Kantrowitz B. Clinical and diagnostic features of portosystemic shunt in a foal. J Am Vet Med Assoc 1988; *192*: 387–390.

Burgess EC, Mattison M. Encephalitis associated with *Borrelia burgdorferi* infection in a horse. J Am Vet Med Assoc 1987; *11*:1457–1458.

Burgess EC, Gilette D, Pickett JP. Arthritis and panuveitis as manifestations of *Borrelia burgdorferi* infection in a Wisconsin pony. J Am Vet Med Assoc 1986; *10*:1340–1342.

Buxton D. Focal symmetrical encephalomalacia in young cattle. Vet Rec 1981; *108*:459.

Cho DY, Leipold HW. Congenital defects of the bovine central nervous system. Vet Bull 1977; *47*:489–504.

Clement SF. Behavioral alterations and neonatal maladjustment syndrome in the foal. Proc 31st Ann Conv Eq Pract 1985; 145–148.

Cook RD, Howel JMcC, Dorling PR, et al. Changes in nervous tissue in bovine generalized glycogenosis type II. Neuropathol Appl Neurobiol 1982; *8*:95–107.

Cordy DR. Pathomorphology and pathogenesis of bacterial meningoventriculitis of neonatal ungulates. Vet Pathol 1984; *21*:587–591.

Crandell RA. Pseudorabies (Aujeszky's Disease). In: Howard JL, ed. *Current Veterinary Therapy: food animal practice*. Philadelphia: WB Saunders, 1981. pp 604–607.

Crowell-Davis SL, Houpt KA. Behavior. Vet Clin North Am [Eq Pract] 1986; *2*:465–671.

Dickie CW, James LF. *Kochia scoparia* poisoning in cattle. J Am Vet Med Assoc 1983; *183*:765–768.

Divers TJ, Blackmon DM, Martin CL, et al. Blindness and convulsions associated with vitamin A deficiency in feedlot steers. J Am Vet Med Assoc 1986; *189*:1579–1582.

Divers TJ, Warner A, Vaala WE, et al. Toxic hepatic failure in newborn foals. J Am Vet Med Assoc 1983; *183*:1407–1414.

Dickson J. Brain damage in dehorned goat kids. Vet Rec 1984; *114*:387.

Dollahite JW, Younger RL, Crookshank HR, et al. Chronic lead poisoning in horses. Am J Vet Res 1978; *39*:961–964.

Donnelly WJC, Sheahan BJ. Bovine GM$_1$ gangliosidosis: an inborn lysosomal disease. Vet Sci Comm 1977; *1*:65–74.

Dubey JP, Perry A, Kennedy MJ. Encephalitis caused by a *Sarcocystis*-like organism in a steer. J Am Vet Med Assoc 1987; *191*:231–232.

Emmons RW, Woodie JD, Lamb RL, et al. Main drain virus as a cause of equine encephalomyelitis. J Am Vet Med Assoc 1983; *183*:555–558.

Ford J, Lokai MD. Complications of Streptococcus equi infection. Vet Clin North Am [Eq Pract] 1980; *2*:41–44.

Foreman JH, Reed SM, Rantanen NW, et al. Congenitial internal hydrocephalus in a Quarterhorse foal. Eq Vet Sci 1983; *3*:154–164.

Fountaine JH, Gasche DG, Oehme FW. Experimental salt poisoning (water deprivation syndrome) in swine. Vet Human Toxicol 1975; *17*:5–8.

Gay CC, Blood DC, Wilkinson JS. Clinical observations of sheep with focal symmetrical encephalomalacia. Aust Vet J 1975; *51*:266–269.

Giles N, Davies FG, Duffus WPH, et al. Bovine cerebral theileriosis. Vet Rec 1978; *102*:313.

Gilmour JS, Buxton D, MacLeod NMS, et al. Bovine spongiform encephalopathy [Letter]. Vet Rec 1988; *122*:142–143.

Gonzalez D, Rodriguez-Carbajal J, Aluja A, et al. Cerebral cysticercosis in pigs studied by computed tomography and necropsy. Vet Parasitol 1987; *26*:55–69.

Gulick BA, Liu IKM, Qualls CW, et al. Effect of pyrrolizidine alkaloid-induced hepatic disease on plasma amino acid patterns in the horse. Am J Vet Res 1980; *41*:1894–1898.

Harper PAW, Walker KH, Healy PJ, et al. Neurovisceral ceroid-lipofuscinosis in blind Devon cattle. Acta Neuropathol 1988; In Press.

Harper PAW, Healy PJ, Dennis JA, et al. Citrullinaemia as a cause of neurological disease in neonatal friesian calves. Aust Vet J 1986; *63*:378–379.

Harshfield GS. Sporadic bovine encephalomyelitis. J Am Vet Med Assoc 1970; *156*:466–477.

Hartley WJ, Blakemore WF. An unidentified sporozoan encephalomyelitis in sheep. Vet Pathol 1974; *11*:1–12.

Hatziolos BC, Sass B, Albert TF, et al. Ocular changes in a horse with gutturomycosis. J Am Vet Med Assoc 1975; *167*:51–54.

Haughey KG, Jones RT. Meningeal haemorrhage and congestion associated with the perinatal mortality of foals. Vet Rec 1976; *98*:518–522.

Healy PJ, Seaman JT, Garner IA, et al. β-mannosidase deficiency in Anglo-Nubian goats. Aust Vet J 1981; *57*:504–507.

Held JP, McGavin MD, Geiser D. Ataxia as the only clinical sign of cerebrospinal meningitis in a horse with equine infectious anemia. J Am Vet Med Assoc 1983; *183*:324–326.

Horner GW, Oliver RE, Hunter R. An epizootic of malignant catarrhal fever. 2. Laboratory investigations. NZ Vet J 1975; *23*:35–38.

Huxtable CR, Dorling PR. Poisoning of livestock by *Swainsona* spp: current status. Aus Vet J 1982; *59*:50–53.

James MP, Neilson JA, Stewart WJ. An epizootic of malignant catarrhal fever. 1. Clinical and pathological observations. NZ Vet J 1975; *23*:9–12.

James LF, Hartley WJ, Van Kampen KR. Syndromes of *Astragalus* poisoning in livestock. J Am Vet Med Assoc 1981: *178*:146–150.

Jolly RD, Hartley WJ. Storage diseases of domestic animals. Aus Vet J 1977; *53*:1–8.

Joyce JR, Russell LH. Clinical signs of rabies in horses. Comp Cont Ed Pract Vet 1981; *3*:S56–S61.

Juck FA, Smith LL. Phycomycotic meningoencephalitis in a neonatal calf. Can Vet J 1978; *19*:75–78.

Keane D, Blackwell T. Hepatic encephalopathy associated with patent ductus venosus in a calf. J Am Vet Med Assoc 1983; *182*:1393–1394.

Kerr LA, Groce AW, Kersting KW. Amoniated forage toxicosis in calves. J Am Vet Med Assoc 1987; *5*:551–552.

Kiley-Worthington M, Wood-Gush D. Stereotypic Behavior. In: Robinson NE, ed. *Current Therapy in Equine Medicine.* 2nd Ed. Philadelphia: 1987. pp 131–134.

King JM, Roth L, Haschek WM. Myocardial necrosis secondary to neural lesions in domestic animals. J Am Vet Med Assoc 1982; *180*:144–148.

Kirkbride CA, Frey RA. Experimental water intoxication in calves. J Am Vet Med Assoc 151 1967; *151*:742–746.

Konno S, Moriwaki M, Nakagawa M. Akabane disease in cattle: congenital abnormalities caused by viral infection. Spontaneous disease. Vet Pathol 1982; *19*:246–266.

Konno S, Nakagawa M. Akabane disease in cattle: congenital abnormalities caused by viral infection. Experimental disease. Vet Pathol 1982;*19*:267–279.

Kosanke SD, Pierce KR, Bay WW. Clinical and biochemical abnormalities in porcine GM_2-gangliosidosis. Vet Pathol 1978; *15*:685–699.

Kumar K, Jones MZ, Cunningham JG, et al. Caprine β-mannosidosis: phenotypic features. Vet Rec 1986; *118*:325–327.

Kurtz HJ, Bergeland ME, Barnes DM. Pathologic changes in edema disease of swine. Am J Vet Res 1969; *30*:791–806.

Kurtz HJ, Short EC Jr. Pathogenesis of edema disease in swine: pathologic effects of hemolysin, autolysate, and endotoxin of *Escherichia coli* (0141). Am J Vet Res 1976; *37*:15–24.

Leadon DP, Jeffcott LB, Rossdale PD. Behavior and viability of the premature neonatal foal after induced parturition. Am J Vet Res 1986; *47*:1870–1874.

Lee JYS, Wilson MR. A review of pseudorabies (Aujeszky's disease) in pigs. Can Vet J 1979; *20*:65–69.

Leipold HW, Smith JE, Jolly RD, et al. Mannosidosis of angus calves. J Am Vet Med Assoc 1979; *175*:457–459.

Lincoln SD, Black B. Halogeton poisoning in range cattle. J Am Vet Met Assoc 1980; *176*:717–718.

Little PB. *Haemophilus somnus* complex: pathogenesis of the septicemic thrombotic meningoencephalitis. Canad Vet J 1986; *27*:94–96.

Little PB, Sorensen DK. Bovine polioencephalomalacia, infectious embolic meningoencephalitis, and acute lead poisoning in feedlot cattle. J Am Vet Med Assoc 1969; *155*:1892–1903.

Little PB, Thorsen J, Moore W, et al. Powassan viral encephalitis: a review and experimental studies in the horse and rabbit. Vet Pathol 1985; *22*:500–507.

Luttgen PJ, Storts RW. Ceroid-lipofuscinosis in Nubian goats. Proc Vth Annual Vet Int Med Forum 1982; p 843.

Lynch J.A., Binnington BD, Artsob H. California serogroup virus infection in a horse with encephalitis. J Am Vet Med Assoc 1985; *186*:389–390.

MacLachlan NJ, Osburn BI. Bluetongue virus-induced hydranencephaly in cattle. Vet Pathol 1983; *20*:563– 573.

McCormack JE. Papilledema related to left cerebral hemisphere abscess in a heifer. Vet Med Sm Anim Clin 1973; 1249–1252.

Marasas WFO, Kellerman TS, Pienaar JG, et al. Leukoencephalomalacia: a mycotoxicosis of equidae caused by *Fusarium moniliforme* Sheldon. Onderstepoort J Vet Res 1976; *43*:113–122.

Markson LM, Wells GAH. Evaluation of autofluorescence as an aid to diagnosis of cerebrocortical necrosis. Vet Rec 1982; *111*:338–340.

Mayhew IG. Observations on vascular accidents in the central nervous system of neonatal foals. J Reprod Fertil 1982; Suppl *32*:569–575.

Mayhew IG. Neurological and neuropathological observations on the equine neonate. Eq Vet J 1988; Suppl 5: 28–33.

Mayhew IG, Jolly RD, Pickett BT, et al. Ceroid-lipoduscinosis (Batten's disease): pathogenesis of blindness in the ovine model. Neuropath Appl Neurobiol 1985; *11*:273–290.

Mayhew IG, Lichtenfels JR, Greiner EC, et al. Migration of a spiruroid nematode through the brain of a horse. J Am Vet Med Assoc 1982; *180*:1306–1311.

Mengeling WL. Encephalitis—Vomiting and Wasting Disease Complex of Swine. In: Howard JL, ed. *Current Veterinary Therapy: food animal practice.* Philadelphia: WB Saunders, 1981. pp 613–616.

Mayer EE, Morris PG, Elcock LH, et al. Hindlimb hyperesthesia associated with rabies in two horses. J Am Vet Med Assoc 1986; *188*:629–632.

Miksch D. Fescue toxicosis update/bovine hysteria from ammoniated forages update. Proc 18th Ann Conf Am Assoc Bov Pract 1985; 124–126.

Molyneux R, James L. Loco intoxication: Indolizidine alkaloids of spotted locoweed (*Astragalus lentiginosus*). Science 1982; *216*:190–191.

Montgomery DL, Lee AC. Brain damage in the epileptic beagle dog. Vet Pathol 1983; *20*:160–169.

Morgan G. Terlecki S, Bradley R. A suspected case of *Sarcocystis* encephalitis in sheep. Brit Vet J 1984; *140*:64–69.

Nation PN, Calder WA. Necrosis of the brain in calves following dehorning. Can Vet J 1985; *26*:378–380.

Neilan MC, McCausland IP, Maslen M. Mycotic pneumonia, placentitis and neonatal encephalitis in dairy cattle caused by *Mortierella wolfii*. Aust Vet J 1982; *59*:48–49.

Osweiler GD, Ruhr LP. Lead poisoning in feeder calves. J Am Vet Med Assoc 1978; *172*:498–500.

Padovan D. Polioencephalomalacia associated with water deprivation in cattle. Cornell Vet 1980; *70*:153–159.

Palmer AC, Leadon DP, Rossdale PD, et al. Intracranial haemorrhage in pre-viable, premature and full term foals. Eq Vet J 1984; *16*:383–389.

Palmer AC, Rossdale PD. Neuropathological changes associated with the neonatal maladjustment syndrome in the thoroughbred foal. Res Vet Sci 1976; *20*:267–275.

Pépin M, Blancou J, Aubert MFA. Rage expérimentale des bovins: sensibilité, symptômes, réactions immunitaries humorales, lésions et excrétion du virus. Ann Rech Vét 1984; *15*:325–333.

Pesanti EL, Nugent KM. Modulation of pulmonary clearance of bacteria by antioxidants. Infect Immun 1985; *48*:57–61.

Pierson RE, Storz J, McChesney AE, et al. Experimental transmission of malignant catarrhal fever. Am J Vet Res 1974; *35*:523–525.

Pierson RE, Jensen R. Polioencephalomalacia in feedlot lambs. J Am Vet Med Assoc 1975; *166*:257–259.

Pritchard D, Eggleston GW, Macadam JF. Nardoo fern and polioencephalomalacia. Aust Vet J 1978; *54*:204.

Raisbeck MF. Is polioencephalomalacia associated with high-sulfate diets? J Am Vet Med Assoc 1982; *180*:1303–1306.

Rammell CG, Hill JH. A review of thiamine deficiency and its diagnosis, especially in ruminants. NZ Vet J 1986; *34*:202–204.

Raphel CF. Brain abscess in three horses. J Am Vet Med Assoc 1982; *180*:874–877.

Read DH. Congenital polymicrogyria in Murray grey calves. In: Alley MR, ed. *Diseases of Muscle and Peripheral Nerve.* Proc. 13th Ann Meet NZ Soc Vet Comp Path. Palmerston North, NZ., 1983; 69–74.

Reid HAC. Outbreak of cattle rabies in the north west region of Guyana. Vet Rec 1985; *117*:641.

Robinson WF, Maxie MG. The Cardiovascular System. In: Jubb KVF, Kennedy PC, Palmer N, eds. *Pathology of Domestic Animals.* 3rd Ed. Vol. 3. Orlando: Academic Press, 1985. pp 24–26.

Ross MW, Lowe JE, Cooper BJ, et al. Hypoglycemic seizures in a Shetland pony. Cornell Vet 1983; *73*:151–169.

Roth IJ, Morrow CJ, Wilkins JF, et al. Holoprosencephaly in Border Leicester lambs. Aust Vet J 1987; *64*:271–273.

Rumbaugh GE. Disseminated septic meningitis in a mare. J Am Vet Med Assoc 1977; *171*:452–454.

Scarratt WK, Collins TJ, Sponenberg DP. Water deprivation—sodium chloride intoxication in a group of feeder lambs. J Am Vet Med Assoc 1985; *186*:977–978.

Scott TW, Olson JG, Gibbs EPJ. Surveillance and rapid diagnosis of eastern equine encephalomyelitis virus by enzyme immunoassay. Ann Meet Am Soc Trop Med Hyg 1986; Abstract 323.

Schillhorn van Veen TW. Parasitic diseases of the bovine nervous system. Vet Clin North Am [Food Anim Pract] 1987; *3*:99–105.

Seaman W. Phycomycosis associated with encephalitis caused by *Haemophilus somnus* in a heifer. J Am Vet Med Assoc 1977; *171*:435–437.

Seiler RJ, Omar S, Jackson ARB. Meningoencephalitis in naturally occurring *Trypanosoma evansi* infection (Surra) of horses. Vet Pathol 1981; *18*:120–122.

Selman IE, Wiseman A, Wright NG, et al. Transmission studies with bovine malignant catarrhal fever. Vet Rec 1978; *102*:252–257.

Sharma HN, Nigam JM, Ramkumar. Successful surgical treatment of the brain abscess in a cow. Indian Vet J 1975; *52*:398–401.

Skerritt GC, Stallbaumer MF. Diagnosis and treatment of coenuriasis (gid) in sheep. Vet Rec 1984; *115*:399–403.

Smith MC. Polioencephalomalacia in goats. J Am Vet Med Assoc 1979; *174*:1328–1332.

Staley EE. An approach to treatment of locoism in horses. Vet Med/Sm Anim Clin 1978; *73*:1205–1206.

Steckel RR, Adams SB, Long GG, et al. Antemortem diagnosis and treatment of cryptococcal meningitis in a horse. J Am Vet Med Assoc 1982; *180*:1085–1089.

Stephan HA, Gay GM, Ramirez TC. Encephalomyelitis, reproductive failure and corneal opacity (blue eye) in pigs, associated with a paramyxovirus infection. Vet Rec 1988; *122*:6–10.

Strain GM, Claxton MS, Turnquist SE, et al. Evoked potential and electroencephalographic assessment of central blindness due to brain abscesses in a steer. Cornell Vet 1987; *77*:374–382.

Stubbings DP, Jeffrey M. Presumptive protozoan (*Sarcocystis*) encephalomyelitis with paresis in lambs. Vet Rec 1985; *116*:373–374.

Sullivan ND. The Nervous System. In: Jubb KVF, Kennedy PC, Palmer N, eds. *Pathology of Domestic Animals.* 3rd Ed. Vol 1. Orlando: Academic Press, 1985. pp 276–290.

Summers BA, Smith CA. Renal encephalopathy in a cow. Cornell Vet 1985; *75*:524–530.

Sweeney CR, Benson CE, Whitlock RH, et al. *Streptococcus equi* infection in horses—Part II. Compend Cont Ed Pract Vet 1987; *9*:845–851.

Thomas KW. The effect of thiaminase-induced subclinical thiamine deficiency on growth of weaner sheep. Vet Rest Comun 1986a; *10*:125–141.

Thomas KW. Oral treatment of polioencephalomalacia and subclinical thiamine deficiency with thiamine propyldisulphide and thiamine hydrochloride. J Vet Pharmacol Therap 1986b; *9*:402–411.

Thompson KG, Lake DE, Cordes DO. Hepatic encephalopathy associated with chronic facial eczema. NZ Vet J 1979; *27*:221–223.

Tirgari M, Howard BR, Boargob A. Clinical and radiographical diagnosis of coneurosis cerebralis in sheep and its surgical treatment. Vet Rec 1987; *120*:173–178.

Vaala WE. Diagnosis and treatment of prematurity and neonatal maladjustment syndrome in newborn foals. Comp Cont Ed Pract Vet 1986; *8*:S211–223.

Valli VEO. The Hematopoietic System. In: Jubb KVF, Kennedy PC, Palmer N, eds. *Pathology of Domestic Animals.* 3rd Ed. Vol 3. Orlando: Academic Press, 1985. pp 210–214.

Wells GAH, Scott AC, Johnson CT, et al. A novel progressive spongiform encephalopathy in cattle. Vet Rec 1987; *121*:419–420.

West GP. Equine rabies. Eq Vet J 1985; *17*:280–282.

Williams ES, Young S. Chronic wasting disease of captive mule deer: a spongiform encephalopathy. J Wildl Dis 1980; *16*:89–98.

Wilson BJ, Maronpot RR. Causative fungus agent of leucoencephalomalacia in equine animals. Vet Rec 1971; *88*:484–486.

Wilson TM, Nelson PE, Ryan TB, et al. Linking leukoencephalomalacia to commercial horse rations. Vet Med 1985; *80*:63–69.

Worthington RW, Mulders MSG. The effect of *Clostridium perfringens* epsilon toxin on the blood brain barrier of mice. Onderstepoort J Vet Res 1974; *42*:25–28.

Wright HJ, Adams DS, Trigo FJ. Meningoencephalitis after hot-iron disbudding of goat kids. Vet Med/Sm Am Clin 1983; *78*:599–601.

CHAPTER 6

Problem 2:
Seizures

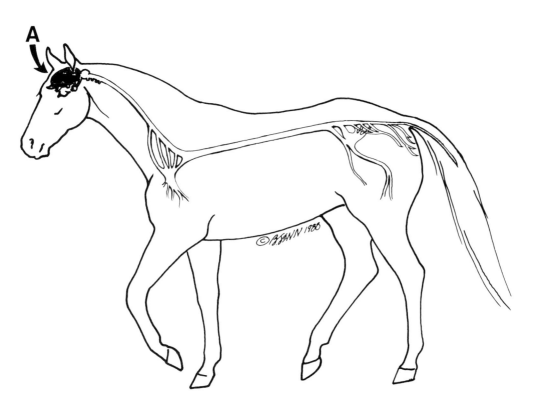

Location of lesions resulting in seizures: focal and diffuse forebrain and thalamus (A).

A seizure, fit, ictus or convulsion is considered abnormal behavior. Seizures are the physical expression of abnormal electrical discharges in forebrain neurons that reach the somatic and visceral motor areas and initiate spontaneous, paroxysmal, involuntary movements. These cerebral dysrhythmias tend to begin and end abruptly and they have a finite duration.

There may be a prodromal phase or aura for minutes to hours when the animal is distracted from its environment and usually is restless (Fig. 6–1A). The beginning of the ictus may be a localizing finding with one part of the body involved (partial seizure). Usually these muscle spasms spread to the whole body (generalized seizure) and the animal usually falls to the ground thrashing rhythmically (Fig. 6–1B,C). The postictal phase of depression and temporary blindness may last for minutes to hours, although blindness may be apparent in foals for several days following severe generalized seizures (Fig. 6–2).

Fortunately, large animals have a relatively high seizure threshold, as it seems to take a considerable insult to the brain to precipitate convulsions. Younger animals, particularly foals, convulse more readily than adults. Foals

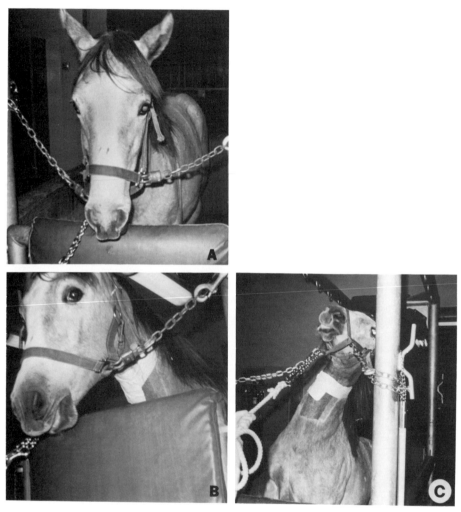

Figure 6–1. Benign epilepsy of foals. This weanling Arabian foal was suffering from bacterial pneumonia and had several seizures. These were characterized by a preictal aura and the foal became detached from its environment, lowered its head, and lost facial expression (A). Within about 10 seconds, the foal would raise its head in a jerky manner and show rapid symmetric twitching of the facial muscles (B). With no restraint the foal would become recumbent and paddle. With restraint the foal's head would jerk back several times with more prominent facial, neck, and body muscle twitching (C). After this, the foal would stand quietly for many minutes before regaining its normal mental attitude. This typifies a mild generalized seizure. The foal recovered totally after the pneumonia resolved.

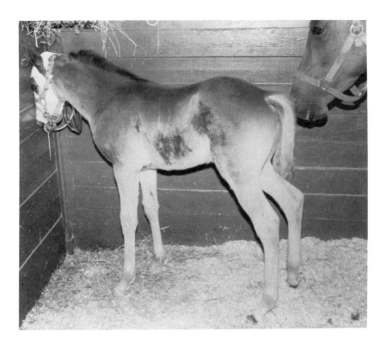

Figure 6–2. Benign epilepsy of foals. This Arabian foal had two severe generalized seizures and injured its head and eyes. No cause for the seizures was determined. The foal remained blind for four to five days, lost its affinity for its dam, and would stand with its head in the corner as shown. These postictal changes in behavior most probably represent neuronal exhaustion and can last several days in foals. On the other hand, it is possible that head trauma, or metabolic derangements occurring during severe convulsive episodes, could have caused further cerebral dysfunction. The foal was treated with phenobarbital for several weeks then weaned from the anticonvulsant drug. No further seizures occurred.

frequently demonstrate mild generalized seizures, seen as periods of jaw chomping ("chewing-gum fits"), tachypnea, tremor of facial muscles, and jerky head movements.

Seizures most frequently occur in conjunction with other signs of brain disease. The syndrome of inherited, recurrent seizures, that continues through life with no underlying morphologic disease process, is true epilepsy. This probably has not been demonstrated in horses, although it is seen in some breeds of cattle.

Large animals, especially horses, often become violent in response to painful processes, and when attempting to regain their footing. These intermittent and sometimes continuous episodes of struggling and thrashing are difficult to distinguish from convulsions. Secondary head trauma often ensues, usually adding to the delirious state. Primary processes that fall in this category include colic, myopathy, vertebral injury, long bone fractures, and acute spinal cord, brainstem, and particularly vestibular disease.

The states of narcolepsy and cataplexy, as well as other causes of acute collapse that are frequently confused with seizures, are discussed in Problem 4.

Table 6–1 suggests therapeutic regimens for seizure medication in a foal and in a horse. Pharmacokinetic studies on phenytoin in horses (Kowalczyk

Table 6–1. Anticonvulsant Drugs Used to Treat Seizure Disorders in Horses[a]

Regimen	Drug	50-kg Foal Dose	450-kg Horse Dose
Initial therapy (including *status epilepticus*)	Diazepam[b]	5–20 mg, IV	25–100 mg, IV
	Pentobarbital	150–1000 mg, IV	To effect
	Phenobarbital	250–1000 mg, IV	2–5 g IV
	Phenytoin	50–250 mg, IV or PO, q4h	—
	Primidone	1–2 g, PO	—
	Chloralhydrate ($\pm$MgSO$_4$, barbiturate)	3–10 g, IV	15–60 g, IV
	Xylazine	25–100 mg, IV or IM	300–1000 mg, IV or IM
	Guaifenesin ($\pm$ barbiturate)	To effect	40–60 g
Maintenance therapy	Phenobarbital	100–500 mg, PO, BID	1–5 g, PO, BID
	Phenytoin	50–250 mg, PO, BID	500–1000 mg, PO, TID (low therapeutic index)
	Primidone	1 g, PO, SID or BID	

[a]Included are suggested dose ranges for both initial therapy of acute convulsions (including *status epilepticus*) and for maintenance therapy in an average sized foal (50-kg) and an adult horse (450-kg). Although these drugs have been used with success, several are not licensed for use in the horse. These doses should be regarded as guidelines only, and drugs should be given to effect. Lower doses may be equally effective and it is most appropriate to monitor blood levels of all maintenance anticonvulsant drugs. Side effects (e.g., marked respiratory depression with xylazine, transient stimulation with phenobarbital given too rapidly) should be given due consideration prior to their use. Also, interactions must be considered when other drugs are to be administered to an animal already on anticonvulsant therapy.

[b]Do not leave in plastic container or syringe for more than a few minutes or diazepam may become inactivated.

Table 6–2. Principles of Maintenance Anticonvulsant Therapy (after Chrisman, 1982)

1. Select a single anticonvulsant drug.
2. Begin at the recommended dose and adjust the dose until the seizures are controlled and there are no toxic side effects (excessive drowsiness with phenobarbital).
3. Give all medication on an empty stomach and do not feed for 1 to 2 hours.
4. If side effects, such as excessive sedation with phenobarbital or collapse with phenytoin, are seen and seizures are not controlled, decrease the dose of the first drug to nontoxic levels and begin a second drug at the recommended dose.
5. If the seizures are controlled with the administration of the two drugs, slowly taper the dose of the first drug over a 1 to 2 week period and discontinue.
6. If the seizures return after the first drug is withdrawn, then begin the first drug again and maintain the animal on the combination of drugs.
7. If no toxic side effects are seen, do not begin decreasing the dose or altering the frequency of medication until after the animal has been seizure-free for 4 weeks. Sudden withdrawal of drugs may precipitate seizures.
8. Monitor blood anticonvulsant concentrations in animals that are difficult to control. Therapeutic anticonvulsant blood concentrations for phenobarbital in men and dogs are 15 to 40 µg/ml; they may be lower than this in horses. In fact we seem to have achieved seizure control in horses at 5 to 15 µg/ml.
9. If the routine anticonvulsants fail, less used anticonvulsants may be tried with caution, as dosages are not standardized and long-term side effects are unknown.
10. Warn owner that a large animal with a seizure disorder may not be safe to be around or to ride; consider this strongly before embarking on permanent anticonvulsant therapy for epilepsy.
11. For economic and practical purposes it is reasonable to attempt to slowly reduce, and finally stop anticonvulsant therapy after 6 to 12 weeks of seizure control. If seizures reappear then another decision as to whether to embark on long-term or lifelong therapy must be made.
12. Beware of interactions when other drugs are used in a patient on anticonvulsant therapy. Tetracyclines and chloramphenicol inhibit hepatic microsomal enzymes, thereby prolonging the effect of phenytoin and phenobarbitone (Davis, 1979). It has been noted that epileptic horses and foals that are successfully controlled with phenobarbitone have had several, severe seizures several hours to days following the use of ivermectin anthelmintics. It is suggested that tetracyclines, chloramphenicol, and ivermectin not be given to patients on anticonvulsant therapy.

et al., 1983) and phenobarbital in the horse (Duran et al., 1987), (Ravis et al., 1987) and foal (Spehar et al., 1984) have been published; use of the other drugs listed is empirically determined. Several other human anticonvulsant drugs may be worth considering if control of seizures is unsatisfactory. Two drugs that have been tried in foals, with unknown results, are carbamazepine at 250 to 500 mg doses and triaziline at 1 g doses. Table 6–2 outlines principles of maintenance therapy (Chrisman, 1982). These regimens may be extrapolated to other species. All ruminants that have seizures should receive gram doses of thiamin immediately after any samples have been drawn for blood glucose and possibly red cell transketolase (thiamin) activity.

Categories of Disease and Differential Diagnosis
*NOTE: Only diseases marked * are discussed in this section.*

I. Congenital and Familial
  *1. Familial Epilepsy
  *2. Benign Epilepsy of Foals (VIII.2)
   3. Congenitial Brain Malformations (Problem 1)
   4. Lysosomal Storage Diseases (Problem 1)
   5. Citrullinemia (Problem 1)
II. Physical
  *1. Lightning Strike
  *2. Intracarotid Injection
   3. Head Trauma (Problem 4)
II. Infectious, Inflammatory, Immune
   1. All Infectious Meningoencephalomyelitides (Problems 1, 6, 9, 10, and 13)
IV. Metabolic
  *1. Hypocalcemia (Problems 2 and 8B)
  *2. Hypomagnesemia (Problems 2 and 8B)
  *3. Hyponatremia
   4. Hypoglycemia (Problem 1)
   5. Hepatic Encephalopathy (Problem 1)
V. Toxic
  *1. Organophosphates and Chlorinated Hydrocarbons
  *2. Strychnine
  *3. Metaldehyde
  *4. Arsanilic Acid and 3-nitro
  *5. Miscellaneous
   6. Lead (Problem 1)
   7. Water and Salt (Problem 1)
   8. Moldy Corn Poisoning (Problem 1)
   9. Bracken Fern (Problem 10)
   10. Plant-Associated Tremor Syndromes (Problem 8B)
   11. Tetanus (Problem 8A)

VI. Nutritional
1. Thiamin Responsive Polioencephalomalacia (Problem 1)
2. Vitamin A Deficiency (Problem 3)
3. Vitamin E Deficiency—Mullberry Heart Disease of Swine (Problem 1)
VII. *Neoplastic (including tumors)
VIII. Idiopathic
*1. Grove Poisoning
*2. Benign Epilepsy of Foals
*3. Nervous Coccidiosis
4. Neonatal Maladjustment Syndrome (Problem 1)

I. Congenital and Familial
1. **Familial Epilepsy**
   Seizures, characterized by lowering of the head, tongue chewing, foaming at the mouth, and collapse, occur in certain Brown Swiss cattle beginning by 1 year of age (Atkeson et al., 1944). The disease has an autosomal dominant mode of inheritance.
   A form of familial epilepsy occurs in certain Swedish Red cattle (Isaksson, 1943).
   Cerebellar ataxia and convulsions occur in Aberdeen Angus calves (also Problem 9).
2. **Benign Epilepsy of Arabian Foals**
   Benign epilepsy is seen in foals of many breeds, but occurs with a much higher frequency in foals of the Arabian breed (Fig. 6–1). With appropriate therapy, affected foals appear to recover. Therefore, this disorder is not true inherited epilepsy and is discussed under Benign Epilepsy of Foals, VIII.2.
II. Physical
1. **Lightning Strike**
   Following acute episodes of recumbency and various neurologic syndromes, which are reportedly caused by lightning strikes, several horses have developed epilepsy. No histopathologic lesions were found in the two cases in which the brain was studied. The possibility that this syndrome is posttraumatic epilepsy is undetermined. In fact, a relationship between the supposed lightning strike and the epilepsy may not exist.
2. **Intracarotid Injection**
   Signalment. Most often this occurs in horses.
   History. A known or suspected intracarotid injection.
   Neurologic Syndrome. Inadvertent intracarotid injection, which frequently occurs in horses, may have little effect, but usually it results in an acute seizure, often followed by recumbency and paddling with degrees of coma (Gabel et al., 1963). Contralateral facial twitching, along with apprehension (wide-eyed appearance) may precede the seizure. The onset of signs is rapid (a few seconds) with ataractic and viscous or irritant drugs. However, a slight delay in

the onset of signs (seconds to a few minutes) may occur. With xylazine, acetylpromazine, and other water soluble drugs, recovery usually occurs; the horse stands in 5 to 60 minutes and is totally normal in 1 to 7 days. Signs of contralateral blindness, facial hypalgesia (nasal septum) and subtle hemiparesis abate during this time. With procaine penicillin, phenylbutazone, and other insoluble and oil-based drugs, recovery usually is unsatisfactory; epilepsy, coma, and stupor often necessitate euthanasia.

Assessment. Varying combinations of cerebral neuronal anesthesia, vasospasm, vasculitis, hemorrhage, and neuronal necrosis occur, depending on the volume and properties of the drug.

Treatment. Treatment usually is not required with the tranquilizers and water soluble agents. Corticosteroids, DMSO, and anticonvulsant therapy may be necessary in other circumstances.

IV. Metabolic

   1. **Hypocalcemia (also Problems 2 and 8B)**

   Signalment. Adult horses, sometimes sheep, and rarely cattle demonstrate seizures with hypocalcemia.

   History. Often the animal has recently given birth and is lactating, but hypocalcemia also occurs before parturition, particularly in stressed ewes and mares.

   Physical Examination. The animal may be hyperexcitable and have a fever of 103° to 106° F. However, cattle and sheep usually have a normal or low temperature. A static rumen, slow, weak heartbeat, and arrhythmias usually occur in ruminants; synchronous diaphragmatic flutter ("thumps") often occurs in horses.

   Neurologic Examination. Cows generally are depressed, paralyzed, and unable to rise. Frequently they adopt a recumbent posture with head and neck turned toward the flank. Horses goose-step, convulse more often than ruminants, and have "thumps."

   Assessment. Hypocalcemia is a common disorder in cattle after calving. Rarely, it occurs in primary parathyroid disorders.

   Diagnostic Aids. Serum Ca^{++} concentration usually is below 5 mg/dl in ruminants and below 8 mg/dl in horses. Concurrent alterations in other electrolyte and glucose concentrations may be detected.

   Therapy. Calcium gluconate, with or without Mg^{++}, PO_4^{---} and glucose, is given slowly IV, to effect. Recurrences can be prevented with further prophylactic therapy.

   Prevention. Balancing input of Ca^{++} with output should be the long-term goal. However, a diet high in Ca^{++} prior to calving predisposes the animal to milk fever because of the relative hypoparathyroid state that is induced.

   2. **Hypomagnesemia (also Problems 2 and 8B)**

   Signalment. Sheep, and particularly cattle, of any age, usually on lush pasture, most often are affected.

   Physical Examination. The patient usually is hyperactive and nervous. There may be fever and usually the heart pounds.

   Neurologic Examination. Whole body tremor, bellowing, and running blindly occur. Eventually, affected animals fall on their side in convulsions.

Assessment. Hypomagnesemia may result from eating lush grasses low in magnesium during periods of heavy lactation. This is grass tetany. Ruminants cannot mobilize magnesium rapidly, thus they depend on a constant dietary intake. Cold weather and lactation can be important precipitating factors in hypomagnesemia.

Diagnostic Plan. Serum magnesium levels usually are less than 1.0 mg/dl and often there is concurrent hypocalcemia. Cerebrospinal fluid magnesium concentrations also may be helpful in diagnosing grass staggers in cattle, even postmortem (Pauli et al., 1974).

Therapy. Give calcium and magnesium salt solutions slowly IV while monitoring the heart. Also give supplemental magnesium in the feed such as 2 oz calcined magnesite/cow, daily.

Prognosis. This is good if daily treatment is given early; however, patients may die with the excitement of therapy.

3. Hyponatremia

Signalment. Foals with severe renal disease or iatrogenic water overload.

History. Seizures may begin abruptly in a healthy foal, or in one that has evidence of systemic illness. Overzealous administration of water enemas have been part of the history in neonatal foals.

Examination. Unremarkable, unless other indications of renal disease are evident. Seizures are generalized and usually severe.

Assessment. Hyponatremia in foals is one pathophysiologic mechanism that mimics benign epilepsy of foals (see VIII. 2).

Diagnosis. Azotemia and particularly hyponatremia (< 110 mEq/L) and hypochloremia (< 90 mEq/L) are present. Degrees of hyperkalemia and other electrolyte derangements occur.

Therapy. Accurate evaluation of any renal disease is necessary. Slow correction of the low serum sodium and low serum osmolality is advisable with normal saline IV. Low dose furosemide with saline administration may be indicated in severe cases of renal failure. Phenobarbitone sodium should be instituted if seizures are repeated (Table 6–1).

Prognosis. If iatrogenic water overload has occurred the outlook is good, but patients with severe renal disease have a guarded prognosis.

V. Toxic

1. Organophosphates and Chlorinated Hydrocarbons

Signalment. Any age and all species.

Primary Complaint. Seizures, tremor, and muscle weakness.

History. Contact with a parasiticide.

Physical Examination. Organophosphates may produce salivation, miotic pupils, diarrhea, and bradyarrhythmia.

Neurologic Examination. Body tremor and apprehension usually are present. Jaw chomping, nystagmus, opisthotonus, tremor, ataxia, and seizures ("running fits") are characteristic of chlorinated hydrocarbon poisoning (Glastonbury et al., 1987). Weakness may be prominent with organophosphates.

Assessment. The organophosphates and chlorinated hydrocarbons are commonly used in therapeutic substances. Organophosphates are found in anthelmintics, and in insecticide sprays and dips. Chlorinated hydrocarbons are also found in sprays and dips.

Diagnostic Aids. With organophosphates, the erythrocyte and serum cholinesterase concentrations are reduced, but this test may not be valid in cattle because values can be low in normal animals. With chlorinated hydrocarbons, fat may be biopsied and analyzed for the drug.

Therapy. Stop the seizure with either 5 to 100 mg doses of diazepam IV in small to large patients, respectively, or pentobarbital to effect. With organophosphates, treatment should include atropine sodium and possibly 2-PAM. Intravenous crystalloid fluids should aid in diuresis and elimination of toxins. Bathe the animal to remove residual toxins in the hair. Gastric (rumen) lavage is sensible for oral intoxication. Saline cathartics (not oily) should be used.

Prognosis. This is good if treatment begins early, but often the syndrome is too profound by the time seizures occur.

2. **Strychnine**

Strychnine toxicity is seen rarely in large animals, although generalized convulsions with *risus sardonicus* (facial spasms) are expected.

3. **Metaldehyde**

Severe *status epilepticus* and death caused by snail bait ingestion has been seen in cattle (Longbottom et al., 1979), sheep (Simmons, et al., 1974), and horses (Harris, 1975). Anticonvulsant therapy, which may entail general anesthesia with pentobarbital, as well as attempted gastric lavage and catharsis, are indicated.

4. **Arsanilic Acid and 3-nitro-4-hydroxyphenylarsonic Acid (3-nitro)**

3-nitro is an arsenical growth promotant used in swine. A syndrome of muscle tremor and convulsions, especially when induced by forced exercise, can be seen with intoxication by 3-nitro (Rice et al., 1985). It should be noted that intoxication with arsanilic acid, another growth promotant and medicament for swine dysentery, results in signs of hyperesthesia, blindness, ataxia, and progressive paraparesis (Rice et al., 1985).

The precise differences between these clinical syndromes and associated lesions is not clear (Gilbert, 1981), although a specific central-peripheral axonopathy has been described in one experiment with 3-nitro (Kennedy et al., 1986). In fact, in this experiment, the evidence suggests that the convulsions are more correctly viewed as a progression from generalized tremor, to tetany, to clonic movements, without seizure discharges occurring on the EEG (see Problem 8).

5. **Miscellaneous Toxins and Toxic Plants**

In addition to *Helichrysum* sp, Nardoo ferns, *Swainsona* sp, and locoweeds, which are discussed in Problem 1, buckeye (*Aesculus* sp—USA) (Edwards et al., 1980), and *Solanum* spp (Problem 9) also cause seizures, ataxia, and other signs.

VII. Neoplastic (Tumors)

Intracranial neoplasms are rare in large animals, particularly in horses. The most frequently occurring equine brain tumor, pituitary adenoma, usually causes hyperadrenocorticism, although rarely induces blindness and severe depression. A hamartoma, and massive choroid plexus cholesterol granuloma, have been associated with epilepsy and with intermittent circling, blindness, and depression, respectively.

VII. Idiopathic

1. **"Grove Poisoning"**

Signalment. Adult horses of all breeds.

History. In south Florida, and possibly other subtropical climatic regions, a syndrome of ataxia, with intermittent episodes that resemble convulsions, occurs in adult horses. Cases appear to be sporadic and signs frequently are fluctuant.

Clinical Syndrome. Signs resemble diffuse, symmetric and fluctuant cerebral, cerebellovestibular, and probably spinal cord signs. Unusual oral membrane congestion and ulceration, as well as corneal edema and sometimes ulceration occur frequently.

Assessment. No consistent neuropathologic lesions exist. "Grove poisoning" occurs in areas where considerable horticultural practices exist, though no direct connection is proven. During the so-called convulsions, affected horses may show nystagmus, be aware of their environment, and have a menace response. Thus, these episodes may not all represent cerebral dysrhythmia, but may be signs of waxing and waning cerebellar-vestibular dysfunction discussed in Problems 8B and 9. Signs do resemble chlorinated hydrocarbon intoxication in other species; however, no particular compound has been consistently detected in tissues from horses suspected of grove poisoning.

Treatment. Therapy with diazepam and atropine, along with saline purgatives may have cured a few patients.

2. **Benign Epilepsy of Foals**

Signalment. Young growing foals, particularly of the Arabian breed, up to 12 months old.

History. The foal may suddenly become recumbent and thrash violently; usually this occurs on more than one occasion, although it may not be seen. A frequent complaint of the client is that the foal has facial (particularly eye) injuries, with no explanation as to the origin (Figs. 6–2 and 6–3).

Physical Examination. Corneal ulcers, with soil impacted in the conjunctival sac and lacerations of the lips and gums, often are found (Fig. 6–3). Concurrent diseases such as pneumonia (Fig. 6–1), arthritis, or diarrhea sometimes are present.

Neurologic Examination. Seizures may not be observed in the early stages of the syndrome, particularly if the foal is taken into a different environment for hospitalization. Postictal depression, loss of affinity for the dam, head pressing, and particularly amaurosis often are present (Fig. 6–2).

Ancillary Aids. Efforts must be made to rule out identifiable

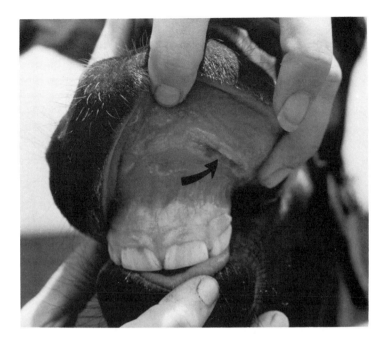

Figure 6–3. Benign epilepsy of foals. Many times the first one or two seizures in this syndrome are not observed, as was the case with this Arabian foal. Such foals can be presented for evaluation of contusions to the gums and lips as shown, (arrow) or for head and eye injuries (Fig. 6–2).

causes of seizures (see Table 6–1). CSF analysis may indicate previous head trauma, which most often is thought to be the result of seizures.

Assessment. A similar syndrome occurs in children (Freeman et al., 1987). The equine syndrome appears to be more frequent in adolescent Arabian foals, and possibly reflects a relatively low seizure threshold present during development. This would allow for the expression of fits in response to many temporary toxic, infectious, metabolic, and physical, cerebral perturbations (see Table 6–1). In this regard it is considered a familial disorder.

This is analogous to benign epilepsy in childhood (Freeman et al., 1987) and is not true, inherited, idiopathic epilepsy.

Treatment. Guidelines for anticonvulsant therapy are outlined in Tables 6–1 and 6–2. Also, any underlying disease must be attended to.

The decision of whether or not to institute maintenance anticonvulsant therapy can be difficult to make because so many foals totally recover from temporary epilepsy without treatment. However, several foals that have not had their seizures controlled well to begin with, have gone on to develop intractable epilepsy. At postmortem examination some of these foals have had hippocampal, dorsal thalamic, laminar cerebrocortical and Purkinje cell neuronal necrosis. These findings are probably the result of prolonged, repeated seizures, but also are likely to act as seizure foci themselves. Thus a vicious cycle can result. Therefore, it is reasonable to consider using maintenance anticonvulsant therapy if multiple, generalized seizures have occurred over several days. One to 3 months is a reasonable period of anticonvulsant therapy, and it has been utilized successfully in many cases. At the end of this period the drug (phenobarbital) is slowly withdrawn (over 1 to 2 weeks). No evidence proves that an affected foal, effectively treated, has any greater chance of having seizures as an adult than any other foal.

3. **Nervous Coccidiosis**

Signalment. Calves and young adult cattle, particularly feedlot calves, are affected.

History. Associated with an outbreak of intestinal coccidiosis, up to 30% of affected calves may demonstrate neurologic signs. Minimal ataxia and tremor may occur, but most have seizures and many die. The disease often occurs in cold climates and during cold seasons.

Physical Examination. Evidence of intestinal coccidiosis usually is apparent.

Neurologic Examination. Ataxia, muscle tremor, blindness, and hyperexcitability may accompany intermittent or continuous seizures. Typical generalized seizures consist of an affected calf becoming recumbent with opisthotonus, tonic-clonic movement, medial strabismus, and snapping of the eyelids (Isler et al., 1987a), (Julian et al., 1976). Seizures may be precipitated by stress and handling.

Assessment. Many aspects of the pathophysiology of the nervous form of coccidiosis have been studied and discussed (Isler et al., 1987a), (Julian et al., 1976). Recently, a heat labile neurotoxin has been identified in the serum of affected calves, but not in the serum of calves with only intestinal signs of coccidiosis or in the serum of control calves (Isler et al., 1987b). Neurotoxicity was determined in experimental mice and neurotoxin activity was associated with a large molecule of over 300,000 MW (Isler et al., 1987c).

Consistently, hyperglycemia and low liver copper and iron stores, and hypochloremia during seizure activity are associated with the syndrome (Isler et al., 1987a). The significance of these findings and their relationship to the putative seizure-inducing toxin has not been determined.

Diagnosis. Microscopic examination of feces will confirm enteric coccidiosis.

Therapy. Sulfonamides, or other anticoccidial drugs, and fluid and electrolyte therapy for enteritis is indicated. Probably, excessive amounts of intravenous dextrose should be avoided. Placing affected calves in a warm, dry, dark, quiet environment (Isler et al., 1987a) and administering anticonvulsant drugs (extrapolated from Table 6–1) should assist in controlling convulsions. Whether or not therapy with copper and iron salts is beneficial is not known.

Prognosis. The prognosis is poor, with 70 to 100% mortality expected (Isler et al., 1987a), (Julian et al., 1976). Death usually occurs within the first 5 days of neurologic signs.

REFERENCES

Atkeson FW, Ibsen HL, Eldridge F. Inheritance of an epileptic type character in Brown Swiss cattle. J Hered 1944; *35*:45–48.

Chrisman CL. *Problems in Small Animal Neurology.* Philadelphia: Lea and Febiger, 1982. pp 173–183.

Davis LE. Important interactions of antibiotic drugs. J Am Vet Met Assoc 1979; *175*:729–730.

Duran SH, Ravis WR, Pedersoli WM, et al. Pharmacokinetics of phenobarbital in the horse. Am J Vet Res 1987; *48*:807–810.

Edwards AJ, Mount ME, Oehme FW. Buckeye toxicity in Angus calves. Bov Pract 1980; *1*:18–20.

Freeman JM, Tibbles J, Camfield C, et al. Benign epilepsy of childhood: a speculation and its ramifications. Pediatrics 1987; 79:864–868.

Gabel AA, Koestner A. The effects of intracarotid artery injection of drugs in domestic animals. J Am Vet Med Assoc 1963; *142*:1397–1403.

Gilbert FR, Wells GAH, Gunning RF. 3-nitro-4-hydroxphenylarsonic acid toxicity in pigs. Vet Rec 1981; *109*:158–160.

Glastonbury JRW, Walker RI, Kennedy DJ, et al. Dieldrin toxicity in housed Merino sheep. Aust Vet J 1987; *64*:145–148.

Harris WF. Metaldehyde poisoning in three horses. Mod Vet Pract 1975; *56*:336–337.

Isaksson A. Genuin epilepsi hos notkreatur. Skand Vet Tidskr 1943; *33*:1. In: Palmer AC. *Introduction to Animal Neurology.* 2nd Ed. Oxford: Blackwell Scientific Publications, 1976. p 167.

Isler CM, Bellamy JEC, Wobeser GA. Pathogenesis of neurological signs associated with bovine enteric coccidiosis: A prospective study and review. Can J Vet Res 1987a; *51*:261–270.

Isler CM, Bellamy JEC, Wobeser GA. Labile neurotoxin in serum of calves with "nervous" coccidiosis. Can J Vet Res 1987b; *51*:253–260.

Isler CM, Bellamy JEC, Wobeser GA. Characteristics of the labile neurotoxin associated with nervous coccidiosis. Can J Vet Res 1987c; *51*:271–276.

James LF, Hartley WJ, Van Kampen KR. Syndromes of *Astralagus* poisoning in livestock. J Am Vet Med Assoc 1981; *178*:146–150.

Julian RJ, Harrison KB, Richardson JA. Nervous signs in bovine coccidiosis. Mod Vet Pract 1976; *57*:711–718.

Kennedy S, Rice DA, Cush PF. Neuropathy of experimental 3-nitro-4-hydroxyphenylarsonic acid toxicosis in pigs. Vet Pathol 1986; *23*:454–461.

Kowalczyk DF, Beech J. Pharmacokinetics of phenytoin (diphenylhydantoin) in horses. J Vet Pharmacol Therap 1983; *6*:133–140.

Longbottom GM, Gordon ASM. Metaldehyde poisoning in a dairy herd. Vet Rec 1979; *104*:454–455.

Pauli JV, Allsop TF. Plasma and cerebrospinal fluid magnesium, calcium and potassium concentrations in dairy cows with hypomagesaemic tetany. NZ Vet J 1974; *22*:227–231.

Ravis WR, Duran SH, Pedersoli WM, et al. A pharmacokinetic study of phenobarbital in mature horses after oral dosing. J Vet Pharmacol Therap 1987; *10*:283–289.

Rice DA, Kennedy S, McMurray CH, et al. Experimental 3-nitro-4-hydroxyphenylarsonic acid toxicosis in pigs. Res Vet Sci 1985; *39*:47–51.

Seawright AA. *Animal Health in Australia,* Vol 2, *Chemical and Plant Poisons.* Canberra, Australia: Australian Government Publishing Service, 1982. pp 100–101.

Simmons JR, Scott WA. An outbreak of metaldehyde poisoning in sheep. Vet Rec 1974; *95*:211–212.

Spehar AM, Hill MR, Mayhew IG, et al. Preliminary study on the pharmacokinetics of phenobarbital in the neonatal foal. Equine Vet J 1984; *16*:368–371.

CHAPTER 7

Problem 3:
Visual Dysfunction

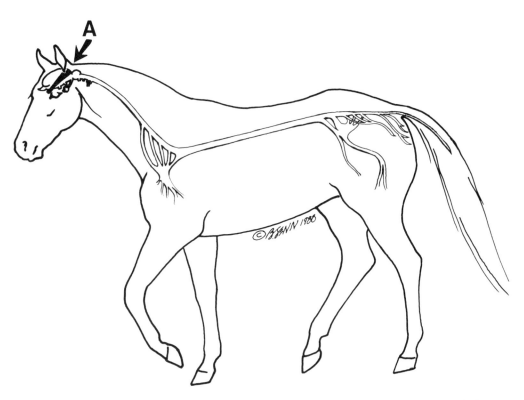

Location of lesions resulting in visual dysfunction: Eye, optic nerve, optic tract, lateral thalamus, optic radiation, and occipital cortex (A).

The visual and pupillary light pathways should be reviewed as well as the discussion on testing for vision in the neurologic examination section (Figs. 2–4 to 2–7).

Often animals with forebrain lesions are blind, with depressed menace responses in one or both eyes. A central blindness, or amaurosis, with pupillary reflexes intact, occurs in an eye contralateral to a thalamic or occipital lobe lesion. An optic nerve lesion results in suppressed direct and consensual pupillary light reflexes when light is shone in the ipsilateral eye; the lesion also causes a dilated ipsilateral pupil, as well as a depressed ipsilateral menace response (Fig. 7–1A and B). The postictal period (Problem 2) may be associated with temporary blindness, and neonates, although they can see, may have poor menace responses in the first weeks of life.

Degrees of blindness occur with many ocular diseases. The reader is referred to texts of ophthalmology such as Moore (1986) and Glaze (1987) for evaluation and treatment of eye disease in large animals.

Categories of Disease and Differential Diagnosis
*NOTE: Only diseases marked * are discussed in this section.*

    I. Congenital and Familial
        *1. Optic Nerve Hypoplasia
        *2. Night Blindness (Nyctalopia)
        3. Various Familial Cerebral Disorders (Problem 1)
        4. Benign Epilepsy of Foals (Problem 2)
    II. Physical
        *1. Head Trauma (Problem 4)
        2. Dehorning Injuries (Problem 1)
        3. Lightning Strike (Problem 2)
        4. Intracarotid Injection (Problem 2)
   III. Infectious, Inflammatory, Immune
        *1. Optic Neuritis
        2. Many Infectious Meningoencephalomyelitides (Problem 1)
        3. Guttural Pouch Mycosis (Problem 5F)
    IV. Metabolic
        *1. Anesthetic Hypoxia—Anoxia
        2. Other Metabolic Encephalopathies (Problem 1)
    V. Toxic
        *1. *Sypandra* sp
        2. Many Toxic Encephalopathies (Problem 1)
    VI. Nutritional
        *1. Vitamin A Deficiency (Problem 1)
        2. Thiamin Responsive Polioencephalomalacia (Problem 1)
        3. Vitamin E Deficiency—Mullberry Heart Disease (Problem 1)
   VII. Neoplastic
        *1. Retrobulbar Neoplasia
        2. Central Neoplasia (Tumors) (Problem 2)
  VIII. Idiopathic
        1. Neonatal Maladjustment Syndrome (Problem 1)
        2. Nervous Coccidiosis (Problem 1)

    I. Congenital and Familial
        1. Optic nerve hypoplasia.
            Degrees of blindness are evident in young animals, and hypoplasia of the optic nerves and neuroretinas are evident on ophthalmic examinations (Gelatt et al., 1969). Eyeball deviations and abnormal movements of the eyeballs and head can be expected.

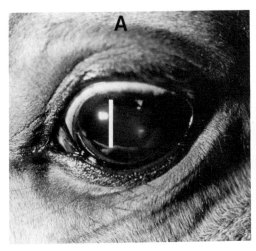
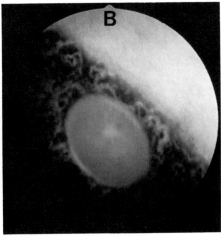

Figure 7–1. Head trauma. Four weeks ago this filly injured its head and was thought to be blind afterwards. It had slightly asymmetric, widely dilated pupils (as shown by white bar in A) and poor pupillary light reflexes. Initially there was a normal fundoscopic examination, but within 4 weeks postinjury optic atrophy, with attenuation of optic vasculature and peripapillary retinal degeneration, was evident (B).

2. **Night blindness (Nyctalopia)**

This disease involves the retina, but is included because the clinical syndrome is suggestive of partial central blindness or amaurosis.

In young, adult, Appaloosa horses the disease is seen as a progressive disability that affects performing in restricted light. It could, for example, cause stumbling at the end of a trail ride at dusk. Scotopic (rod) degeneration of the retina occurs. The disease is nonprogressive and probably is inherited (Witzel et al., 1977a and b). Severely affected foals and horses may show a dorsal or dorsomedial eye deviation (Problem 5B) when attempting to visually fix on an object (Rebhun et al., 1984).

Nyctalopia is one of the early signs of vitamin A deficiency in cattle and horses (see section VI.1 below).

II. Physical

1. **Head Trauma**

Syndrome. Following recovery from head trauma, some horses show visual impairment and develop optic and retinal degeneration. Peripapillary, then generalized retinal degeneration, along with optic nerve atrophy, will become apparent in the days or weeks following the traumatic event (Fig. 7–1). Both partial and asymmetric lesions occur. It can take 2 to 4 weeks for the optic atrophy and peripapillary retinal degeneration to become prominent by fundic examination.

Assessment. A compressive-type lesion occurs to the optic nerve(s) within the bony optic canal, or more frequently, where the nerve enters the canal about 1 to 1.5 in. behind the globe, just distal to the optic chiasm. Hemorrhage, neuronal fiber degeneration, and frank necrosis occur to a variable degree, followed by astrogliosis (Martin et al., 1986). Many reported cases of acquired optic degeneration and associated blindness in horses most likely represent this pathogenesis (Platt et al., 1983), (Glastonbury et al., 1985), (Gelatt, 1979). However, the direct effects of severe blood loss (Gelatt, 1979), (Platt, 1983) and of intracarotid injections (Helper et al., 1980) cannot be excluded totally from etiologic considerations.

Prognosis. If vision does not return within 7 days the prognosis is poor. The chances of recovery from vestibular damage caused by head trauma, if accompanied by this syndrome, are poor (Problem 6).

III. Infectious, Inflammatory, Immune

1. Optic neuritis.

Syndrome. This condition, which is unassociated with head injury, is presumed to occur in horses that develop acute blindness with dilated pupils and some evidence of papilledema.

Assessment. Nonsuppurative inflammation of the optic nerves may be seen histologically (Hieronymi, 1914). One case of granulomatous optic neuritis, possibly resulting from verminous migration, has been reported (Slatter et al., 1983). Suppurative optic neuritis occurred in a 9-year-old Quarterhorse mare as a consequence of bacterial endocarditis and *Actinobacillus equuli* septicemia (Hatfield et al., 1987). In other horses the cause is unknown, but possibly is an immune mediated process.

Treatment and Prognosis. Some affected horses have recovered with glucocorticosteroid therapy. If no response is seen in 1 week the outlook for return of vision is bad.

IV. Metabolic

1. Anesthetic hypoxia—anoxia

Syndrome. If an animal survives an episode of cardiac or respiratory failure under anesthesia (anesthetic accident) there may be residual signs of blindness with normal pupils, and degrees of depression and behavioral changes.

Assessment. Signs result from neuronal necrosis, particularly in the cerebral cortex, hippocampus, thalamus, caudal colliculi, and cerebellar Purkinje cells (Palmer et al., 1970). A similar pattern of involvement occurs in humans dying of hypoxic brain damage (Adams, 1975). The clinical course and histologic findings in a few severe cases of neonatal maladjustment syndrome (Problem 1) strongly resemble diffuse ischemic-hypoxia.

Therapy. In this disease DMSO therapy is probably indicated (1 g/kg, 10% in D5W, slowly IV). This is because there is a global ischemic-hypoxia with oxygen-derived free radicals causing tissue damage during reperfusion/reoxygenation (McCord, 1985); the treatment can be started at the time of reperfusion. Supportive care and anticonvulsant therapy as needed are indicated.

Outcome. The initial quality of survival can be assessed on recovery from anesthesia. Even with dense periods of semicoma, treatment should be continued for 2 to 4 days. Considering some remarkable long-term recoveries in other species, if the client can handle such a "dummy" animal it might be worth persisting with nursing care for several weeks to months before euthanasia is elected.

V. Toxic

1. *Sypandra* sp

Sheep and horses eating this grass-like plant in Western Australia can develop ataxia and weakness and may die. If they survive, permanent blindness may result because of optic nerve degeneration (Sulivan, 1985).

VI. Nutritional

1. Vitamin A deficiency

Clinical Syndrome. Experimental and naturally occurring vitamin A deficiency in calves and adult cattle can result in neurologic syndromes. In calves, signs include blindness, ill thrift, diarrhea, dermatitis, and pneumonia. In cattle, signs include blindness, convulsions, diarrhea, and generalized edema (Divers et al., 1986), (Booth et al., 1987). Night blindness, ill thrift, and seizures have occurred in young horses fed a vitamin A-deficient diet (Schryver et al., 1987), (Howell et al., 1941).

Blindness in calves is peripheral, with absent menace responses, absent pupillary light reflexes, and dilated pupils in severe cases. Blindness is apparent if the animal becomes confused when moving, is unable to negotiate its pen, or adopts a star-gazing attitude (Booth, 1987). Signs are more evident at night (Booth et al., 1987). Fundic examination reveals pale tapeta lucidum, papilledema, indistinct disk margins, and tortuous retinal vasculature (Booth et al., 1987), (Divers, et al., 1986).

Assessment. The syndrome is associated with papilledema and retinal and optic nerve degeneration. These changes are thought to be the result of decreased CSF absorption and increased intracranial pressure causing hydrocephalus and optic nerve compression (Booth et al., 1987). Deformed bones of the skull may be found in vitamin A deficient calves. Serum vitamin A concentrations are low (2 to 15 μg/dl).

Therapy. Affected animals should receive 440 IU vitamin A/kg parenterally.

Prognosis. Prominent blindness probably is not reversible, although signs of other organ involvement may regress rapidly with vitamin A supplementation (Booth et al., 1987).

VII. Neoplasia

1. Retrobulbar neoplasia

This is uncommon in cattle and rare in horses.

One of the sites of predilection for bovine multicentric lymphosarcoma is retrobulbar, when degrees of blindness and particularly exophthalmos occur (Rebhun, 1982).

Rarely do other retrobulbar tumors occur in all species and most result in orbital lesions and funduscopic abnormalities (Moore, 1986), (Glaze, 1987), (Bistner et al., 1983), (Eagle et al., 1978).

REFERENCES

Adams JH. Hypoxic brain damage. Br J Anaesth 1975; *47*:121–129.

Bistner S, Campbell RJ, Shaw D, et al. Neuroepithelial tumor of the optic nerve in a horse. Cornell Vet 1983; *73*:30–40.

Booth A, Reid M, Clark T. Hypovitaminosis A in feedlot cattle. J Am Vet Med Assoc 1987; *190*:1305–1308.

Divers TJ, Blackmon DM, Martin CL, et al. Blindness and convulsions associated with vitamin A deficiency in feedlot steers. J Am Vet Med Assoc 1986; *189*:1579–1582.

Eagle RC Jr., Font RL, Swerczek TW. Malignant medulloepithelioma of the optic nerve in a horse. Vet Pathol 1978; *15*:488–494.

Gelatt KN, Leipold HW, Coffman JR. Bilateral optic nerve hypoplasia in a colt. J Am Vet Med Assoc 1969; *155*:627–631.

Gelatt KN. Neuroretinopathy in horses. J Equine Med Surg 1979; *3*:91–96.

Glastonbury JRW, Gill PA, Day DG. Degenerative optic neuropathy in a horse. Aust Vet J 1985; *62*:243–244.

Glaze MB, consulting ed. Ocular diseases. In: *Current Therapy in Equine Medicine.* 2nd Ed. Robinson NE ed. Philadelphia: WB Saunders, 1987. pp 427–464.

Hatfield CE, Rebhun WC, Dietze AE, et al. Endocarditis and optic neuritis in a Quarterhorse mare. Comp Cont Ed Pract Vet 9187; *9*:451–454.

Helper LC, Lerner D. Unilateral retinopathy and blindness in a horse following intracarotid injection of phenylbutazone. Equine Pract 1980; *2*:33–35.

Hieronymi E, 1914. Cited in Platt et al. 1983.

Howell CE, Hart GH, Ittner MR. Vitamin A deficiency in horses. Am J Vet Res 1941; *2*:6074.

McCord JM. Oxygen-derived free radicals in postischemic tissue injury. N Engl J Med 1985; *312*:159–163.

Martin L, Kaswan R, Chapman W. Four cases of traumatic optic nerve blindness in the horse. Equine Vet J 1986; *18*:133–137.

Moore CP. Guest editor. Large Animal Ophthalmology. Vet Clin North Am [Large Anim Pract] 1984; *6*:433–703.

Moore CP, consulting ed. Diseases of the eye. In: *Current Veterinary Therapy: food animal practice.* 2nd Ed. Howard JL, ed. Philadelphia: WB Saunders, 1986. pp 819–847.

Palmer AC, Walker RG. The neuropathological effects of cardiac arrest in animals: a study of five cases. J Small Anim Pract 1980; *11*:779–790.

Platt H, Barnett KC, Barry DR, et al. Degenerative lesions of the optic nerve in Equidae. Equine Vet J 1983; Suppl *2*:91–97.

Rebhun WC. Orbital lymphosarcoma in cattle. J Am Vet Med Assoc 1982; *180*:149–152.

Rebhun WC. Traumatic optic neuropathy: how to prevent permanent blindness. Vet Med 1986; *81*:350–353.

Rebhun WC, Loew ER, Riis RC, et al. Clinical manifestations of night blindness in the Appaloosa horse. Comp Cont Ed Pract Vet 1984; *6*:S103–S106.

Schryver HF, Hintz HF. Vitamins. In: *Current Therapy in Equine Medicine.* 2nd Ed. Robinson NE, ed. Philadelphia: WB Saunders, 1987. pp 405-412.

Slatter DH, Huxtable CR. Retinal degeneration and granulomatous optic neuritis in a horse. Equine Vet J 1983; Suppl *2*:98–100.

Sulivan ND. The nervous system. In: *Pathology of Domestic Animals.* Jubb KVF, Kennedy PC, Palmer N (eds.). 3rd Ed., Vol 1, Orlando: Academic Press, 1985; Ch 3, p 265.

Witzel DA, Joyce JR, Smith SL. Electroretinography of congenital night blindness in an Appaloosa. J Equine Med Surg 1977; *1*:226–229.

Witzel DA, Riis, Rebhun WC, Hillman RB. Night blindness in the Appaloosa: Sibling occurrence. J Equine Med Surg 1977; *1*:383–386.

CHAPTER 8

Problem 4:
Coma and Altered States of Consciousness

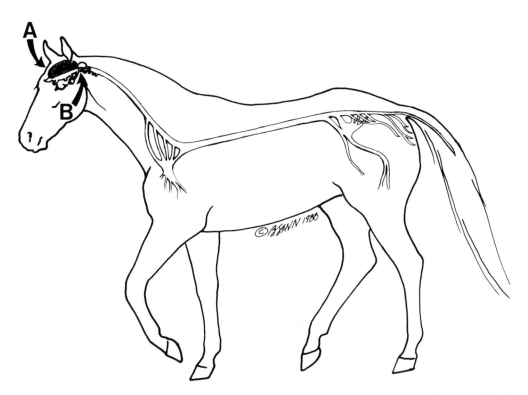

Location of lesions resulting in coma and altered states of consciousness: diffuse and focal forebrain and diencephalon (A) and recticular activating system in the brain stem (B).

Stages of depression, semicoma, and coma represent a progressive lack of awareness of the environment. An alert state is maintained through multiple sensory inputs to the ascending reticular activating system (ARAS) in the rostral brainstem and subsequently in the thalamus and cerebral cortex, where consciousness presumably is attained. Diffuse cerebral disease and severe lesions involving just the thalamus, internal capsule, or frontal regions can result in a severely depressed mental attitude, often expressed as "dummy syndrome."

Additional signs of behavioral disturbances (Problem 1), seizures (Problem 2) and visual disturbances (Problem 3) frequently accompany this condition. Coma can result from acute damage to these regions of the forebrain, but particularly from midbrain (ARAS) lesions. Almost all of the diffuse brain diseases discussed in Problems 1 and 2 can ultimately result in coma prior to death.

Severely depressed animals do not respond well or appropriately to noxious stimuli, such as loud noises and prodding with an instrument. Also, lesions involving the thalamus, internal capsule, or sensory parietal lobe of the cerebrum can be associated with decreased sensation on the contralateral side of the face, most prominent on the nasal septum. This exceeds degrees of non-responsiveness that can be expected from any associated depressed state.

Sleep is an active, complex phenomenon that involves many areas of the central nervous system. Rare sleep disorders do affect animals, and usually present as cataplexy. Episodes of partial or complete collapse into a flaccid and usually areflexic paralysis (from which the animal completely recovers) occur. The term narcolepsy (sleep attacks) often is used to describe this episodic phenomenon, which must be differentiated from cardiovascular syncope and particularly from seizures. Thus the differential diagnosis of sudden collapse involves more than morbid neurologic diseases and often it is regarded, rightly so, as a crisis by the client. Thus, a discussion of sudden collapse follows.

To witness a large animal suddenly collapse, or to be called urgently to evaluate a patient that has suffered one or more episodes of collapsing, can be confusing for the clinician and certainly distressing for the owner or manager. On most occasions the situation resolves quickly to one of sudden death, recovery with recumbency, a gait abnormality, another neurologic syndrome, recovery with or without evidence of a non-neurologic problem, or repetitive episodes of collapsing.

Poorly informed clients and children must be reminded of their own safety and should be advised to keep clear of a collapsing large animal until the veterinarian arrives. The client may be directed to stop any massive bleeding, or roll a heavy animal that might be cast. In the event that the animal arises, the client can guide it, if it is ambulatory, to soft ground, away from potentially harmful objects.

Upon arriving at the scene of a collapsed patient the "ABCs" of acute care must be attended to concurrently.

*A*irway. Determine that the patient has a patent airway and is breathing adequately. Oxygen or assisted ventilation may be necessary. Obstructing fluids or objects should be removed from the airway and 10 ml 50% ethanol can be given intratracheally if pulmonary edema is evident.

*B*leeding. Hemorrhage should be stopped by packing, suturing, and bandaging.

*C*irculation. Briefly evaluate cardiovascular function and institute cardiac resuscitation with thoracic massage and intravenous or intracardiac epinephrine (0.5 to 1.0 ml of 1:1000 in 10 ml H_2O for adult horse) if asystole or anaphylaxis is evident. Intravenous volume expansion with polyionic fluids, plasma, or blood is used as indicated and when available.

The presence of any fractures that may mean a hopeless prognosis (femur), that may be life-threatening (ribs), or that may require splinting (metacarpus) must be identified and appropriate measures should be taken.

A thrashing patient may require sedation or anticonvulsant therapy (also Problem 2). If shock or respiratory depression are not problems, and there is no evidence of seizure activity, then xylazine, detomidine, chloral hydrate, pentobarbitone or acetylpromazine can be instituted. Diazepam in 5 to 10 mg (foal) to 25 to 100 mg (horse) doses should be given IV to control seizures. A horse recumbent for any reason can become terribly violent in its frantic attempts to rise, and in response to pain, and it may be impossible to distinguish this behavior from true seizures. With the latter, the horse is in a state of unconsciousness and its attention cannot be attracted. Also, the jaw and facial muscles usually become spastic, the eyeballs move, opisthotonus tends to occur and sometimes urine and feces are voided.

Information as to the duration and repetition of the episodes of collapse, exposure to various environmental factors (heat, poisonous plants, injections, previous or prodromal illness, different feeds) and whether other herdmates have been affected, all should be noted.

A brief physical examination can then be undertaken. The general aim at this stage is to determine which basic category of acute collapse best fits the particular case. These general categories include: syncope, seizure, sleep disorders, coma, motor paralysis, and generalized and metabolic disorders. Some of the characteristics of each of these is given to assist in an accurate diagnosis.

Syncope. A small number of animals that experience one or more episodes of acute collapse are suspected of having syncope or a fainting condition. Usually, this is because of the presence of a cardiac arrhythmia or a cardiac murmur. Definitive cardiac disease is confirmed in a small proportion of these cases. Such documented disorders include atrial fibrillation, ruptured chordae tendineae, myocardial infarction, myocardial fibrosis, aortic endocarditis, and pericarditis.

With syncopal attacks, usually there is little or no premonitory warning of collapse; because of cerebral hypoxia, a temporary, quiet, comatosed state ensues. Some struggling may occur during recovery, before the patient regains its footing. Other overt signs of cardiac failure may become evident.

Seizures. A seizure, convulsion, or fit is the physical expression of bizarre electrical neuronal discharges in all or part of the cerebrum. Often a preictal aura of a few seconds to minutes occurs; then the ictus or seizure lasts a few seconds to minutes; this is followed by a postictal phase lasting several minutes to days. The aura may cause the animal to be distracted from its environment, to have a blank expression, and to occasionally become restless. If the seizure becomes generalized, the patient usually becomes recumbent and lies rigid for a while before paddling or thrashing for several seconds to minutes. With status epilepticus this phase is repeated continually and is fatal unless chemical, anticonvulsant-restraint is used. A postictal animal usually regains its footing relatively easily then may pace, act blind, constantly drink or eat, and may not recognize its handler. Depending on the underlying cause, other neurologic signs may be evident.

Anticonvulsant therapy (also Problem 2) may be required if more than one generalized seizure has occurred.

Sleep Disorders. Narcolepsy is characterized by uncontrolled episodes of sleep. Unlike seizures and many metabolic disorders, such as hyperkalemia, there are no warning signs. With multiple attacks the patient may appear sleepy between episodes. Adult animals do not always drop to the ground and may catch themselves after the head suddenly lowers and the thoracic limb stay apparatus begins to fail. Most often prominent cataplexy, which entails sudden loss of all voluntary motor effort occurs and the animal collapses to the ground. Petting about the head and neck, hosing down after exercise, beginning to eat or drink, and resting quietly in a barn at night, all seem to have been associated or precipitating factors with various cases. Sleep attacks do not usually occur while an animal is exercising vigorously.

Coma. Coma is a state of recumbency with unconsciousness and total unresponsiveness. It is primarily associated with profound changes in the forebrain or midbrain. Head trauma, birth asphyxia, bacterial meningoencephalitis, thiamin-responsive polioencephalomalacia, parasitic infarction/migration, spontaneous hemorrhage, moldy corn intoxication, liver disease, intracarotid injections, and many poisons (Problem 1) are some of the more frequent causes of acute coma. Consequently, it is important to determine if the animal has a history or evidence of trauma or other premonitory neurologic signs. Immediately following head trauma a temporary period of coma often ensues. Thus, the animal should not be euthanized during the first 24 hours; at this time appropriate diagnostic and therapeutic approaches should be instituted.

Motor Paralysis. Collapse without loss of consciousness can be caused by loss of motor function. Motor pathways may be interrupted at the level of the brainstem, vestibular apparatus, spinal cord, peripheral nerve, neuromuscular junction, or muscle. A neurologic examination is needed to identify where the lesion(s) is (are). Trauma is the most frequently occurring mechanism at the first three of these sites (this Problem and Problem 10). Acute collapse without loss of consciousness is also caused by botulism (including the shaker-foal syndrome), postanesthetic myasthenic syndrome, postanesthetic neuromyopathy, exercise-associated rhabdomyolysis, and hyperkalemic periodic paralysis (Problem 10).

Generalized and Metabolic Disorders. This category of acute collapse includes miscellaneous disorders such as hyperthermia, shock, hypoglycemia, hypocalcemia, hyperkalemia, hypokalemia, endotoxemia, anaphylaxis, anaphylactoid reaction, acute exotoxemia, and snake envenomation. Usually, several systems are found to be abnormal after a physical examination, and subsequent, appropriate system examinations and therapy can be undertaken.

Categories of Disease and Differential Diagnosis
*NOTE: Only diseases marked * are discussed in this section.*

    I. Congenital and Familial
        *1. Narcolepsy and Cataplexy
        2. Hydrocephalus, Hydranencephaly (Problem 1)
        3. Lysosomal Storage Diseases (Problem 1)
        4. Citrullinemia (Problem 1)
        5. Miscellaneous Forebrain Malformations

II. Physical
   *1. Head Trauma
   *2. Heat Stroke
    3. Dehorning Injuries (Problem 1)
    4. Lightning Strike (Problem 2)
    5. Intracarotid Injection (Problem 2)
III. Infectious, Inflammatory, Immune
    1. All Listings, Problem 1
IV. Metabolic
   *1. Shock
    2. All Listings, Problem 1
 V. Toxic
    1. All Listings, Problem 1
VI. Nutritional
    1. All Listings, Problem 1
VII. Idiopathic
    1. Neonatal Maladjustment Syndrome (Problem 1)
    2. Grove Poisoning (Problem 2)
    3. Nervous Coccidiosis (Problem 2)

I. Congenital and Familial
   1. Narcolepsy and Cataplexy

Signalment. Sleep attacks (narcolepsy), usually accompanied by profound loss of muscle tone (cataplexy), rarely occur in large animals (Fig. 8–1). It has been reported in Suffolk foals, Shetland and Welsh ponies, a miniature horse, crossbred ponies, thoroughbreds, a Quarterhorse, and a Morgan horse (Sweeney et al., 1987), (Dreifuss et al., 1984), (Sweeney et al., 1983), (Sheather, 1924), (Palmer, et al., 1980), and in a Guernsey and a Brahman bull (Palmer et al., 1980), (Strain et al., 1984). Possibly, it is familial in Shetland pony foals and Suffolk horses. Also we have seen it in newborn thoroughbred, Appaloosa and miniature foals (Fig. 8–1D), and in adult thoroughbred and standardbred horses.

Neurologic Examination. Between attacks there are no neurologic abnormalities (Fig. 8–1A). An attack may progress from buckling at the knees without falling (Fig. 8–1B), to sudden and total collapse and areflexia, usually with maintenance of some eye and facial responses and normal cardiorespiratory function (Fig. 8–1C,D). The clinical diagnosis of narcolepsy with cataplexy is best substantiated by observing rapid eye movements and by demonstrating the absence of spinal reflexes during repeated episodes of inappropriate recumbency (Fig. 8–1D). The animal can be aroused from this state with varying degrees of difficulty and can regain its footing quietly.

Assessment. Deep, rapid-eye-movement sleep, with its associated atonic, areflexic state, occurs at inappropriate times with no morphologic lesion to account for this sleep dysrhythmia. A bio-

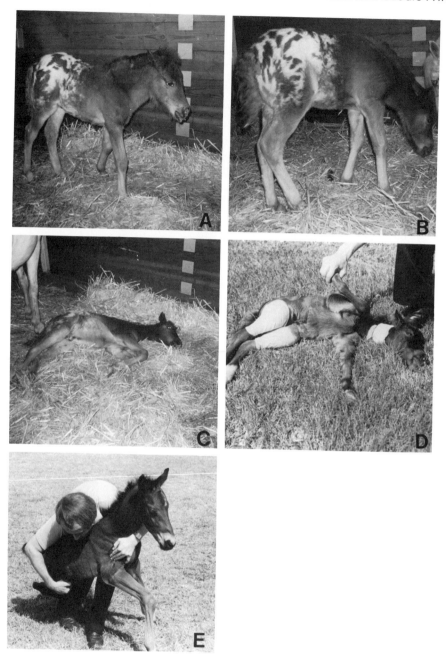

Figure 8–1. Narcolepsy and cataplexy. The syndrome of collapse may occur spontaneously or with a stimulus such as walking or manipulation. This affected Shetland × Appaloosa foal is shown alert (A), beginning to buckle on its limbs with head lowered (B), and totally collapsed (C). The syndrome persisted in this foal. Another American Miniature foal is shown in a state of cataplexy with no spinal reflexes present (D), only slight facial muscle movements, and rapid eye movements. This foal had undergone bilateral stifle surgery but grew out of these "sleep attacks." This syndrome of temporary narcolepsy may be a persistence of the cataplectic state that can be induced in newborn foals by applying firm restraint to a large part of the foal's body (E).

chemical defect is probably operative in the brainstem, sleep-wake centers.

Outcome. Some of these syndromes appear to resolve and others persist. A few newborn thoroughbred and miniature foals have temporarily shown prominent, repeated narcoleptic and cataplectic attacks, but they recover fully (Fig. 8–1D). These episodes are similar to the cateplectic state that can be induced in most newborn foals by tight manual restraint applied on a large surface area of the foal's body (Fig. 8–1E). It has been suggested that this phenomenon is operative in utero to prevent violent movements from occurring, particularly during birth (Mayhew, 1988). Aged horses have had relentless persistence of the syndrome to the point of severe knee and face trauma. In Shetland and Suffolk foals (fainting foals) the disease persists (Dreifuss et al., 1984), (Sheather, 1924). In young (1 to 3-year-old), light-bred horses one or several episodes may occur, occasionally triggered by specific stimuli (e.g., hosing down), with no permanent consequences.

Diagnosis. Attacks may be induced with 0.05 to 0.1 mg/kg physostigmine, given slowly IV, at least to adult animals (Sweeney et al., 1983), (Strain et al., 1984). Caution is required in this provocative test, as the drug can cause colic and other cholinergic responses. The clinical syndrome, however, is distinctive once epilepsy and cardiorespiratory causes of collapse have been excluded from the diagnosis.

Therapy. Doses of 20 to 60 mg atropine IV, and 250 mg IV, to 750 mg orally of imipramine have resolved signs for many hours in adult horses (Sweeney et al., 1983); 0.5 mg/kg imipramine IV probably prevented attacks in one Brahman bull for several hours (Strain et al., 1984).

II. Physical

1. Head Trauma

History. Cranial injury occurs in horses of all ages and commonly results from direct kicks by other horses, from running into solid objects, and from rearing up and falling over backwards, thereby striking the poll. The neurologic signs resulting from brain trauma depend on the site and degree of concussion, contusion, laceration, and hemorrhage. Brain trauma in food-producing animals is far less common than in horses, partly because of their temperaments, the relatively slower speeds they attain, and the size and strength of their calvaria. For this reason most of the following remarks pertain to the horse.

Assessment. Closed head injuries (i.e., no skull fractures) often result in brainstem hemorrhages and in subarachnoid bleeding. With trauma to the caudal part of the head hemorrhage involving the medulla oblongata occurs, and frequently the occipital and temporal bones fracture. True subdural hematomas, which occur frequently in man, are not common in large animals. However, large hematomas may form in the cerebral hemispheres, usually in conjunction with fractures of the frontal bones; such hematomas do not necessarily form at the site of impact.

Injury to the frontal area results in skull fractures, which often are compound, and direct cerebral laceration and hemorrhage (Fig. 8–2). Skull fractures resulting from injury to the occipital region usually are through the occipital, sphenoid, and temporal bones, particularly their basillar regions (Fig. 8–3). Hemorrhage from the venous sinuses often occurs around the medulla and often into the inner and middle ear cavities (Fig. 8–4).

With severe brain injury the so-called brain-heart syndrome can result in cardiac arrhythmias, elevated serum activities of heart specific enzymes (BB-CPK, HBD*), myocardial necrosis, and sudden death due to heart failure (King, 1982). This syndrome can occur with other profound intracranial disorders, such as fulminant Eastern equine encephalitis (EEE) (see Problem 1).

Syndromes. Following head injuries patients often have degrees of depression and dementia. Often, horses develop optic nerve and retinal damage that usually is the result of shearing forces of the bony optic canals on the optic nerves (Problem 3) (Martin et al., 1986).

With prominent cerebral injury there is a period of coma from which the horse usually recovers in minutes to hours. Then depression, wandering in circles (toward the damaged cerebral hemisphere), and occasionally seizures occur (Fig. 8–5A). Characteristically the horse is blind and has decreased facial sensation on the side opposite the lesion. If the cerebrum swells it directly compresses the thalamus. Such cerebral swelling, which may be asymmetric, may result in the occipital lobe(s) herniating caudally under the tentorium cerebelli to press on the midbrain. This in turn compresses the oculomotor nerves (CNIII) ventral to the midbrain (Figs.

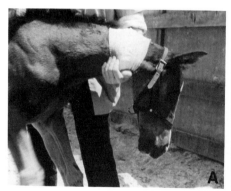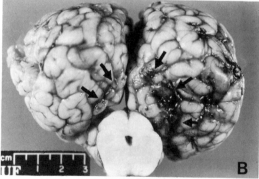

Figure 8–2. Cerebral trauma. This foal suffered a presumed episode of head injury and presented in a severely depressed state (A). Asymmetric pupillary dilatation and progressive semicoma ensued. Aggressive, medical, antiedema therapy (dexamethasone and DMSO) was utilized and the signs began to resolve. Unfortunately the foal died of fulminant enterocolitis. The caudal surfaces of its occipital lobes and midbrain are seen in B. Mild, partly resolved, occipital lobe herniations are evident (arrows), with mild midbrain compression on the right.

———————————

*BB-isomer of creatine phosphokinase = BB-CPK. Hydroxybutyrate dehydrogenase = HBD

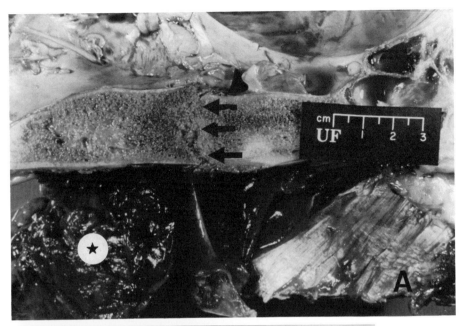

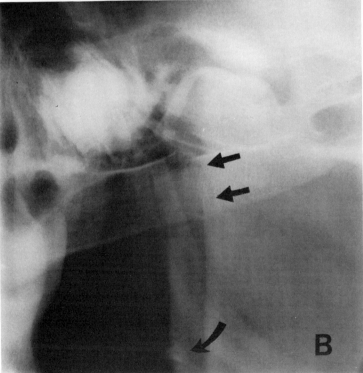

Figure 8–3. Basillar skull fracture. With a blow to the poll, as occurs when a horse flips over backward, fractures of the basillar bones frequently occur. A close-up view of the basillar bones (A) and a radiograph of the area (B) are shown; the horse's nose being to the right in each case. Such a fracture (arrows) frequently occurs between the basioccipital and basisphenoid bones (A). These fractures (arrows), when not displaced, can be difficult to document on radiographs of the head (B). Sometimes the rectus capitis ventralis muscle can tear from its insertion on the basillar bones (star). This is suggested from radiographs (B) of the area, which indicate that a piece of bone (curved arrow) has been avulsed and distracted away from the basillar bones. Such a complication might add to the difficulty a horse has in maneuvering its head and in getting up.

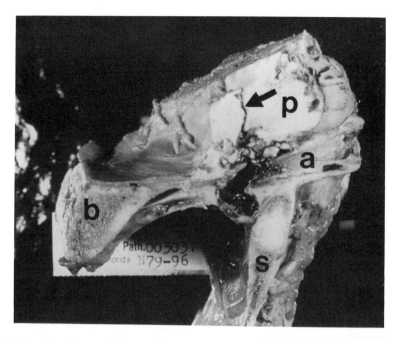

Figure 8–4. Fractured temporal bone. Also with injury to the poll, fractures of the temporal bones frequently occur. A transverse section of the caudal left part of this region of a horse's cranium is seen from a cranial view. The basioccipital bone is to the left (b), the petrous temporal bone (p) with fracture line visible (arrow) is dorsal, and the stylohyoid bone (s) is ventral. A blood clot fills the medial part of the external auditory canal (a). These lesions most often result in signs of peripheral vestibular disease and in facial paralysis.

5–6; 5–9; 8–2). These movements of brain tissue result in deepening depression, asymmetric pupils, dilation of the pupil with depressed pupillary light reflex on the same side as the lesion (usually), and eye deviations and vestibular signs (sometimes). Affected animals have marked ataxia and weakness that may progress to recumbency.

With midbrain hemorrhage usually a period of coma ensues, followed by marked depression, and an abnormal gait or tetraplegia. Usually there is no blindness or menace deficit, but asymmetric pupils with decreased pupillary light reflexes do occur. The pupils may be smaller than normal, and pupillary size often fluctuates. Progression to bilateral pupillary dilation and coma warrants a grave prognosis. This syndrome does not occur frequently.

Hemorrhage into the middle and inner ear cavities (Fig. 8–4) results in facial (also Problem 5E) and vestibular nerve (also Problem 6) signs, respectively. This consists of facial paralysis on the same side as the lesion, a head tilt toward the side of the lesion, and horizontal or rotary nystagmus with the fast phase away from the side of the lesion. If hemorrhage occurs around or in the medulla oblongata there are additional central signs—such as depression, ataxia, and weakness—with additional vestibular and other cranial nerve signs.

Diagnosis. Many times there is direct or circumstantial evidence

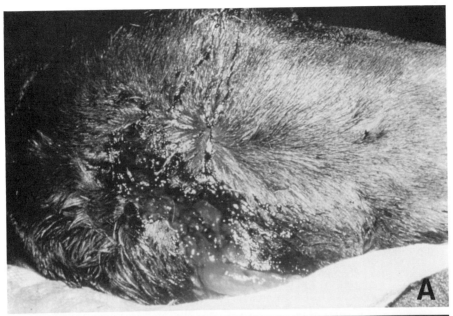

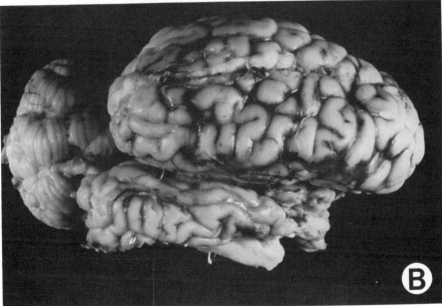

Figure 8–5. Head trauma. A suckling thoroughbred foal suffered head trauma with a depressed, comminuted, compound fracture of the right frontal bone. The foal was comatose. Its forehead is viewed with the foal lying on its right side with its nostrils to the right (A). Because of deteriorating neurologic status the area was surgically explored (Dr. Ted Stashak). A large volume of lacerated right cerebral hemisphere was removed along with bone fragments and blood. Following an uneventful recovery, the foal grew to be a normal looking horse in training. Some facial deformity and a depressed menace response in the left eye were the only permanent abnormalities. For other reasons the horse was euthanized and the remaining "brain," with little right cerebrum remaining, is viewed from its dorsal surface (B).

that head injury has occurred. Sometimes the clinician has to perform CSF collection to help confirm a diagnosis of occult trauma in large animals. This must be done with considerable caution because of the risk of suddenly lowering CSF pressure at the foramen magnum and precipitating herniation of brain tissue caudally as a consequence of brain swelling or hematoma formation. Collection of CSF from the cisterna magna must not be undertaken when signs of brain herniations, such as dilated pupils, are evident. Lumbosacral CSF collection is safer than atlanto-occipital collection under these circumstances, but in the immediate post-trauma phase a sample obtained from the former site may not reflect a change in intracranial CSF.

A decision should be made as to the need for skull radiographs. These should be obtained in cases with severe or progressive neurologic signs, in cases with blood discharge from the ears or nostrils, and in cases with lacerations and fractures of the forehead (Figs. 8–3, 8–4, and 8–5).

Therapy. The immediate care of head injury patients progresses from attending to preservation of a patent airway, stopping bleeding, and then treating shock. If no other major damage needs to be evaluated, such as fractured long bones, fractured ribs, and ruptured lungs, then therapy for CNS injury should be instituted. Sedation of a delirious, thrashing patient is best done with low doses of glyceryl guaiacolate, chloral hydrate, pentobarbitone, or acetylpromazine. Xylazine and detomidine should be used cautiously because they cause transient hypertension, which may exacerbate CNS hemorrhage, and then respiratory depression.

If seizures are evident, diazepam at 5 mg (foal) to 25 to 100 mg (horse) doses, repeated as necessary, is useful. Intractable seizures may necessitate anesthesia with glyceryl guaiacolate and thiamylal sodium, chloral hydrate (adult), or pentobarbitone 5 to 10 mg/kg (foal).

All large animals with substantial neurologic signs following cranial trauma probably should receive glucocorticosteroids; however, the risk of laminitis in adult horses warrants concern. A dose of 0.1 to 0.2 mg/kg dexamethasone probably is adequate to decrease elevated intracranial pressure and decrease CNS edema. This dose can be repeated every 4 to 6 hours, for 1 to 4 days. In spite of the continued use of glucocorticosteroids in patients suffering from brain injury, little proof exists that their use is necessarily beneficial. Indeed some clinical evidence shows dexamethasone at either high (1.3 mg/kg, daily) or low (0.22 mg/kg, daily) doses has no significant effect on the morbidity or mortality following severe head injury (Cooper et al., 1979). Perhaps a rational approach is to begin glucocorticoid therapy but discontinue in 2 to 3 days if there is no evidence that the patient is benefiting from its use (Saul et al., 1981).

If a horse is in a coma or semicoma and recumbent then intravenous hyperosmolar fluids probably are indicated. The best of these appears to be 20% mannitol given IV at 0.25 to 1.0 g/kg over 20 minutes. This also may be repeated every 6 to 12 hours for 24 hours if there is neurologic improvement following its use. One g/kg, 10% DMSO in 0.9% saline or D5W, slowly IV, repeated 1 to 6 times in 72 hours, appears to be helpful. This drug is not licensed for use in animals by this route of administration.

Renal diuretics, such as furosemide, probably are not as effective as glucocorticosteroids and mannitol in the therapy of swollen CNS tissue and are not recommended in the therapy of brain injured patients (Gaab et al., 1979). Prostaglandin synthetase inhibitors (phenylbutazone and flunixin) symptomatically appear to be useful in alleviating depression believed to be the result of pain in these patients. Because they are powerful antiedema and anti-inflammatory agents in horses, their use is recommended provided the toxic effects of gastrointestinal ulceration and renal disease are considered, especially in dehydrated patients.

Many large animal neurologists are conservative with this type of medical management. Complications of recumbency and drug therapy, including laminitis, necrotic cystitis, decubital sores, gastroduodenal ulceration, nephrosis and superinfections, frequently are lethal. Thus, one should be reluctant to use large, repeated doses of glucocorticoids, furosemide, DMSO, and mannitol unless the situation is critical.

Surgical decompressive craniotomy is indicated when bone fragments penetrate the brain from an open skull fracture and also in horses that clinically deteriorate or fail to respond to medical management. Such deterioration, associated with hematoma formation and brain edema, progresses until the animal is in a comatosed state with dilated, unresponsive pupils. These signs are related to caudal cerebral (occipital) herniation under the tentorium cerebelli causing compression of the midbrain (Fig. 8–2). The procedures for these surgical approaches are given in textbooks on large animal surgery (Stashak et al., 1984).

Prognosis. Some amazing recoveries occur following brain trauma, especially in horses with cerebral damage (Fig. 8–5). Repeated evaluations, with documentation of signs, intensive fluid, nutrient, metabolic and nursing support, judicious medical therapy, and time, are the basis of successful management of these cases.

   2. Heat Stroke (See Shock, IV.1)
IV. Metabolic
   1. Shock (including Heat Stroke)
      Cardiocirculatory collapse and diffuse organ dysfunction frequently is associated with degrees of depression and finally coma. Such complications may accompany the systemic component of neurologic disorders, such as many encephalitides, neurotoxicities and metabolic disturbances with neurologic signs. Also, profound comatosed states may occur in the terminal stages of shock; these are associated with disseminated intravascular coagulation, septicemia, blood loss, gastrointestinal crises, fulminant liver and renal disease, and heat stress.

      In all cases, cardiovascular support, including maintenance of adequate circulating blood volume and maintenance of a physiologic body temperature, as well as therapy aimed at the primary process, must be undertaken. Texts on general medicine should be consulted.

REFERENCES

Cooper PR, Moody S, Clark WK, et al. Dexamethasone and severe head injury. A prospective double-blind study. J Neurosurg 1979; *51*:307–316.

Dreifuss FE, Flynn DV. Narcolepsy in a horse. J Am Vet Med Assoc 1984; *184*:131–132 (Letter).

Gaab M, Knoblich OE, Schupp J, et al. Effect of furosemide (Lasix) on acute severe experimental cerebral edema. J Neurol 1979; *220*:185–197.

King JM, Roth L, Haschek WM. Myocardial necrosis secondary to neural lesions in domestic animals. J Am Vet Med Assoc 1982; *180*:144–148.

Martin L, Kaswan R, Chapman W. Four cases of traumatic optic nerve blindness in the horse. Equine Vet J 1986; *18*:133–137.

Mayhew IG. Neurological and neuropathological observations on the equine neonate. Equine Vet J 1988; Suppl *5*:28–33.

Palmer AC, Smith GF, Turner SJ. Cataplexy in a Guernsey bull. Vet Rec 1980; 421 (Letter).

Saul TG, Ducker TB, Salcman M, et al. Steroids in severe head injury. A prospective randomized clinical trial. J Neurosurg 1981; *54*:596–600.

Sheather AL. Fainting in foals. J Comp Path Ther 1924 ; *37*:106–113.

Stashak TS, Mayhew IG. The Nervous System: In: *The Practice of Large Animal Surgery,* Jennings PB. Philadelphia: WB Saunders, 1984. Ch. 17, p 983–1008.

Stick JA, Wilson T, Kunze D. Basilar skull fractures in three horses. J Am Vet Med Assoc 1980; *176*:228–231.

Strain GM, Olcott BM, Archer RM, et al. Narcolepsy in a Brahman bull. J Am Vet Med Assoc 1984; *185*:538–542.

Sweeney CR, Hendricks JC, Beech J, et al. Narcolepsy in a horse. J Am Vet Med Assoc 1983; *183*:126–128.

Sweeney CR, Hanson TO. Narcolepsy and epilepsy. In: *Current Therapy in Equine Medicine—2.* Robinson NE, ed. Philadelphia: WB Saunders, 1987. pp 349–353.

CHAPTER 9

Problem 5:
Cranial Nerve [III–VII, IX, X, XII] Dysfunction and Horner's Syndrome

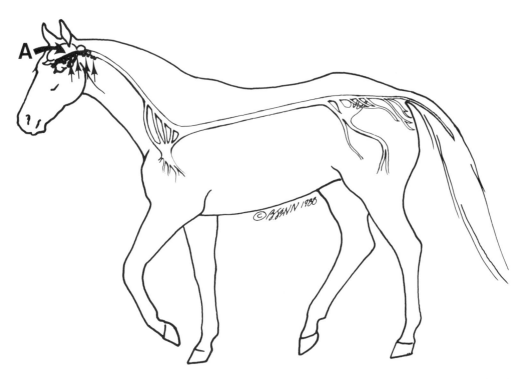

Location of lesions resulting in cranial nerve (III–VII, IX, X, XII) dysfunction: diffuse and focal brain stem (A) and peripheral cranial nerves (small arrows).

Examination for cranial nerve (CN) dysfunction is described in the examination section (Ch 2) and should be consulted. Lesions can involve specific single or multiple peripheral cranial nerves resulting in one or more of the problems discussed below. Often the central nuclei of these nerves are affected when other signs of brain disease usually are present. Additional signs include combinations of degrees of depression (also Problem 4), vestibular dysfunction (Problem 6), ataxia and weakness (also Problem 10), and sometimes cerebellar dysfunction (Problem 7). Thus, the identification of signs of specific cranial nerve dysfunction greatly assists in localizing signs that result from the diseases that can cause focal, multifocal, and diffuse involvement of the brainstem. Therefore, the differential diagnoses of syndromes discussed herein include most of the diffuse, focal, and multifocal diseases listed in the Problems covering cerebral and vestibular syndromes (Problems 1, 2, 3, 4, 6).

Specific syndromes involving olfaction (CNI) are not described. Problems affecting vision are covered in the examination section (Ch 2) and in Problem 3. Cranial nerve VIII is discussed in the section on vestibular disorders (Problem 6) and deafness (Problem 7). Accessory nerve (XI) neurectomy in the horse produces little in the way of a clinical syndrome. This section discusses problems arising from lesions affecting cranial nerves III–VII, IX, X, and XII and their central nuclei and pathways in the brainstem from the midbrain to the caudal medulla oblongata and the sympathetic supply to the head. These problems are:

    5A: Miosis, Mydriasis, Anisocoria, and Horner's Syndrome
    5B: Strabismus
    5C: Dropped Jaw and Muscle Atrophy of the Head
    5D: Decreased or Increased Facial Sensation
    5E: Facial Paralysis
    5F: Dysphagia
    5G: Megaesophagus
    5H: Laryngeal Paralysis and Roaring
    5I: Tongue Paralysis

Problem 5A:

Miosis, Mydriasis, Anisocoria, and Horner's Syndrome (CNIII, Ocular Sympathetic Supply)

Degrees of miosis (constricted pupil), mydriasis (dilated pupil), and anisocoria (asymmetric pupils) occur in many ocular diseases, often accompanied by degrees of visual impairment. Texts discussing the evaluation and treatment of eye problems in large animals should be consulted for these diseases (Moore, 1986), (Glaze, 1987).

The pupillary constriction (CNIII) and dilation (ocular sympathetic) pathways have been reviewed (Figs. 2–5 and 2–6).

Large animal patients infrequently are presented because of these problems alone. However, finding these on a neurologic examination helps to localize the lesion.

Many asymmetric infectious, traumatic, and vascular brain diseases discussed under other problems can result in midbrain oculomotor involvement and anisocoria. A dilated pupil (mydriasis), normal vision and usually no eye deviation, is seen with parasympathetic (CNIII) involvement in large animals. When this is found with no other neurologic abnormalities, particularly in a horse, the possibility of previous atropine therapy must be considered.

The constricted pupil (miosis) seen in Horner's Syndrome is not dramatic in large animals. Horner's Syndrome in horses consists of miosis, enophthalmos, and protruding nictitating membrane as in other species (Fig. 9–1). In addition, hyperemic mucous membranes of the head, hyperthermia of the face, and sweating of the face and neck to C_2 may be evident. These latter findings are caused by the interruption of sympathetic fibers to the blood vessels and sweat glands of the head (Smith et al., 1977). If the sympathetic fibers are affected at the level of, or distal to, the cranial cervical ganglion in the wall of the guttural pouch, the sweating projects only to the level of about the atlas.

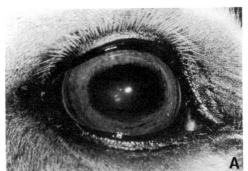
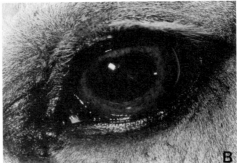
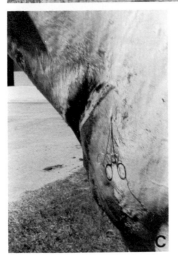

Figure 9–1. Signs of Horner's syndrome include ptosis, miosis and slight protrusion of the nictitating membrane, seen in the left eye (B) of this horse compared with the normal right eye (A). The cause of this Horner's syndrome was a deep, caudal cervical wire cut (C) that injured the left cervical sympathetic trunk. Also, branches of caudal, segmental cervical nerves were damaged, as evidenced by the hemostat indicating analgesia caudal to the wound.

Preganglionic lesions caudal (proximal) to this level result in sweating further down the neck to about the level of C_2 to C_3 (Usenik, 1957) (Fig. 9–2).

Horner's syndrome in cattle includes eye signs, with dilated vessels on the pinnae, warm face and ears, and an *absence* of droplets of "sweat" forming in the muzzle (Smith, 1977), (Rebhun, 1979), (Guard, 1984) (Fig. 9–3). Eye signs in Horner's syndrome are not prominent in other large animal species (Smith et al., 1977). It may be reasonable to expect ectoparasites, such as ticks, to be attracted to skin with altered temperature (Samuel et al., 1987).

The cranial cervical ganglion is beneath C_1, in the wall of the guttural pouch in horses, and can be involved in guttural pouch lesions. Third order sympathetic neuronal fibers may not pass through the petrosal bone as in small animal species. Thus, Horner's syndrome usually is not recognized with otitis media in large animals or with petrosal bone fractures.

In the horse, a first order sympathetic neuron lesion in the descending, cervical spinal cord, tectotegmentospinal tract, results in sweating on the whole side of the body as well as Horner's Syndrome (Mayhew, 1980). This is discussed further below (II.1). Finally, many systemic toxins, such as those mediated by atropine-like alkaloids, and those acting with anticholinesterase activity, cause degrees of mydriasis and miosis, respectively.

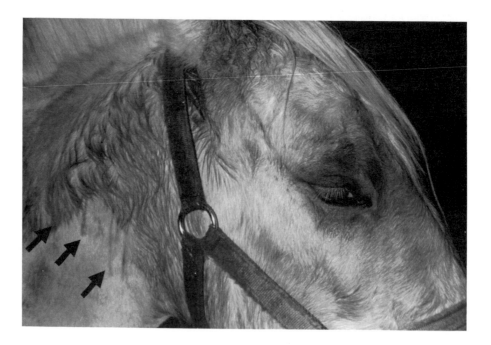

Figure 9–2. Horner's syndrome in the horse includes eye signs (such as ptosis as shown); in addition there usually is sweating on the skin of the face and cranial neck. With central lesions and preganglionic cervical lesions (shown), sweating occurs down to the level of C_{2-3} (arrows). Postganglionic sympathetic lesions result in sweating cranial to about C_1.

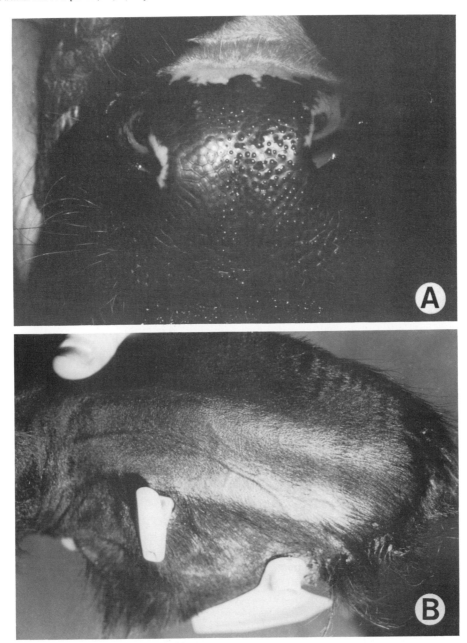

Figure 9–3. Horner's syndrome in cattle includes the ophthalmic signs described, as well as a *lack* of sweat production on the affected (right) side of this cow's muzzle (A), and a prominence of cranial vasculature, which are particularly evident on the ear (B).

Categories of Disease and Differential Diagnosis
NOTE: Only those diseases marked * are discussed in this section.

I. Physical
   *1. Neck Trauma (also Problem 10)
   2. Head Trauma (Problem 4)
II. Infectious, Inflammatory, Immune
   *1. Equine Protozoal Myeloencephalitis (also Problem 10)
   2. Other Brainstem and Cervical Spinal Cord Diseases (Problems 1, 10)
   3. Guttural Pouch Mycosis and Empyema (Problem 5F)
   4. Basillar Empyema/Pituitary Abscess (Problems 5D, 6)
   5. Listeriosis (Problem 6)
III. *Neoplastic

───────────

I. Physical
   1. Neck Trauma (also Problem 10)
   Neck trauma occurs frequently, particularly in horses (Fig. 9–1C). Not often does the cervical sympathetic trunk, traveling with the vagus nerve adjacent to the carotid artery, become damaged and result in Horner's Syndrome (Mayhew, 1980).
   Horner's syndrome occurs during attempts at intravascular (jugular and carotid) placement of needles and catheters. Resulting carotid hematoma formation, as well as extravascular deposition of drugs such as xylazine, both can result in (usually temporary) Horner's syndrome, which is most often seen in the horse (Sweeney et al., 1984).
   Surgical trauma to the ventral neck can cause Horner's syndrome. Usually this occurs during guttural pouch exploration, cervical myectomies, and procedures involving the larynx, trachea, and esophagus.
II. Infectious, Inflammatory, Immune
   1. Equine Protozoal Myeloencephalitis (also Problem 11)
   Although equine protozoal myeloencephalitis (EPM) is discussed fully in Problem 11, it is one of the few brainstem and spinal cord diseases that causes Horner's syndrome in the horse. In each case signs of asymmetric gait abnormalities, and signs of cranial nerve involvement in one case, were evident, along with hyperhidrosis on the entire side of the body ipsilateral to the lesion (Mayhew, 1980). This remarkable syndrome results from damage to the tectotegmentospinal tract descending through the brainstem and cervical spinal cord. This tract contains first order upper motor neurons to the sympathetic second order neurons in the thoracolumbar spinal cord. These in turn are the origin of the peripheral sympathetic fibers innervating (sweat) glands and blood vessels on one entire side of the body. Thus, damage to this tract which only occurs with massive or selective lesions in the brainstem and cervical spinal cord, such as EPM, results in dilated cutaneous blood vessels over the entire ipsilateral side of the body. This appears to be the major factor that causes more circulating epinephrin to reach the sweat glands, re-

sulting in excessive sweating. Spinal cord lesions caudal to the cranial thoracic segments may damage the descending sympathetic neuronal fibers and cause excessive sweating caudal to the lesion, but would not be expected to cause Horner's syndrome.

III. Neoplastic

Retrobulbar neoplasia may cause a dilated pupil because of involvement of the oculomotor nerve or ciliary ganglion. Often exophthalmos and degrees of blindness occur due to optic nerve involvement (Rebhun, 1979). Occasionally, retrobulbar and paraorbital neoplasms have been associated with Horner's syndrome. These include respiratory epithelial adenocarcinoma and squamous cell carcinoma in cattle (Guard et al., 1984) and parotid adenocarcinoma in a horse.

Caudal cervical and cranial intrathoracic neoplasia, including carcinoma (Mayhew, 1980), melanoma (Milne, 1986) and lymphosarcoma (Firth, 1978), have caused Horner's syndrome in horses because of involvement of the thoracic sympathetic ganglion and cervical sympathetic trunk.

Problem 5B:

Strabismus (CNIII, IV, VI, VIII, cerebrum)

Strabismus refers to abnormal deviation of the axis of the eyeball. Because of the loss of specific extraocular muscle function, paralysis of the oculomotor (III), trochlear (IV), or abducens (VI) nerves should result in lateral, dorsomedial, or medial strabismus, respectively. In each case the eyeball cannot be moved out of the deviated position and can be considered fixed strabismus. These are rarely seen as acquired syndromes in large animal neurology (Fig. 9–4). An eyeball deviation, particularly when it moves ventral or dorsal and is able to return to its normal position, is seen frequently. Usually this is because of diseases of the vestibular system, and is referred to as vestibular strabismus. This is discussed further in Problem 6.

Congenital blindness can be associated with abnormal eyeball positions (also Problem 3). Also, Appaloosa horses severely affected with night blindness (also Problem 3) can have dorsomedial strabismus, which may be noticed when they attempt to visually fix on an object. There is no resting strabismus (Rebhun et al., 1984).

Although many inflammatory, physical, metabolic, toxic, and nutritional disorders discussed in Problem 1 may affect the regions of the brainstem where the oculomotor, trochlear and abducens nuclei are, prominent signs of fixed strabismus are not usually seen (Fig. 9–4).

However, many severe cerebral diseases result in deviated eye postures, particularly directed toward the same side as the lesion if it is unilateral (part

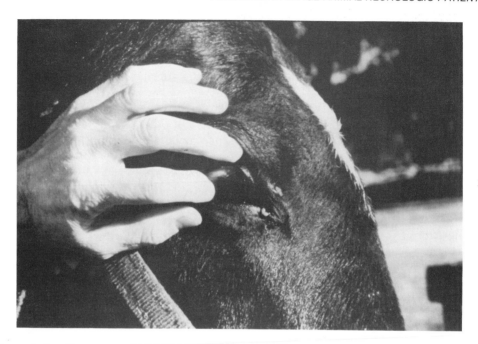

Figure 9–4. Abnormal eyeball retraction characterized by an inability to retract the eyeball when the cornea is touched, along with a fixed, slightly ventral, strabismus as shown in this horse, is rarely seen in large animals. This depressed horse had normal eyelid movement and could clearly feel from the side of the face and cornea, yet had these signs. No normal vestibular nystagmus could be induced. There was asymmetric ataxia and tetraparesis. The horse was euthanized and found to have EPM with prominent lesions involving the brain stem, including the right abducens (VI) nucleus. Loss of function in most, or all, of the oculomotor (III), trochlear (IV), and abducens (VI) cranial nerves is probably required to produce such a syndrome.

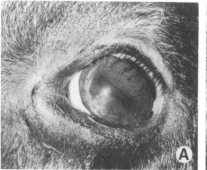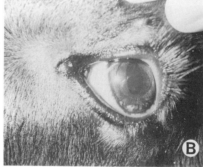

Figure 9–5. Dorsomedial or rotational strabismus often occurs in large animals suffering various diffuse and severe cerebral diseases. These examples show the left eye of a calf suffering from water intoxication (A) and that of one with *Salmonella* sp meningitis/ventriculitis (B).

of adversive phenomenon). The relative dorsomedial rotation of the eyeball seen in polioencephalomalacia, lead and water intoxication, and bacterial meningitis in ruminants and with the neonatal maladjustment syndrome in foals [Problem 1] may not be a specific cranial nerve IV (trochlear) paralysis (Fig. 9–5). This might reflect severe forebrain disease with involvement of the upper motor pathways controlling eyeball posture.

Categories of Diseases and Differential Diagnosis
*NOTE: Only those diseases marked * are discussed in this section.*

I. Congenital and Familial
  *1. Hydrocephalus (Problem 1)
  *2. Convergent Strabismus and Exophthalmos
   3. Congenital Blindness (Problem 3)
II. Physical
   1. Head Trauma (Problem 4)
III. Infectious, Inflammatory, Immune
  *1. Retrobulbar Abscess and Inflammation
   2. Various Encephalitides (Problem 1)
IV. Toxic
   1. Lead (Problem 1)
   2. Water and Salt (Problem 1)
V. Nutritional
   1. Thiamin-Responsive Polioencephalomalacia of Ruminants (Problem 1)
VI. Neoplastic
  *1. Retrobulbar Neoplasia

I. Congenital and Familial
  1. Hydrocephalus (also Problem 1)
     In association with the deformed forehead associated with marked congenital hydrocephalus a down and out deviation of the eyeballs can also occur. Presumably, this is the result of a change in shape and position of the bony orbits. Normal eyeball movements can occur.
  2. Convergent Strabismus and Exophthalamos
     This disease of cattle is described as an inherited trait in Jersey (Regan et al., 1944) and Shorthorn (Holmes et al., 1957) breeds and less often in Holstein (Fig. 9–6), Ayrshire, and Brown Swiss breeds (Rebhun, 1979) and several European breeds (Schütz-Hänke et al., 1979). No blindness occurs, although defective vision is referred to, and the syndrome may not be noticed until the first lactation (Holmes et al., 1957).
     Detailed cytonumeric studies on the abducens nuclei and nerves and the extraocular muscles in the autosomal recessive form seen in black and white cattle in Germany have revealed a paucity of abducens neurons and hypoplasia of the retractor oculi and lateral rectus muscles (Schütz-Hänke et al., 1979).

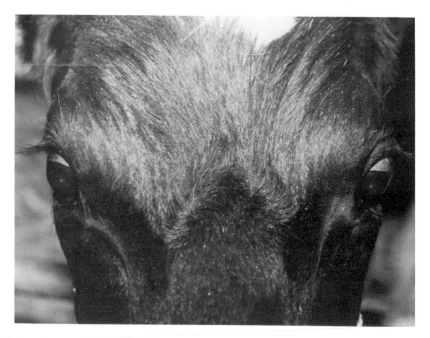

Figure 9–6. Congenital convergent strabismus in a mature Holstein dairy cow.

II. Infectious, Inflammatory, Immune
  1. Retrobulbar Abscess and Inflammation
    The mechanical pressures and perhaps extraocular neuromuscular damage associated with retrobulbar abscesses often result in strabismus. Such abscesses may originate from abscessed pharyngeal lymph nodes, and from a pharyngeal phlegmon. In addition, strabismus and exophthalmos may accompany chronic sinusitis and actinomycosis and actinobacillosis in cattle (Rebhun, 1979).
III. Neoplastic
  1. Retrobulbar Neoplasia
    Exophthalmos almost always occurs with retrobulbar neoplasia and can be accompanied by strabismus. Lymphosarcoma is the most frequently occurring type in cattle (Rebhun, 1979); various carcinomas also have been identified (Guard et al., 1984).

Problem 5C:

Dropped Jaw and Masseter Muscle Atrophy (CNV motor)

Sudden onset of a dropped jaw in a large animal patient should prompt the clinician to suspect trauma to the jaws, with or without fracture of the mandible. Neurologic diseases resulting in a dropped jaw, with no other neurologic signs, occur rarely in large animals. In the eastern part of the United States however, a syndrome of masseter muscle atrophy is seen somewhat frequently with equine protozoal myeloencephalitis (also Problem 11) (Fig. 9–7).

Many encephalitides (also Problem 1) that may involve the pontomedullary region where the motor nucleus of CNV and the trigeminal nerve reside, can effect this syndrome. Degrees of weakness, ataxia, depression, and other cranial nerve palsies are evident.

With denervation of the muscles of mastication, the masseter, temporalis, and distal belly of the digastricus muscles on the affected side atrophy rapidly (within 1 to 2 weeks). Unilateral atrophy is not associated with any major difficulty in chewing food; however, bilateral atrophy can result in a horse showing ponderous eating habits and dropping food from its mouth. Total jaw paralysis in all large animals causes the jaw to hang down with food and saliva present in the mouth; usually the tongue hangs out over the incisor teeth (Fig. 9–10).

Marked masseter and temporalis muscle atrophy also results in slight degrees of enophthalmos and drooping of the upper eyelid, at least in cattle (Rebhun, 1979) and horses. This appears to be caused by the loss of muscle mass behind the globe, which is seen as a sinking in of the retrobulbar tissues in the supraorbital fossa. A presumed (idiopathic) trigeminal neuritis that is

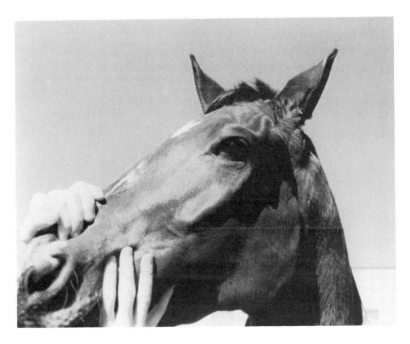

Figure 9–7. Severe, unilateral atrophy of the muscles innervated by the trigeminal nerve in eastern North American horses is almost always due to equine protozoal myeloencephalitis, as was the case in the horse shown here. Temporalis and masseter atrophy causes the supraorbital fossa to become prominent. It also causes a degree of ptosis, which results from the eyeball receding within the bony orbit. Distal digastricus muscle atrophy is palpable on the medial surface of the mandible.

transient, seen in dogs as a sudden onset of inability to close the jaws, does not appear to have been seen in large animals.

To be differentiated from this problem is the trismus seen with tetanus (Problem 8A), and the dystonia of jaw and tongue muscles seen with nigro-pallidal encephalomalacia (Problem 5F).

Categories of Disease and Differential Diagnosis
*NOTE: Only those diseases marked * are discussed in this section.*

   I. Congenital and Familial
      *1. Dropped Jaw Syndrome in Newborn Calves and Lambs
  II. Physical
      *1. Squeeze-Shute Accidents in Cattle
      *2. Fractured Stylohyoid Bone in Horses
      *3. Temporomandibular Luxation in the Horse
 III. Infectious, Inflammatory, Immune
      1. Equine Protozoal Myeloencephalitis (Problem 10)
      2. Listeriosis (Problem 6)
      3. Basillar Empyema (Problems 5D and 6)
      4. Polyneuritis Equi (Problem 13)
      5. Woody Tongue (*Actinobacillus lignieresii*) (Problem 5I)
 IV. Idiopathic
      *1. Masseter Myopathy in Horses

   I. Congenital and Familial
      1. Congenital Dropped Jaw in Newborn Calves and Lambs
         Usually following anterior presentation, dystocia and assisted delivery, a calf or lamb may have a dropped jaw. Some recover completely. It is assumed that a neuromyopathy, associated with degrees of edema of the head, usually accompanies the syndrome. However, one newborn calf that was seen with masticatory muscle atrophy and a dropped jaw had a degenerative myopathy consistent with white muscle disease involving the masseter muscles (Fig. 9–8).
  II. Physical
      1. Squeeze-Shute Accidents in Cattle
         Following the use of a neck clamp, or in a squeeze-shute during cattle processing, an occasional animal has been seen to have a dropped jaw (Fig. 9–9). The tongue protrudes from the front of the mouth, perhaps because of its weight and the animal is unable to prehend and chew food. Signs may abate in days to weeks. Fracture of the mandible and luxation of the temporomandibular joint have not been detected, although previous luxation of this joint may play a role in the syndrome, along with degrees of masseter trauma and perhaps trigeminal neurapraxia.
      2. Fractured Stylohyoid Bone in Horses
         Prominent symmetric masseter atrophy has been associated with fractures of the stylohyoid in horses (Hertsch et al., 1975). The precise relationship between these findings is not clear.

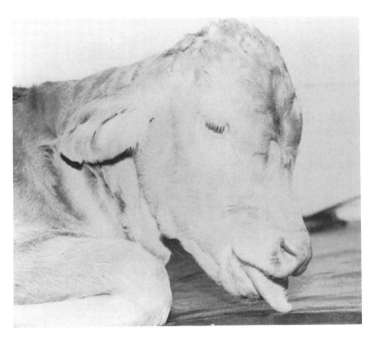

Figure 9–8. Dropped jaw syndrome in newborn calves and lambs usually is associated with dystocia and a degree of edema of the head. However, in this calf it appeared to be due to masticatory myopathy, which is histologically consistent with white muscle disease.

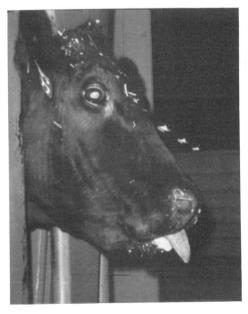

Figure 9–9. Following restraint in a squeeze-shute, cattle can develop a dropped jaw even in the absence of temporomandibular fractures or luxation. The heavy tongue usually hangs over the incisor teeth as shown.

3. Temporomandibular Luxation in the Horse

This injury occurs in association with fractures of the mandible and is reported to occur alone (Hurtig et al., 1984). Inability to prehend and chew food is seen, and the mandible may protrude and the teeth cannot be manually apposed. Even with correction of the luxation under anesthesia, total resolution of the problem may not occur.

II. Idiopathic

1. Masseter Myopathy in Horses (Myopathy of muscles of mastication and deglutition)

Signalment. This is a rare disease affecting adult horses and ponies of all breeds, particularly those stabled and in poor condition.

History. There is usually a sudden onset of complete anorexia or of swollen masseter muscles. Foals with diffuse myodegeneration and steatitis (also Problem 10B) may have a swollen, painful tongue in conjunction with generalized stiffness and reluctance to move.

Examination. This may be part of the more generalized polymyopathy seen in nutritional myodegeneration (also Problem 10B) (Hulland, 1985). Firm, apparently painful muscles of mastication and deglutition are found. Cardiac involvement, as evidenced by arrhythmias, may result in sudden death. Affected horses are unable to eat, and manipulation of the swollen affected muscles appears to be painful.

Assessment. Histologically, there is a degenerative myopathy with few inflammatory cells. The disorder is related (questionably) to vitamin E and selenium deficiency and to poor nutrition. Differential diagnoses include tetanus (Problem 8A), nigropallidal encephalomalacia (Problem 5F), brainstem disease, and snake bite.

Treatment. Alimentation and maintenance of fluid and electrolyte requirements are important aspects of therapy. Vitamin E and selenium probably are worth administering. Phenylbutazone and aspirin for pain is reasonable therapy.

Prognosis. If the condition is associated with debility then the prognosis is poor. The prognosis is bad if the heart is involved. Muscle atrophy is likely if the animal survives.

Problem 5D:

Decreased Facial Sensation (CNV sensory, cerebrum)

Many animals, depressed because of marked systemic illness and particularly severe brain disease, are slow to respond to noxious stimuli anywhere on the body, including the face. In comparison, this particular problem of decreased facial sensation is identified when the degree of hypoalgesia detected is greater than that to be expected by any accompanying depressed or moribund state.

In defining this problem, care must be taken to separate facial hyporeflexia from facial hypoalgesia (see Neurologic Examination). The facial reflex (V sensory, VII motor) can be depressed with lesions involving the trigeminal nerve, ganglion or nucleus, or the facial nerve or nucleus. With trigeminal nerve (sensory branch) involvement degrees of facial hypoalgesia also occur and the animal does not pull its head away from the stimulus. With lesions affecting the sensory pathways from the face, above the medulla oblongata, in the thalamus, and in the contralateral internal capsule and frontal cortex, there can be degrees of facial hypoalgesia but no interruption to the facial (V sensory—VII motor) reflexes. This facial hypoalgesia or analgesia is most evident when the noxious stimulus is applied to the sensitive nasal membranes. Several severe, particularly focal, diseases of the forebrain, such as cerebral abscess, do result in this syndrome and thus have been itemized.

It is interesting to note that facial analgesia (and paralysis) was seen in a cow that had an ocular squamous cell carcinoma invading the trigeminal nerve. Part of the syndrome included a specific and dense infestation of ticks only on the denervated skin of the face (Samuel et al., 1987).

Equine protozoal myeloencephalitis and rabies have caused facial hypoalgesia with extensive brainstem involvement. A star-gazing attitude, bradycardia, blindness, dilated pupils, dropped jaw, and facial, tongue, and pharyngeal paralysis, along with facial analgesia can be seen in cattle with pituitary abscesses (see Fig. 9–10 and Problem 6, Basillar Empyema).

Facial (and body) hyperesthesia due to trigeminal (and diffuse) nerve root irritation occurs in early stages of diffuse bacterial meningitis (also Problem 1). Idiopathic trigeminal neuritis, or head rubbing in horses, is the presumed diagnosis, with acquired, profound irritation on the side of the face. This has been seen in association with asymmetric, fluctuating signs of facial paresis and masseter atrophy, which have all resolved spontaneously (also Problem 14).

Partial facial analgesia resulting from trauma to single branches of CNV is not common and usually is associated with trauma to the face, nasal region, and sinuses.

Finally, massive retrobulbar tumors, including lymphosarcoma, squamous cell carcinoma, and parotid adenocarcinoma have caused facial hypoalgesia, usually with other overt evidence of face and eye lesions (Rebhun, 1979), (Guard, 1984).

Categories of Disease and Differential Diagnosis

   I. Physical
       1. Head Trauma (Problem 4)
       2. Intracarotid Injection (Problem 2)
  II. Infectious, Inflammatory, Immune
       1. Rabies (Problem 1)
       2. Brain Abscess (Problem 1)
       3. Basillar Empyema (Problem 6)

Problem 5E:

Facial Paralysis and Facial Spasm (CNVII, cerebrum)

Paralysis of the muscles of facial expression (facial paralysis) is a common problem in large animals with neurologic disorders. Dysfunction of the facial nerve produces decreased spontaneous and reflex movements of the ear, eyelids, lips, and external nares. The ear and lips on the side of the lesion droop and the muzzle tends to be pulled to the opposite side with a unilateral lesion. Ptosis of the upper lid, perhaps because of the bulk of atonic supraorbital muscles and paralysis of the frontalis muscle, also occurs (Figs. 9–10, 9–11, 10–5).

Damage to the upper motor pathways, which control the facial nucleus and nerve, and which are in the frontal, motor cerebral cortex, internal capsule, crus cerebri, and brainstem, can result in abnormal facial expression. This occurs without flaccid, facial paralysis, or facial areflexia, at least in the horse. Large, focal, cerebral lesions, such as hematoma, equine protozoal myeloencephalitis, and abscess have produced such a supranuclear paralysis. There is still tone in the muscles of facial expression, and facial (V-VII) reflexes are present, but the expression may be bland or grimacing (Fig. 9–12) on one or more sides. Needle electromyographic examination of the facial muscles does not reveal denervation because lower motor neuron disease has not occurred.

In the early phase of irritative lesions, such as meningitis, neuritis, and trauma involving the facial nerve, facial muscles can twitch and even spasm prior to paralysis that often ensues.

Permanent facial paralysis may necessitate enucleation of the eyeball because of keratitis sicca and exposure ophthalmitis; exercising horses may require false nostril surgery as a result of an obstruction to inspiratory airflow.

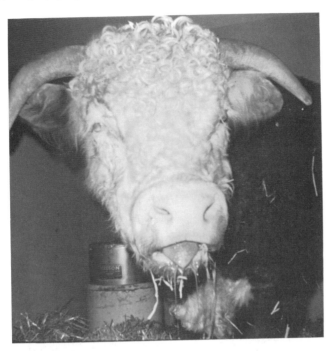

Figure 9–10. Basillar empyema originating in the region of the pituitary fossa (pituitary abscess) can involve multiple cranial nerves. The bull shown here had signs of bilateral damage to the optic (II), trigeminal (V), facial (VII), glossopharyngeal (IX), vagal (X), and hypoglossal (XII) nerves.

Bilateral facial paralysis results in profound dysphagia in horses. Chronic paralysis, with muscle atrophy and fibrous contracture of the face, can cause (hemi) facial spasm.

With distal, peripheral, facial nerve involvement usually one or two branches of the nerve, not all three nerve branches (auricular, palpebral, buccal), are involved. Pressure on the side of the face as a result of a tight halter or recumbency damages buccal branches, paralyzing just the nares and lips; however, the ear and upper eyelid may droop because of direct auricular and palpebral nerve trauma (Fig. 9–11). Brainstem lesions, particularly those caused by equine protozoal myeloencephalitis and listeriosis, can selectively involve the facial nucleus in the brainstem and can mimic a peripheral lesion by producing a selective, partial, facial paresis.

Categories of Disease of Differential Diagnosis
NOTE: Only the diseases marked * are discussed in this section.

    I. Physical
       *1. Facial Nerve Trauma
       2. Head Trauma (Problem 4)
       3. Osteoarthrosis and Fractures of the Temporohyoid Region (Problem 6)
    II. Infectious, Inflammatory, Immune
       1. Equine Protozoal Myeloencephalitis (Problem 10)
       2. Listeriosis (Problem 6)

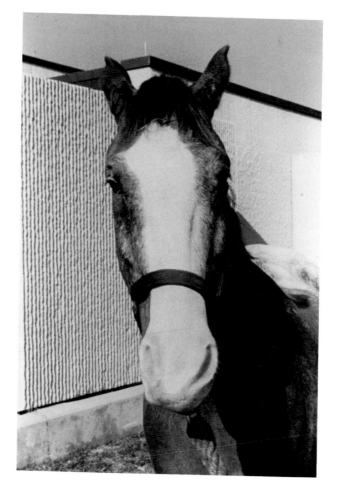

Figure 9–11. Temporary, distal, facial paralysis (neurapraxia) seen here in a horse following general anesthesia in left lateral recumbency resulted from halter pressure on the buccal branches of the facial nerve. Degrees of ptosis (also present) can result from pressure on the auriculo-palpebral nerve or direct periorbital injury. A drooped ear (not seen) can result from direct auricular trauma.

      3. Otitis Media and Interna (Problem 6)
      4. Granulomatous Facial and Vestibulocochlear Neuritis in Calves (Problem 6)
      5. Basillar Empyema (Problem 6)
      6. Verminous Encephalitis (Problem 1)
      7. Cerebral Abscess (Problem 1)
      8. Polyneuritis Equi (Problem 12)
      9. Other Encephalitides (Problem 1)
  III. Toxic
      1. Lead Poisoning in Horses (Problem 5H)
  IV. Neoplastic
      1. Peripheral Neoplasms (Problems 5A and 11)
      2. Central Neoplasms (Problem 6)

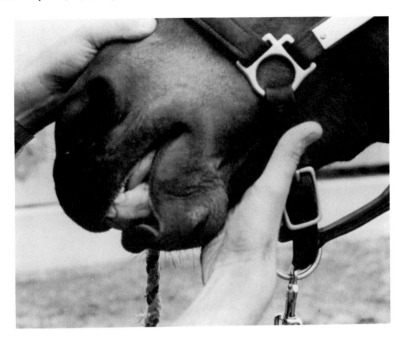

Figure 9–12. Facial grimacing is rarely present with acute inflammatory diseases involving the facial nucleus or nerve. More often it is seen in horses with various, focal forebrain lesions, such as EPM as seen in this horse. This is an upper motor neuron lesion to the facial nucleus and facial reflexes.

I. Physical
   1. Facial Nerve Trauma
      This can occur in any animal, but it occurs particularly in heavy animals that become recumbent for any reason and bang their face on the ground. It also occurs in horses that have excessively tight halters and pull back on a lead rope attached to a halter (Fig. 9–11).

      As with any peripheral nerve, the facial nerve can be injured to various degrees of severity: neurapraxia is loss of function only; axonotmesis is loss of axons; and neurotmesis is severance of axons and their nerve sheaths (see Pathology, Ch. 4).

      Closed trauma to the side of the face usually results in degrees of neurapraxia and axonotmesis. With the former, function normally returns within 14 days, and often does so abruptly. Axonotmesis requires that the damaged axons regrow down the Schwann cell sheaths, a process occurring at about 1 inch per month. Thus, it can take 6 months for recovery from this type of injury; the quality of recovery is never 100%. Fortunately, when no skin is lacerated, functional recovery usually is obtained. Degrees of neurotmesis occur with open wounds to the side of the face and with fractured temporal bones (see Problem 4). Depending on alignment of the damaged nerve fibers and depending on the degree of local tissue reaction, a proportion of the damaged fibers may regrow to their respective muscles of facial expression in 6 to 12 months; however, this does not result in full return of function.

   The same principles for managing peripheral nerve trauma can be applied to the facial nerves (see Problem 11).

Problem 5F:

Dysphagia (CNIX, and X, cerebrum)

   Dysphagia in large animals is common. It is often caused by non-neurologic disorders. Neurologic dysphagia primarily involves either the brainstem nuclear regions, the pharyngeal branches of the glossopharyngeal and vagus nerves, or the neuromuscular junctions or muscles of the pharynx (Fig. 9–13). Motor trigeminal (Problem 5C), bilateral facial (Problem 5E), or hypoglossal (Problem 5I) paralyses also result in neurologic dysphagia.

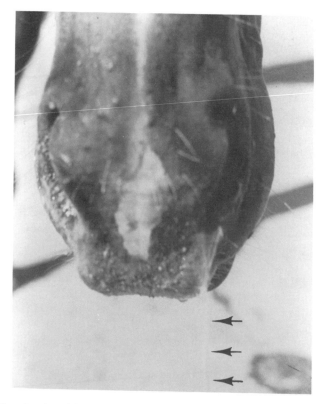

Figure 9–13. Dysphagia, with spillage of saliva (arrows) and even food out the nostrils, often is seen in animals with botulism. This particular horse suffered from postanesthetic myasthenic syndrome (Problem 10) which mimics botulism.

Severe forebrain diseases, including viral encephalitides, abscesses, trauma, polioencephalomalacia, water intoxication, equine protozoal myeloencephalitis, and neonatal maladjustment syndrome, can result in poor initiation and completion of chewing and swallowing maneuvers. Again, this is a supranuclear (above the nucleus ambiguus and solitary tract nucleus) paralysis, without loss of the swallowing reflexes. Yellow star thistle poisoning is a selective example of such a syndrome.

Passing a stomach tube, auscultating the chest for evidence of inhalation, taking appropriate radiographs, and using a fiberoptic endoscope to see the pharynx and larynx and the structures surrounding the guttural pouches, are helpful ancillary aids. In particular, this should exclude the non-neurologic, obstructive disorders, including esophageal choke, pharyngitis, pharyngeal abscess (phlegmon), and neoplastic masses.

When evaluating animals that have had signs of this problem for less than 2 weeks, the clinician must give consideration to the possibility of rabies.

Categories of Disease and Differential Diagnosis
NOTE: Only those diseases marked * are summarized here.

I. Physical
    1. Caudal Brainstem Trauma (Problem 4)
    2. Fractured Stylohyoid Bone (Problem 5C)
II. Infectious, Inflammatory, Immune
    *1. Guttural Pouch Mycosis and Empyema
    2. Basillar Empyema—Pituitary Abscess (Problem 6)
    3. Bacterial Meningitis (Problem 1)
    4. Listeriosis (Problem 6)
    5. Equine Viral Encephalitides (EEE) (Problem 1)
    6. Rabies (Problems 1, 12, 13)
    7. Equine Protozoal Myeloencephalitis (EPM) Problem 10)
    8. Verminous Encephalitis (Problems 1, 10)
    9. Masseter Myopathy of Horses (Problem 5C)
III. Toxic
    *1. Nigropallidal Encephalomalacia
    *2. Botulism (Problem 10)
    3. Postanesthetic, Myasthenic Syndrome (Fig. 9–13, and Problem 10)
    4. Lead Poisoning (Problem 1 and 5H)
IV. Idiopathic
    *1. Grass Sickness

I. Infectious, Inflammatory, Immune
    1. Guttural Pouch Mycosis and Empyema
        Signalment. These conditions, especially empyema, are relatively common in horses of all ages, though neurologic signs accompanying the diseases occur less frequently.
        History. Bilateral or unilateral mucopurulent nasal discharge with (mycosis) or without (empyema) epistaxis, are frequent primary complaints made by owners of affected horses (Fig. 9–14).

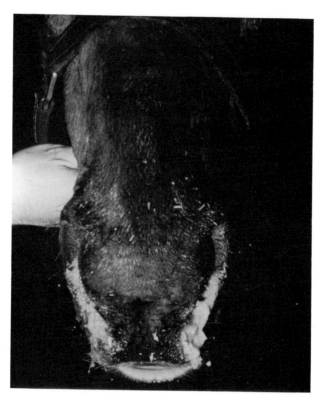

Figure 9-14. Dysphagia with saliva, food, and mucopurulent nasal discharge was present in this horse suffering from left guttural pouch mycosis. At postmortem examination there was histologic involvement of the pharyngeal nerves.

Physical Examination. This may reveal filling or tenderness in the area of the guttural pouch, which is called "parotid pain." Combinations of purulent exudate and food, which often is foul smelling, appear out the nostrils. Neck stiffness, pharyngeal swelling, abnormal head posture, colic, and cough may also occur (Greet, 1987), (Freeman, 1980), (Church et al., 1986).

Neurologic Examination. This reveals varying deficits in swallowing ability, occasionally with Horner's syndrome. Laryngeal and facial hemiplegia, and blindness sometimes are present (Greet, 1987), (Freeman, 1980), (Cook et al., 1968), (Hatziolos et al., 1975).

Assessment. Aspergillus sp colonizes in the guttural pouch, particularly in the dorsocaudal region of the medial compartment adjacent to the temporohyoid articulation. Lesions can involve the internal carotid artery, vagus and glossopharyngeal nerves, and cranial cervical sympathetic trunk (Cook et al., 1968). Further extension of the lesion into the carotid artery may explain some other signs, such as blindness (Hatziolos et al., 1975); postsurgical carotid embolization may result in cerebral infarction (Greet, 1987).

Guttural pouch bacterial catarrh or empyema may accompany *Aspergillus* sp infection or occur separately and produce dysphagia. Empyema occurs in about 50% of strangles (*Streptococcus equi*) infections following rupture of abscessed retropharyngeal lymph nodes into one or both guttural pouches.

Diagnosis. The diagnosis is confirmed with endoscopy, radiography, and culture.

Therapy. Surgical removal or cauterization of *Aspergillus* lesions has been successful, but recent surgical techniques to block the internal carotid artery with combinations of surgical ligation (proximal) and balloon catheterization (distal) appear to be more successful than other methods. Overall, surgical cures are reported to be about 80% (Greet, 1987), (Freeman, 1980), (Freeman et al., 1980), (Church et al., 1986), (Caron et al., 1987). When used alone, isotonic fungicidal and antiseptic lavage of affected guttural pouches have not been successful for mycotic infections. Flushing with large volumes of saline and dilute povidone-iodine or hydrogen peroxide (H_2O_2), along with systemic antibiotics, usually resolves empyema and catarrh. Strong irritant solutions must be avoided.

Prognosis. Generally, the prognosis is poor for mycotic disease. However, although surgery is difficult, newer vascular occlusive techniques are hopeful. Prognosis is good for empyema if it is treated early, before pharyngeal paralysis is complete, but chronic cases still can be frustrating to treat.

II. Toxic
   1. **Nigropallidal Encephalomalacia (yellow star thistle poisoning)**
      Signalment. Horses of any age, gender, or breed.

      Primary Complaint. Difficulty eating and chewing and weight loss most often are seen first.

      History. There is evidence of direct (pasture) or indirect (hay) access to yellow star thistle [*Centaurea solstitialis*], (also known as yellow burr in Australia) or Russian Knapweed [*Centaurea repens*] and a history of an acute onset of rigidity of the muscles of mastication. The plants grow predominantly in the Western United States and also in Australia.

      Physical Examination. Weight loss is evident early in the disease.

      Neurologic Examination. Excessive muscle tone (dystonia) is present in the jaws resulting in a grinding movement, without the ability to close or open the mouth completely or chew (Fig. 9–15A). The tongue may be drawn into a longitudinal trough. Affected muscles show prominent fasciculations. Affected horses may circle, wander aimlessly, or occasionally be ataxic (Cordy, 1954), (Young et al., 1970), (Gard, 1973).

      Assessment. This is a toxicity produced by eating the unpalatable-looking thistles, which results in necrosis of the substantia nigra and globus pallidus; nigropallidal encephalomalacia (Fig. 9–15B). Horses have to eat the plants for several weeks, and it is believed that they may become addicted to them. Sheep thrive on a diet of only these plants (Cordy, 1954).

      Diagnosis. The diagnosis is based on signalment, history, physical, and neurologic findings.

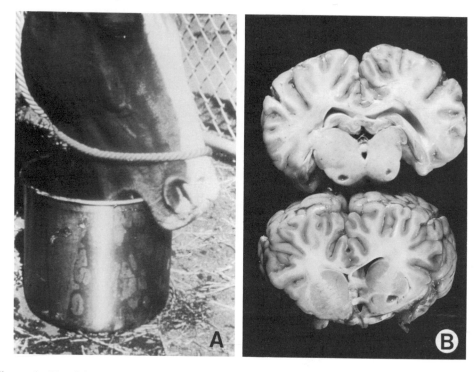

Figure 9–15. A horse suffering from yellow star thistle poisoning has dystonia of the muscles of prehension and mastication, causing the jaws to be fixed in a partially open position (A). The horse is unable to fully open or close its mouth. The lesions (B) often are grossly visible in the substantia nigra (upper) and globus pallidus (lower). (Fig. 9–15A courtesy of Dr. A. Koterba.)

Therapy. Horses can be maintained with feeding through a nasogastric tube, but no specific treatment exists (Gard et al., 1973).

Prognosis. The outlook is grave; affected horses starve to death.

2. Botulism (also Problem 10)

In addition to degrees of tetraparesis to tetraplegia (Problem 10), ruminants, and particularly horses and foals, with botulism frequently are unable to prehend, chew, and swallow food and water because of neuromuscular blockade of cranial musculature. On occasion, dysphagia is the major presenting complaint; limb weakness and other signs of motor paralysis are apparently better compensated for to begin with.

Assessment, diagnosis, treatment, and prevention are discussed under Problem 10.

VI. Idiopathic

1. Grass Sickness

Signalment. Horses of all breeds and nondomestic equidae can be affected. Most often, this disease occurs in 3 to 8-year-old horses that are kept outside during late spring and summer. The disease occurs commonly in Western Europe, particularly in Scotland and England (Gilmour, 1974), (Ashton, 1977).

History. This varies from acute colic and death to chronic cachexia.

Clinical syndrome. Difficulty swallowing, excessive salivation, depressed gastrointestinal sounds, abdominal distension, and usually mild colic are present to varying degrees. Muscular tremor and patchy sweating may be primary signs or may reflect the dehydration, electrolyte imbalances, and colic that occur.

Assessment. Degenerative changes found in many autonomic neurons, particularly in the thoracic and abdominal ganglia (Gilmour, 1975), are presumed to be the pathologic substrate of this form of dysautonomia.

The disease does not seem to be contagious, but multiple cases do occur in certain districts and even on particular farms. Attempts at transferring the disease through blood transfusions may have reproduced the neuropathologic changes, but not the clinical signs (Gilmour et al., 1977).

Diagnosis. No definitive clinical diagnostic test exists. Exploratory laparotomy reveals colonic impaction. The degree of esophageal dilatation usually is significant; radiographically, a contrast-swallow esophagram, demonstrating ineffective peristalsis in the absence of obstruction, is the best diagnostic tool available (Greet et al., 1986).

Treatment. There is no treatment except palliative nursing care.

Prognosis. Most (if not all) horses die or have to be destroyed because of chronic ill thrift. Mildly affected horses suspected of having grass sickness have survived with degrees of ill thrift remaining.

Problem 5G:

Megaesophagus

Megaesophagus is not frequently seen in large animals; however, it has been observed with chronic esophageal obstruction, lower esophageal sphincter scarring and ulceration, severe pneumonia with dyspnea, and with gastroesophageal ulceration and associated bruxism, retching, and aerophagia. It is seen in several diffuse myasthenic syndromes, many of which defy specific diagnosis, and is one of the hallmarks of the paralytic gastrointestinal syndrome in Europe known as Grass Sickness (Problem 5F).

Categories of Disease and Differential Diagnosis

I. Toxic
   1. Botulism (Problem 10)
   2. Organophosphate Toxicity (Problems 2, 5H, and 10)
   3. Postanesthetic Myasthenic Syndrome (Problem 10)
   4. Lead Poisoning (Problem 5H)

II. Idiopathic
    1. Grass Sickness (Problem 5F)

Problem 5H:

Laryngeal Paralysis or Paresis: Roaring (CNX)

This is a common problem in most light and draft breeds of horses (idiopathic disease). Also, it accompanies a wide variety of other diseases.

Many families of horses have a high frequency of roaring, although no specific hereditary malformation has been determined. Congenital alterations (which may be pathologic) in the left recurrent laryngeal nerves of foals are believed to occur. One previously popular hypothesis for the idiopathic disorder in horses involves physical forces. The syndrome occurs most commonly on the left side in large, mature thoroughbreds and draught breeds with long necks and deep chests. The left recurrent laryngeal nerve has a longer course around the aortic arch than the right nerve does around the costocervical artery. The leverage effect created by neck movement could then result in tension on the nerve and its blood supply with ischemia resulting in local and distal nerve fiber degeneration. This hypothesis is no longer popular. Thus, the exact pathogenesis of the most frequently seen cases of laryngeal hemiplegia is unknown.

Misplaced injections in the neck can damage the vagus and recurrent laryngeal nerve, which results in laryngeal hemiplegia.

Retropharyngeal abscesses can result in degeneration of laryngeal nerves and roaring, as can guttural pouch mycosis (also Problem 5F).

Horses with severe liver disease have had bilateral laryngeal paralysis with inspiratory dyspnea. The pathophysiologic basis of this is not understood.

Categories of Disease and Differential Diagnosis
NOTE: Only those diseases marked * are discussed here.

I. Infectious, Inflammatory, Immune
    1. Guttural Pouch Mycosis and Empyema (Problem 5F)
II. Toxic
    *1. Lead (also Problem 1)
    *2. Organophosphates (also Problems 2 and 10)
    3. Botulism (also Problems 5F and 10)
III. Metabolic
    1. Hepatoencephalopathy (Problem 1)
IV. Idiopathic
    *1. Equine Idiopathic Laryngeal Hemiplegia

I. Toxic
  1. Lead (also Problem 1)

   One of the more consistent findings in cases of lead poisoning is inspiratory stridor caused by laryngeal paralysis. Other motor nerves can be involved, resulting in pharyngeal, esophageal, facial, and anal paralysis. Weakness and ataxia are reported, but most severely affected horses become depressed, lose weight, and develop inhalation pneumonia making interpretation of these signs difficult (Burrows, 1982), (Knight et al., 1973).

  2. Organophosphates (also Problems 2 and 10)

   Organophosphates can produce seizures (Problem 2) and a delayed ataxic syndrome (Problem 10). In the horse, repeated doses of certain organophosphates, such as haloxon, have been associated with bilateral laryngeal paralysis (Rose et al., 1981), (Duncan et al., 1985). Signs partly improved in some affected horses with supportive care that included tracheostomy.

II. Idiopathic
  1. Equine Idiopathic Laryngeal Hemiplegia

   Signalment. Idiopathic laryngeal hemiplegia, as a singular problem, frequently is recognized in mature, light breed, long-necked horses used for performance (Cahill et al., 1987).

   History. While exercising, the horse is noticed to make an excessive respiratory noise (roaring) during inspiration. The horse may "fade" or "quit" near the end of a race.

   Examination. It can be possible to induce the horse to "grunt" if

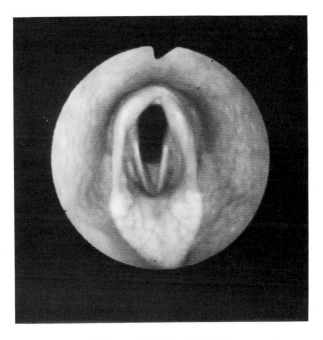

Figure 9–16. Endoscopic view of a horse with idiopathic, left recurrent laryngeal paresis (roarer). At full inspiration little or no abduction of the left arytenoid cartilage and vocal fold can be seen.

frightened, as it cannot abduct the vocal folds when it gasps or keep the laryngeal os closed when it breath-holds. There often is a palpable loss of dorsal and lateral musculature on the left side of the larynx, and the projection of the muscular process of the arytenoid cartilage is prominent. Endoscopy reveals an asymmetric position of the arytenoid cartilages (Fig. 9–16) and a failure to abduct the vocal fold on (forced) inspiration. Poor adduction of the vocal fold is demonstrated with the laryngeal adductor ("slap") test.

Assessment. Distal axonal degeneration occurs in the recurrent laryngeal nerves and is worse on the left side. Thus, nerve fiber atrophy is worse close to the larynx; degrees of demyelination and remyelination accompany the axonal disease (Cahill et al, 1986). Similar, milder, nerve fiber loss may occur in other long peripheral nerves in affected horses, suggesting that the syndrome is an expression of a diffuse, peripheral, distal, axonopathy. All intrinsic laryngeal muscles (except the cricothyroid muscle), and particularly the dorsal cricoarytenoid muscle, show denervation atrophy (Cahill et al., 1986). The distal axonopathy that is documented in idiopathic roarers is similar to that seen from the effects of several selective neurotoxins. Thus, chemicals, drugs, mycotoxins, and biotoxins are suggested etiologies. The neural lesions are likened to those seen in many cases of stringhalt (also Problem 12), i.e., a distal axonopathy of long nerve fibers (Cahill et al, 1986).

Diagnosis. Endoscopy reveals poor abduction of the left vocal fold and a negative laryngeal adductor response (slap) test on the left side of the larynx. The latter is performed by slapping the horse behind the withers on the right side and either looking for adduction of the left arytenoid cartilage with an endoscope, or feeling for contraction of the left dorsal and lateral laryngeal musculature externally. Either of these is a positive response. With laryngeal hemiplegia, and sometimes with many different forms of cervical spinal cord disease, often a poor or absent response ipsilateral to the lesion, contralateral to the stimulus (slap), occurs. This is an ancillary aid, but is not a definitive diagnostic test for cervical spinal cord disease or for laryngeal paralysis. The interpretation of partial responses to the slap test and asymmetric movement of arytenoid cartilages is controversial.

Treatment. Laryngeal ventriculectomy and laryngeal muscle prosthesis are performed regularly.

Prognosis. Probably 50% of early cases respond to ventriculectomy, and more complicated surgery may give better results.

Problem 5I:

Tongue Paralysis (CNXII)

This problem rarely occurs alone.
Fractured hyoid bones can cause protrusion of the tongue with dysphagia

in the horse, although this probably can resolve when the hyoid bones heal. Cattle in squeeze-shute accidents can develop a dropped jaw and protrusion of the tongue, with or without a fractured mandible or luxated temporomandibular joint (Fig. 9–9 and Problem 5C). Whether or not the hypoglossal nerves are involved is not known. Calves and lambs born following dystocia can have edematous heads; a swollen, protruded tongue can be a prominent impairment associated with this (Fig. 9–8 and Problem 5C).

The neuromuscular paralysis caused by *Clostridium botulinum* neurotoxins can result in prominent tongue paralysis (Problems 5F and 10).

Central lesions, such as equine protozoal myeloencephalitis (Fig. 9–17), brainstem trauma, and listeriosis, usually result in depression, ataxia, and tetraparesis in addition to cranial nerve deficits, such as tongue paralysis. Equine protozoal myeloencephalitis is unusual because it can produce extremely focal lesions, which only affect individual cranial nerve nuclei, and it has caused hemiatrophy of the tongue, with no other signs of brainstem disease.

Diffuse and focal forebrain disease including cerebral abscess and hematoma, polioencephalomalacia, Eastern equine encephalitis, and hepatoencephalopathy, may result in weakness of the tongue when the patient allows it to remain out of the mouth even though it can be retracted (also Problem 1). There is no lower motor neuron (flaccid) paralysis, no atrophy, and the needle electromyogram does not indicate denervation. These signs indicate that the lower motor neuron is intact and that this is an upper motor neuron, or supranuclear, paralysis.

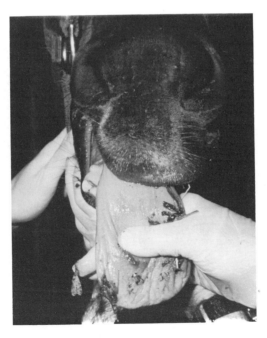

Figure 9–17.   Brain stem lesions that involve the hypoglossal nucleus, such as equine protozoal myeloencephalitis, can result in a weak, flaccid tongue that is easily pulled from the mouth and that will atrophy.

Categories of Disease and Differential Diagnosis
*NOTE: Only those diseases marked * are discussed in this section.*

   I. Congenital and Familial
      1. Dropped Jaw Syndrome in Newborn Calves and Lambs (Problem 5C)
  II. Physical
      1. Squeeze-Shute Accidents (Problem 5C)
      2. Fractured Hyoid Bones (Problem 5C)
      3. Temporomandibular Luxation in the Horse (Problem 5C)
 III. Infectious, Inflammatory, Immune
     *1. Bacterial Glossitis (Woody Tongue)
      2. Listeriosis (Problem 6)
      3. Equine Protozoal Myeloencephalitis (Problem 10)
      4. Basillar Empyema (Problems 5D and 6)
      5. Other Encephalomyelitides (Problem 1)
 IV. Toxic
      1. Botulism (Problems 5F and 10)
      2. Nigropallidal Encephalomalacia (Problem 5F)
  V. Idiopathic
     *1. Tongue Sucking
     *2. Glossal Weakness in Neonatal Foals

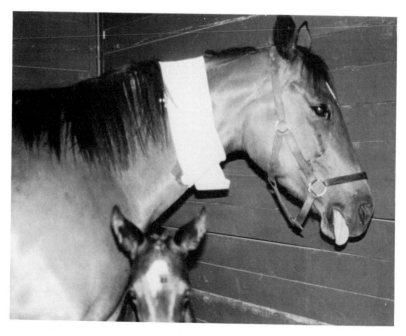

Figure 9–18. This mare was regarded as a "tongue-sucker," which is a form of stereotypic behavior. Interestingly, her newly born foal, shown with her, was seen to mimic its dam.

I. Infectious, Inflammatory, Immune

 1. Bacterial Glossitis (Woody Tongue)

 Bacterial glossitis, or woody tongue, is common in cattle at pasture. Most often, it is a pyogranulomatous myositis caused by *Actinobacillus lignieresii,* but it can be caused by many organisms (Barker et al., 1985). It responds well to antibiotics, such as streptomycin, and to systemic sodium iodide therapy.

 Occasionally it occurs in horses (Baum et al., 1984).

II. Idiopathic

 1. Tongue Sucking

 Some adult horses and foals that are "tongue suckers" often are seen leaving the tongue out of the mouth (Fig. 9–18). In addition, they do not seem to mind having their tongue pulled from the mouth; the tongue may appear to be flaccid, although no dysphagia or other neurologic signs are present. This can be regarded as a vice or as stereotypic behavior (Problem 13).

 2. Glossal Weakness in Neonatal Foals

 Newborn foals up to a week of age have been seen with a protruding tongue that cannot be retracted into the mouth and degrees of dysphagia. With alimentation through a nasogastric tube and nursing care these foals can do well and the problem can be completely resolved.

REFERENCES

Ashton DG, Jones DM, Gilmour JS: Grass sickness in two non-domestic equines. Vet Rec 1977; *100*:406.

Barker IK, van Dreumel AA. The Alimentary System. In: *Pathology of Domestic Animals.* Jubb KVF, Kennedy PC, Palmer N, eds. 3rd Ed. Vol 2, Orlando: Academic Press, 1985: Ch 1, pp 1–237.

Baum KH, Shin SJ, Rebhun WC, et al. Isolation of *Actinobacillus lignieresii* from enlarged tongue of a horse. J Am Vet Med Assoc 1984; *185*:792–793.

Burrows GE. Lead poisoning in the horse—a review. Equine Pract 1982; *4*:30–36.

Cahill JI, Goulden BE. The pathogenesis of equine laryngeal hemiplegia—a review. NZ Vet J 1987; *35*:82–90.

Cahill JI, Goulden BE. Equine laryngeal hemiplegia. Parts I–V. NZ Vet J 1986; *34*:161–175, 181–193.

Caron JP, Fretz PB, Bailey JV, et al. Balloon-tipped catheter arterial occlusion for prevention of hemorrhage caused by guttural pouch mycosis: 13 cases (1982–1985). J Am Vet Med Assoc 1987; *191*:345–349.

Church S, Wyn-Jones G, Parks AH, et al. Treatment of guttural pouch mycosis. Equine Vet J 1986; *18*:362–365.

Cook WR, Campbell RSF, Dawson C. The pathology and aetiology of guttural pouch mycosis in the horse. Vet Rec 1968; *83*:422–428.

Cordy DR. Nigropallidal encephalomalacia in horses associated with ingestion of yellow star thistle. J Neuropath and Exp Neurol 1954; *13*:330–342.

Duncan ID, Brook D. Bilateral laryngeal paralysis in the horse. Equine Vet J 1985; *17*:228–233.

Firth EC. Horner's syndrome in the horse: experimental induction and a case report. Equine Vet J 1978; *10*:9–13.

Freeman DE. Diagnosis and treatment of diseases of the guttural pouch (Parts I and II). Comp Cont Ed Pract Vet 1980; *2*:S3–S11, S25–S31.

Freeman DE, Donawick WJ. Occlusion of internal carotid artery in horse by means of a balloon-tipped catheter: clinical use of a method to prevent epistaxis caused by guttural pouch mycosis. J Am Vet Med Assoc 1980; *176*:236–240.

Gard GP, deSarem WG, Ahrens PJ. Nigropallidal encephalomalacia in horses in New South Wales [letter]. Aust Vet J 1973; *49*:107–108.

Gilmour JS, Mould DL. Experimental studies of neurotoxic activity in blood fractions from acute cases of grass sickness. Res Vet Sci 1977; *22*:1–4.

Gilmour JS. Chromatolysis and axonal dystrophy in the autonomic nervous system in grass sickness of equidae. Neuropathol Appl Neurobiol 1975; *1*:39–47.

Gilmour JS, Jolly GM. Some aspects of the epidemiology of equine grass sickness. Vet Rec 1974; *95*:77.

Glaze MB, consulting ed. Ocular diseases. In: *Current Therapy in Equine Medicine—2*. Robinson NE ed. Philadelphia: WB Saunders, 1987, pp 427–464.

Greet TRC. Outcome of treatment in 35 cases of guttural pouch mycosis. Equine Vet J 1987; *19*:483–487.

Greet TRC, Whitwell KE. Barium swallow as an aid to the diagnosis of grass sickness. Equine Vet J 1986; *18*:294–297.

Guard CL, Rebhun WC, Perdrizet JA. Cranial tumors in aged cattle causing Horner's syndrome and exophthalmos. Cornell Vet 1984: *74*:361–365.

Hatziolos BC, Sass B, Albert TF, et al. Ocular changes in a horse with gutturomycosis. J Am Vet Med Assoc 1975; *167*:51–54.

Hertsch VB, Wibdorf H: Contribution to the therapy of fractures of the head in horses. 2nd communication: stylohyoid fractures. Dtsch Tierärztl Wschr 1975; *82*:473–512.

Holmes JR, Young GB. A note on exophthalmos with strabismus in shorthorn cattle. Vet Rec 1957; *69*:148–149.

Hulland TJ. Muscles and Tendons. In: *Pathology of Domestic Animals*. Jubb KVF, Kennedy PC, Palmer N, eds. 3rd Ed. Vol 1. Orlando: Academic Press, 1985. Ch 2, 173.

Hurtig MB, Barber SM, Farrow CS. Temporomandibular joint luxation in a horse. J Am Vet Med Assoc 1984; *185*:78–80.

Knight HD, Burau RG. Chronic lead poisoning in horses. J Am Vet Med Assoc 1973; *162*:781–786.

Mayhew IG. Horner's syndrome and lesions involving the sympathetic nervous system. Equine Pract 1980; *2*:44–47.

Milne JC. Malignant melanomas causing Horner's syndrome in a horse. Equine Vet J 1986; *18*:74–78.

Moore CP. Guest editor. Large Animal Ophthalmology. Vet Clin North Am [Large Anim Pract] 1984; *6*:433–703.

Rebhun WC, Loew ER, Riis RC, et al. Clinical manifestations of night blindness in the Appaloosa horse. Comp Cont Ed Pract Vet 1984; *6*:S103–S106.

Rebhun WC. Diseases of the bovine orbit and globe. J Am Vet Med Assoc 1979; *175*:171–175.

Regan WM, Gregory PW, Mead SW. Hereditary strabismus in Jersey cattle. J Hered 1944; *32*:233–234.

Rose RJ, Hartley WJ, Baker W. Laryngeal paralysis in Arabian foals associated with oral haloxon administration. Equine Vet J 1981; *13*:171–176.

Samuel JL, Kelly WR, Vanselow BA. Intracranial invasion by bovine squamous cell carcinoma via cranial nerves. Vet Rec 1987; *121*:424–425.

Schütz-Hänke VW, Stöber M, Drommer W. Clinical, genealogical, and pathomorphological studies in black-and-white cattle with bilateral exophthalmus and convergent strabismus. Dtsch tierärztl Wschr 1979; *86*:185–191.

Smith JS, Mayhew IG. Horner's syndrome in large animals. Cornell Vet 1977; *67*:529–542.

Sweeney RW, Sweeney CR. Transient Horner's syndrome following routine intravenous injections in two horses. J Am Vet Med Assoc 1984; *185*:802–803.

Usenik EA. Sympathetic innervation of the head and neck of the horse; neuropharmacological studies of sweating in the horse. Doctoral Thesis. St. Paul: University of Minnesota, 1957.

Young S, Brown WW, Klinger B. Nigrophallidal encephalomalacia in horses caused by ingestion of weeds of the genus *Centaruea*. J Am Vet Med Assoc 1970; *157*:1602–1605.

CHAPTER 10

Problem 6:
Head Tilt, Circling, Nystagmus, and Other Signs of Vestibular Abnormalities

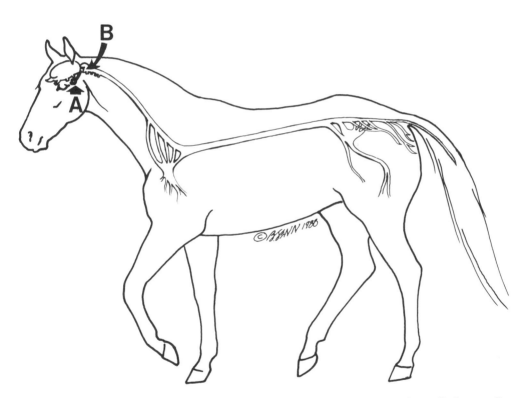

Location of lesions resulting in vestibular abnormalities: membranous labyrinth, vestibular ganglion and nerve (A), and the vestibular nuclei in the medulla oblongata and flocculonodular lobe and fastigial nucleus of the cerebellum (B).

The vestibular system (see Figs. 1–4, 1–5, 2–5) is a special proprioceptive system that helps the animal maintain orientation in its environment, with respect to gravity. The system helps to maintain the position of the eyes, trunk, and limbs in relationship to movements and positioning of the head.

The receptor end organ is located in the inner ear, consisting of the three semicircular canals, the utricle, and saccule. Movement of endolymph in the semicircular canals, caused by movement of the head and by the effects of gravity, stimulates receptors that transmit impulses to the vestibular nuclei by way of the vestibular nerve and its ganglion in the lateral wall of the fourth ventricle of the medulla oblongata. There is a direct afferent connection to a small part of the cerebellum. Importantly, the facial nerve travels next to the middle ear and its nucleus is close to the vestibular nuclei in the medulla oblongata.

From the vestibular nuclei, the vestibulospinal tracts descend ipsilaterally through the length of the spinal cord. These neurons are facilitatory to ipsilateral motor neurons going to extensor muscles of the limbs, are inhibitory to ipsilateral flexor muscles, and are inhibitory to contralateral extensor muscles. Thus, the principal effect of unilateral stimulation of this system on the limbs is a relative ipsilateral extensor tonus and contralateral flexor tonus, which promotes ipsilateral support of the trunk against gravity. Conversely, a unilateral vestibular lesion usually results in ipsilateral flexor and contralateral extensor tonus, forcing the animal toward the side of the lesion.

The nuclei of cranial nerves III, IV, and VI, which control eye movement, are connected with the vestibular system by way of a brainstem tract—the medial longitudinal fasciculus (see Fig. 2–5). Through this tract, coordinated eye movements occur with changes in positioning of the head. Lesions of the vestibular system, or of this tract, can result in the eyes being drawn into abnormal positions (strabismus).

There are other vestibular efferent projections to the reticular formation, cerebellum, and cerebral cortex.

Through these various pathways, the vestibular system coordinates movement of the eyeballs, trunk, and limbs, with head movements. It maintains equilibrium of the entire body during motion and rest.

Signs of vestibular disease vary depending on whether there is unilateral or bilateral involvement, and whether the disease involves peripheral or central components of the system.

General signs of vestibular system dysfunction are staggering, leaning (even rolling), circling, drifting sideways when walking and a head tilt, and various changes in eye position (strabismus) and movement (nystagmus) (see Figs. 10–1, 10–2, 10–4, 10–5, 10–7, 10–8). Horses with peracute vestibular disease can be violent because of profound disorientation, which is described as vertigo in humans.

In the case of unilateral involvement, an asymmetric staggering occurs. The animal has a tendency to drift, roll, or lean toward the side of the lesion. In some cases the animal circles to the affected side. A head tilt is a relatively constant sign (Figs. 10–1, 10–5, 10–7), along with nystagmus. The nystagmus tends to regress, but changes in head position may restimulate it. With unilateral, peripheral vestibular disease, nystagmus is horizontal (or rotary or arc-shaped) with the fast phase directed away from the side of the lesion. With bilateral peripheral vestibular disease, vertical nystagmus has rarely been recognized, and, as in man, it is temporary (Peele, 1977). In central disturbances the nystagmus may be horizontal, rotary, or vertical. Head elevation also exaggerates any tendency for eye deviations. These often are seen as a ventral

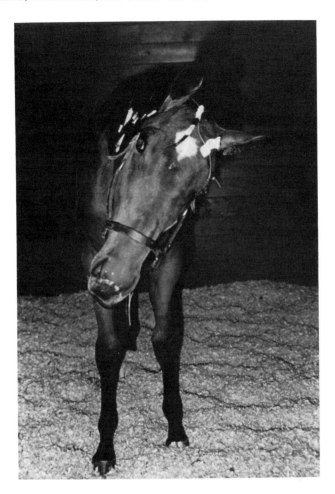

Figure 10–1. A head tilt is the most common sign of acute asymmetric vestibular disease. This yearling thoroughbred filly fractured its left temporal bone and developed a left head tilt, left facial paralysis, eye deviations, and a staggery gait with tendency to move to the left, which was worse when the horse was placed in a stall. Although the filly did well following therapy and convalescence, clear fluid with characteristics of CSF drained from the left ear for several days.

deviation of the eye on the same side as the lesion (Figs. 10–2, 10–4, 10–8). True limb weakness does not occur with peripheral disease, but can occur in the case of central disease because of involvement of the descending motor tracts. In addition, evidence of depression, caused by involvement of the reticular formation (Figs. 10–6, 10–7), and signs of involvement of other cranial nerves indicate central disease.

Occasionally, large animals with central vestibular disease have been noted to have a head tilt away from the side of a cerebellomedullary lesion. This is the same as the paradoxical vestibular syndrome described in small animals (Palmer et al., 1976); the side of the lesion is defined by the side of hemiparesis and of other cranial nerve involvement.

Bilateral vestibular lesions are characterized by more symmetric signs, which strongly resemble generalized cerebellar disease with wide swaying movements of the head and sometimes the trunk. Significantly, no inducible vestibular nystagmus occcurs in dense, bilateral, vestibular disease (Fig. 10–6).

Asymmetric forebrain lesions frequently cause an animal to hold its head and neck turned to one side, usually the same side as the lesion. This can be difficult to distinguish from a vestibular head tilt where there is rotation of the poll around the muzzle. In a more prominent form a head turn due to vestibular or cerebral disease may involve bending of the whole neck and head toward the flank. The presence or absence of a vestibular head tilt is only evaluated when the head and neck are held along a median plane. Sometimes this turning to one side involves the eyes and whole body with spinning in circles, and may be precipitated by any stimulus to either side of the animal, when it can be regarded as an adversive movement. This sign of cerebral disease is seen mostly with prominently asymmetric lesions, such as forebrain abscess, parasitic thromboembolism or verminous migrations, and head trauma.

The most common causes of vestibular disease in all large animals are otitis media-interna and head trauma. Cases in which significant facial paralysis is found are more serious and carry a more unfavorable prognosis. Special attention should be paid to the eye if a facial palsy is present because keratitis and corneal ulceration rapidly occur in these cases.

Hemorrhage into the middle and inner ear cavities results in vestibular and facial nerve signs consisting of a head tilt toward the lesion, facial paralysis on the same side as the lesion, and a horizontal or rotary nystagmus with the fast phase away from the lesion. If the hemorrhage has occurred around or in the medulla, or if meningitis results from an open fracture of the calvarium, additional central signs such as depression, ataxia, weakness, and other vestibular and cranial nerve signs often appear. Hemorrhage or leakage of cerebrospinal fluid from the external ear or nares usually is an indication that the petrosal or ethmoid bones have been fractured. Chronic osteochondroarthrosis of the temporohyoid articulation may be associated with acute hemorrhage into the middle and inner ear cavities.

Treatment of vestibular disease can be discouraging at times. Otitis media-interna should be treated vigorously with antibiotics and anti-inflammatory drugs. Many neglected cases develop granulomata of the ear cavities and these cases are irreversible. Sclerosis of the ear cavities has been found on radiographs of the skull of animals with vestibular disease, but the precise significance of this is not known. The cases attributed to trauma respond better as a whole than those cases attributed to an otitis media-interna or those associated with proliferative bony lesions of the hyoid and temporal bones. Trauma cases also are treated for brain concussion-contusion, and should probably receive 0.1 to 0.2 mg/kg dexamethasone IM repeated every 4 to 6 hours for 1 to 4 days. Some cases do not fully regress but appear to compensate, presumably using vision and general proprioceptive modalities, and are able to function almost normally. Concurrent blindness that may often accompany head trauma (also Problems 3 and 4) does not allow visual compensation to occur, thus worsening the prognosis.

Large animals can be presented with asymmetric central vestibular signs caused by listeriosis, equine protozoal myeloencephalitis (EPM), and by migrating metazoan parasites (*Parelophostrongylus tenuis, Strongylus vulgaris, Draschia megastoma,* and *Hypoderma* spp larvae). In a horse, evidence of multifocal disease would make EPM more likely than larval migrans. In ruminants, listeriosis is the most common cause of vestibular syndromes due to medullary disease. Also a temporary, idiopathic, acute, usually unilateral vestibular syndrome occurs in horses. It mimics a peripheral vestibular lesion, without any associated signs such as facial paralysis, and is assumed to be a viral- or immune-mediated labyrinthitis or neuritis. Horses appear to recover completely, irrespective of therapy.

Symmetric, central vestibular signs can accompany the diffuse cerebellar signs of rye grass and Dallis grass intoxication. These vestibular signs include eye deviations and rapid, variable eyeball tremor or nystagmus. Central vestibular signs also can accompany many diffuse brain diseases, such as rabies, eastern and western equine encephalomyelitis, and hepatoencephalopathy. Space-occupying lesions, such as neoplasms, abscesses, or cholesterol granulomata involving the choroid plexus of the fourth ventricle, could also affect the vestibular system.

An exaggerated eye drop, and slight head tilt when blindfolded, often are the last residual signs following recovery from vestibular disease. Vision is a major input modality to the vestibular system and vision is required to accommodate for vestibular deficits; thus, blind animals do not accommodate well.

Categories of Disease and Differential Diagnosis
*NOTE: Those diseases marked * are summarized in this problem.*

   I. Congenital and Familial
      *1. Pendular Nystagmus in Dairy Cattle
  II. Physical
      *1. Osteoarthrosis and Fractures of Temporohyoid Region
      *2. Lightning Strike
      3. Trauma (Problem 4)
 III. Infectious, Inflammatory, Immune
      *1. Otitis Media-Interna
      *2. Basillar Empyema
      *3. Listeriosis
      *4. Granulomatous Facial and Vestibulocochlear Neuritis in Calves
      5. Equine Protozoal Myeloencephalitis (Problem 11)
      6. Diffuse Inflammatory Encephalomyelitides (Problem 1)
      7. Neuritis of the Cauda Equina (Problem 12)
      8. Verminous Encephalitis (Problems 1, 10)
 IV. Toxic
      1. Plant-Associated Tremor Syndromes (Problem 8B)
      2. Grove Poisoning (Problem 2)
      3. Aminoglycoside Toxicity (Problem 7)
 *V. Neoplastic
 VI. Idiopathic
      *1. Idiopathic Vestibular Syndrome of Horses

I. Congenital and Familial

1. Pendular Nystagmus in Dairy Cattle

About 1 in 200 Holstein and Jersey dairy cows in a survey in New York were afflicted with pendular nystagmus with no other evident signs. The nystagmus most often was vertical, but in some cases it was horizontal or rotary, and sometimes (one case) it was unilateral (McConnon et al., 1983). Some cattle are affected at birth. The same, presumably inherited, syndrome also has been seen in Ayrshire bulls, Guernsey cows, and Holstein bulls.

The condition appears to be stable and has no clinical consequences, thus, it should not be taken as evidence of more serious vestibular disease.

II. Physical

1. Osteoarthrosis and Fractures of Temporohyoid Region

Signalment. Only adult horses have been seen with this disease.

History. Occasionally the animal has a history of head trauma (Firth, 1977), head rubbing, or neck pain. There is an acute onset of a vestibular syndrome or facial paralysis (Fig. 10–2).

Neurologic Signs. Acute peripheral vestibular disease or facial paresis is present. Central (medullary) signs are rarely present.

Assessment. Chronic proliferative osteochondrosis and fusion of the temporohyoid joint, often with fractures of the hyoid, basillar, or temporal bones are found (Blythe et al., 1984), (Power et al., 1983) (Figs. 10–2, 10–3). Signs are the result of hemorrhage into the middle

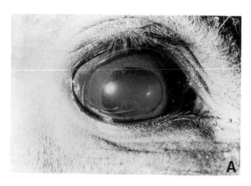

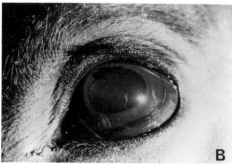

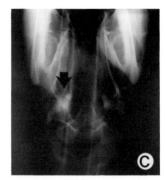

Figure 10–2. Eye deviations commonly are present with asymmetric vestibular disease. In this case there was a ventral deviation of the right eye (A) and dorsal deviation of the left eye (B) in a horse with a right head tilt. This is associated with sclerosis (arrow) of the right temporohyoid region shown on a ventrodorsal radiograph of the skull (C)

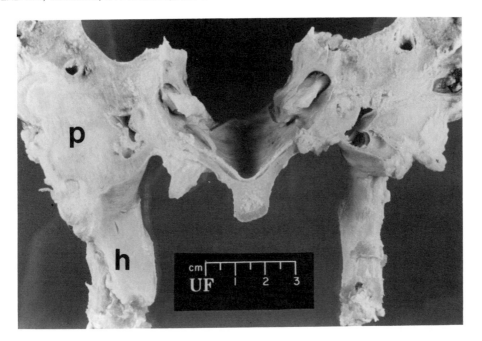

Figure 10–3. Acute, left, peripheral vestibular signs and left facial paralysis occurred in an aged mare. One year later, after recovering almost totally with no therapy, the mare was euthanized for other reasons. Residual, chronic, temporohyoid osteopathy was evident in the left petrosal (p) and proximal stylohyoid (h) bones when a transverse section of the skull through the petrosal and basillar bones was viewed. There was no evidence of suppuration on histologic examination of these tissues.

and inner ear compartments and direct trauma to cranial nerves VII and VIII. Pathogenesis of the proliferative and degenerative bone and cartilage disease is unknown, but physical forces probably play a role, at least in the onset of acute neurologic signs. Occasionally, a (presumably) secondary, suppurative, basillar meningitis may exist (Blythe et al., 1984). Some controversy exists as to whether bacterial otitis precedes the chronic bone and joint changes.

Diagnostic Aids. Guttural pouch endoscopy and skull radiographs (Fig. 10–2C) are essential to making the diagnosis. Myringotomy and aspiration or lavage of the middle ear cavity, with culture of the material obtained, should help define the role of primary otitis in this disorder. The normal bacterial flora of the ear cavities must be taken into account, however, when interpreting culture results.

Prognosis. With time and anti-inflammatory drugs, with or without antibiotics, some horses survive with little or no residual deficits. The initial prognosis, however, should only be fair.

2. **Lightning Strike**

Although lightning strike is a relatively common problem in some areas of the world, the usual result is sudden death. After a thunderstorm passes and other livestock have perhaps been killed by lightning, horses sometimes have been found to show only neurologic signs. The most frequent syndrome is unilateral vestibular disease, with or without facial paralysis. No evidence of cranial trauma, such as blood in the external ear, is evident in these cases (Fig. 10–4). Some horses have recovered, while more still have degrees of residual vestibular signs. Histologically, in one chronic case (Fig. 10–4D) there was hemorrhage and necrosis of temporal bone, vestibular nerve, and adjacent tissue; however, the exact mechanism relating electrocution or trauma to the lesions is unknown.

III. Infectious, Inflammatory, Immune

   1. Otitis Media-Interna

      Signalment. Most often otitis media and otitis interna are seen in feedlot cattle (Jensen et al., 1983) and sheep (Jensen et al., 1982),

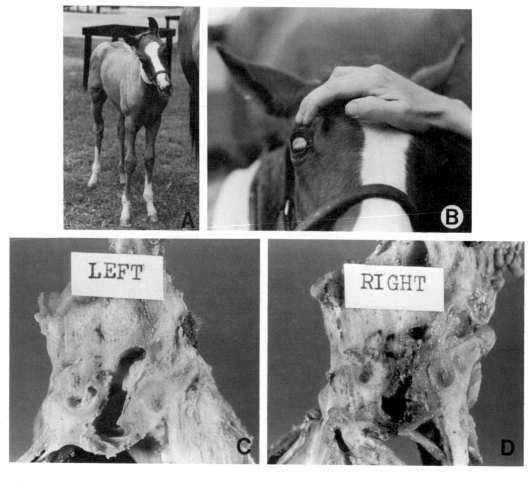

Figure 10–4. Immediately following a lightning storm, the foal shown here had severe signs of right peripheral vestibular disease and facial paralysis. Right head tilt (A) and ventral deviation of the right eyeball (B) were prominent. The foal was ultimately euthanized and transverse sections of the left (C) and right (D) temporohyoid regions are shown. The left middle and inner ear cavities are normal. There are no fractures located in the right petrosal bone but there is hemorrhagic necrosis within the right ear cavities.

feeder pigs (Cheli, 1969), and goats (Wilson, 1984). It is rare in horses (Figs. 10–5, 10–6).

History. Otitis externa, rhinitis, pharyngitis, or head trauma can be pathologically significant factors if present in the history.

Physical Examination. This may reveal an aural or nasal discharge or evidence of other of the above historical conditions. In addition, concurrent "hardware" disease, foot abscess, pneumonia, or sinusitis is occasionally present.

Neurologic Examination. Peripheral vestibular signs including a head tilt, circling, and a pronounced eye droop all occur on the same side as the lesion, with nystagmus having the fast phase to the opposite side. Facial paralysis usually is present (Figs. 10–5, 10–6). Horner's syndrome does not seem to occur with uncomplicated otitis media-interna in large animals.

Assessment. Hematogenous spread, and ascending infection from rhinitis, pharyngitis, and guttural pouch empyema, frequently are the routes of infection, rather than otitis externa, with rupture of the tympanic membrane. Extension of guttural pouch mycosis (*Aspergillus*) to involve the vestibular (or facial) nerves is extremely rare, although temporohyoid osteoarthrosis can be associated with inflammation involving these nerves (see II.1 above). In at least the pig and calf rupture of otitis interna through the internal acoustic meatus can occur, resulting in medullary empyema (abscess) with depression, weakness, and other cranial nerve signs (Cheli, 1969) (Fig. 10–6). In

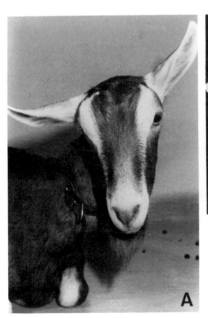
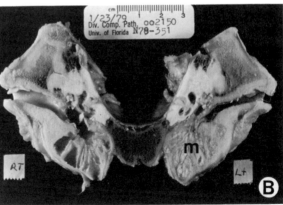

Figure 10–5.   Peracute otitis media-interna can be difficult to prove clinically. However, a sudden onset of facial paralysis and signs of peripheral vestibular disease in a febrile patient (as shown here) is strongly suggestive. This goat (A) recovered completely with penicillin therapy. In a chronic case, purulent material fills the middle ear cavity. This is shown (m) in a case of left otitis media-interna in a calf whose skull has been sectioned transversely through the ear cavities (B).

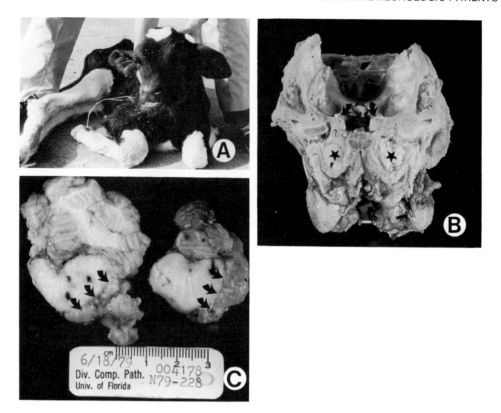

Figure 10–6. Bilateral otitis media-interna in this calf has resulted in bilateral facial paralysis with droopy ears, ptosis, and flaccid lips (A). There is no head tilt but the calf had a staggering gait and no normal vestibular nystagmus could be elicited (i.e., the eyeballs were in a fixed position in the bony orbits). The purulent exudate in the middle ears (stars) has ruptured through the internal acoustic meatus and has protruded into the caudal fossa (arrows), which compressed the medulla oblongata (B). Consequently the calf became depressed and tetraparetic (A). In a different case the subsequent basillar empyema (arrows) and medullary compression can be seen (C).

lambs and cattle *Pasturella* sp, *Streptococcus* sp and *Corynebacterium* sp (Jensen et al., 1982, 1983), and in horses *Streptococcus* sp, *Actinobacillus* sp and *Staphylococcus* sp have been isolated from infected ears. In pigs, *Streptococci,* particularly *Strep. suis* types I and II in suckling and weanling piglets respectively (Jubb, 1985), are usually the cause. Ear mites (*Psoroptes cuniculi*) rarely cause otitis media-interna in goats (Wilson et al., 1984).

Diagnostic Aids. Aural, pharyngeal, and guttural pouch endoscopy, as well as x-ray and cultural examinations are helpful in confirming a diagnosis. Analysis of CSF collected from the cisterna magna can be used to rule out central disease.

Therapy. Probably penicillin or trimethoprim-sulfa are initially the drugs of choice. Ideally, the antimicrobial drug should be chosen following culture and sensitivity results. Myringotomy and aspiration of the exudate in the middle ear is a sensible, relatively noninvasive (though overlooked) procedure in evaluating this condition. However, this is not an easy procedure in horses because they have a narrow, long, bony, horizontal ear canal.

Prognosis. The outlook is good if treatment begins early and is continued for 2 to 4 weeks. Residual signs are common in chronic cases. In pigs, and occasionally in calves, death is usual when the disease leads to a medullary empyema (Fig. 10–6).

2. **Basillar Empyema**

This may occur as described in the previous section (Fig. 10–6), secondary to otitis interna (Cheli, 1969). In cattle it also can result from rupture of a pyogenic mass that can form in the basillar venous sinuses as a sequel to a pyogenic lesion in the head, such as post-dehorning sinusitis or rhinitis. If the pyogenic mass involves the pituitary gland, so-called pituitary abscess results (see Problem 5D).

3. **Listeriosis**

Signalment. Neurologic listeriosis is commonly seen in adult cattle (Rebhun et al., 1982), sheep (Barlow et al., 1985), (Scarratt, 1987) and goats (Wood, 1972), but is extremely rare in horses (Clark et al., 1978).

History. Frequently there is a gradual or sudden onset of dullness, head tilt, and circling (Fig. 10–7). Animals may isolate themselves from the rest of the herd.

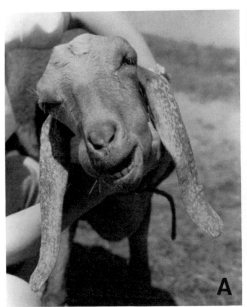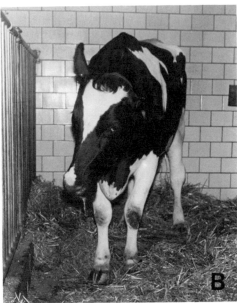

Figure 10–7. Listeriosis in ruminants frequently results in central vestibular disease. This mature goat (A) has right head tilt and bilateral facial weakness, worse on the right, with feed collecting in the right cheek, as well as tetraparesis and depression. The Holstein dairy cow (B) has left-sided head tilt and facial weakness with saliva drooling from the left side of the mouth. Both patients survived with nursing care and antibiotic therapy.

Physical Examination. Ocular and nasal discharge, ophthalmitis, fever, and bloat can be evident.

Neurologic Examination. Head tilt, circling, tetraparesis or paralysis, and ataxia are consistent findings. Later progressive midbrain signs of depression, coma and death develop. Other cranial nerves frequently affected include V, VII, IX, X, and XII (see Problem 5). Signs related only to spinal cord involvement rarely occur (Wood, 1972).

Assessment. Bacterial infection occurs in the form of microabscesses and meningitis of the brainstem, which is produced by *Listeria monocytogenes.* The organism is a motile, gram-positive bacillus and enters the brainstem via the facial and trigeminal nerves and possibly other nerves (Barlow et al., 1985), (Charlton et al., 1977).

Diagnostic Aids. Cerebrospinal fluid analysis reveals increased numbers of large and small mononuclear cells and occasional neutrophils, and increased protein concentrations (Rebhun et al., 1982), (Grotter, 1985), (Scarratt et al., 1983). Culturing *Listeria monocytogenes* from CSF is difficult, but may be easier from an inflamed eye. The sample should be refrigerated for several days prior to culture. The organism can be seen in brain tissue (Charlton et al., 1977) and is readily retrieved from the brainstem following cold incubation and culture.

Therapy. Penicillin, sulfonamides, tetracyclines, or ampicillin for 2 to 4 weeks, when begun while the animal is ambulatory, can result in a total cure. Relieving bloat and administering fluids, electrolytes, and an energy source into the rumen is often a necessary part of nursing care (Rebhun et al., 1982).

Prognosis. The outlook is guarded if the animal is recumbent or cannot swallow, but is approximately 50 to 75% if the animal can stand, and swallow, and is treated appropriately (Scarratt, 1987).

A bacterial vaccine is available but is of unknown efficacy (Scarratt, 1987).

4. Granulomatous Facial and Vestibulocochlear Neuritis in Calves

This unusual syndrome was reported in Europe where 15, 2- to 3-month-old calves were affected in 1 year (Maenhout et al., 1984). Signs consisted of facial paralysis and asymmetric vestibular (peripheral) disease. Fever, leukocytosis, and neutrophilia were detected in some calves, most of which had been recently dehorned with caustic soda, including all those studied pathologically. Nonspecific elevations in CSF protein and cell counts were reported. With and without antibiotic treatment calves recovered completely.

The lesions were nodules of granulomatous neuritis involving cranial nerves VII and VIII. In one calf similar nodular lesions were found on the cornual nerve and the skin around the previously necrotic dehorning site.

The etiopathogenesis of the space-occupying granulomatous masses on cranial nerves was not determined. Whether these cases represent an unusual form of otitis media-interna, with partial rupture through the internal acoustic meatus, is unclear.

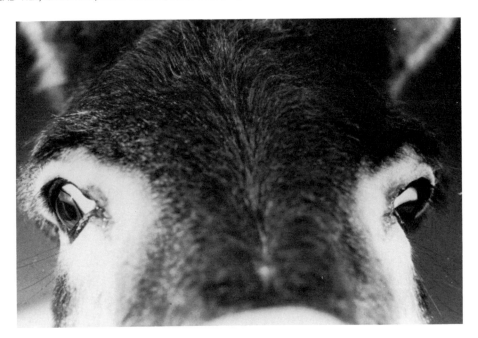

Figure 10–8. Idiopathic left vestibular syndrome was suspected in this young donkey that presented with a left head tilt and ventral deviation of the left eye (shown) with no other signs. There was an acute onset of signs that abated over several days with no therapy and radiographs of the head and analysis of CSF were normal.

IV. Neoplastic

Although neoplasms affecting the central nervous system are rare in large animals, numerous cases report that neoplasms result in various vestibular syndromes. These have included primary neuroectodermal intracranial tumors (Rees and Evans et al., 1960), (Scarratt et al., 1983), intracranial peripheral nerve tumor (Mitcham et al., 1984), and metastatic intracranial tumors affecting the vestibulocochlear nerve and pontomedullary region of the brain (Summers, 1979), (Sweeney et al., 1986).

V. Idiopathic

1. Idiopathic Vestibular Disease in Horses

An acute, temporary, vestibular disorder with no other signs occurs sporadically in adult equids (Fig. 10–8). The cause is unknown, although a viral vestibular neuritis is hypothesized. These animals appear to recover irrespective of medication. Some cases may be undiagnosed examples of other diseases discussed in this problem.

REFERENCES

Barlow RM, McGorum B. Ovine listerial encephalitis: Analysis, hypothesis and synthesis. Vet Rec 1985; *116*:233–236.
Blythe LL, Watrous BJ, Schmitz JA, et al. Vestibular syndrome associated with temporohyoid joint fusion and temporal bone fracture in three horses. J Am Vet Med Assoc 1984; *185*:775–781.
Charlton KM, Garcia MM. Spontaneous listeric encephalitis and neuritis in sheep. Light microscopic studies. Vet Pathol 1977; *14*:297–313.

Cheli R. Su di una particolare sindrome nervosa del suino (oto-encefalite). La Clinica Vet 1969; 92:78–116.

Clark EG, Turner AS, Boysen BG, et al. Listeriosis in an Arabian foal with combined immuno-deficiency. J Am Vet Med Assoc 1978; 172:363–366.

Firth EC. Vestibular disease, and its relationship to facial paralysis in the horse: a clinical study of 7 cases. Aust Vet J 1977; 53:560–565.

Grottker Von S. Liquor-untersuchungen bei der listerienbedinten meningoenzephalitis des rindes. Dtsch Tieärztl Wschr 1985; 92:257–259.

Jensen R, Maki LR, Lauerman LH, et al. Cause and pathogenesis of middle ear infection in young feedlot cattle. J Am Vet Med Assoc 1983; 182:967–972.

Jensen R, Pierson RE, Weibel JL, et al. Middle ear infection in feedlot lambs. J Am Vet Med Assoc 1982; 181:805–807.

Jubb KVF, Kennedy PC, Palmer N. Pathology of Domestic Animals. 3rd Ed, Vol 1, Orlando: Academic Press, 1985. Ch 1, pp 114–115.

Maenhout D, Ducatell R, Coussement W, et al. Space-occupying lesions of cranial nerves in calves with facial paralysis. Vet Rec 1984; 115:407–410.

Mayhew IG, MacKay RJ. The nervous system. In.: Equine Medicine and Surgery. Mansmann RA, McAllister ES, Pratt PW, eds. 3rd Ed, Vol 2, Santa Barbara: American Veterinary Publications, 1982. Ch 21, pp 1159–1252.

Mitcham SA, Kasari TR, Parent JM, et al. Intracranial schwannoma in a cow. Can Vet J 1984; 25:138–141.

McConnon JM, White ME, Smith MC, et al. Pendular nystagmus in dairy cattle. J Am Vet Med Assoc 1983; 182:812–813.

Palmer AC, Malinowski W, Barnett KC. Clinical signs including papilloedema associated with brain tumours in twenty-one dogs. J Small Anim Pract 1974; 15:359–386.

Peele TL. The Neuroanatomic Basis for Clinical Neurology. 3rd Ed. New York: McGraw-Hill Books, 1977. Ch 10, pp 230–267.

Power HT, Watrous BJ, de Lahunta A. Facial and vestibulocochlear nerve disease in six horses. J Am Vet Med Assoc 1983; 183:1076–1080.

Rebhun WC, de Lahunta A. Diagnosis and treatment of bovine listeriosis. J Am Vet Med Assoc 1982; 180:395–398.

Rees Evans ET, Palmer AC. Ependymoma in a cow. J Comp Path 1960; 70:305–307.

Saunders GK. Ependymoblastoma in a dairy calf. Vet Pathol 1984; 21:538–529.

Scarratt WK, Gamble DA. Cerebellar medulloblastoma in a calf. Comp Cont Ed Pract Vet 1983; 5:S627–S630.

Scarratt WK. Ovine listeric encephalitis. Comp Cont Ed Pract Vet 1987; 9:F27–F32.

Summers BA. Squamous cell carcinoma metastatic to the brain in a cow. Vet Pathol 1979; 16:132–133.

Sweeney RW, Divers TJ, Ziemer E, et al. Intracranial lymphosarcoma in a Holstein bull. J Am Vet Med Assoc 1986; 189:555–556.

Wilson J, Brewer BD. Vestibular disease in a goat. Comp Cont Ed Pract Vet 1984; 6:S179–S182.

Wood JS. Encephalitic listeriosis in a herd of goats. Can Vet J 1972; 13:80–82.

CHAPTER 11

Problem 7:
Deafness

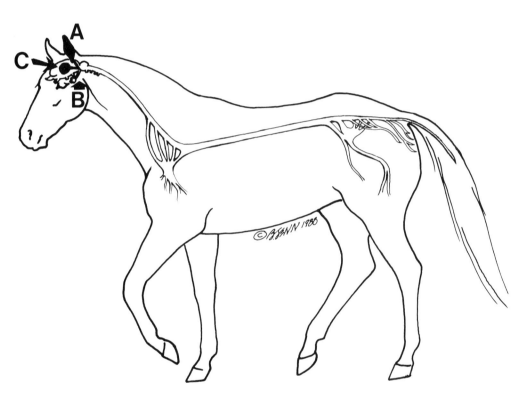

Locations of lesions resulting in deafness: external ear (A); middle ear, spiral organ and ganglion and auditory nerve (B); cochlear nuclei, other brain stem nuclei, and auditory (temporal lobe) cortex (C).

This problem is rarely recognized alone in large animal neurology.

Several diffuse brain diseases, including those discussed in Problem 1, cause an animal to be poorly responsive to external stimuli, including auditory cues; this may represent degrees of deafness. Two frequently occurring examples of this are ruminant polioencephalomalacia and equine neonatal maladjustment syndrome. The unresponsive state seen early in the course of neuronal ceroid lipofuscinosis in South Hampshire lambs probably includes deafness as well as visual loss. Calves with bilateral, severe, otitis-media and interna have been found to be clinically deaf. One filly with bilateral, ponto-medullary, equine protozoal myeloencephalitis became clinically deaf.

Auditory brainstem response (ABR) testing is ideal for evaluation of the auditory pathways in animals and has been studied in calves (Crowell et al., 1981) and horses (Marshall et al., 1981), (Marshall, 1985), (Rolf et al., 1987). The ABR waveforms from a normal horse are shown in Figure 11–1A. Abnormal ABRs have been documented in a horse with temporohyoid osteoarthropathy

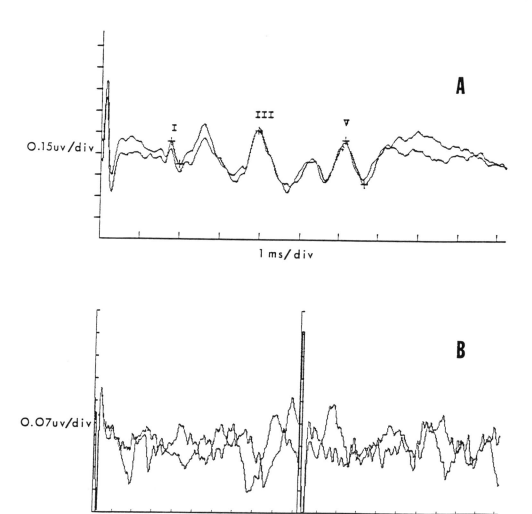

Figure 11–1.   Auditory brainstem response (ABR) recording from a normal mare (A) and a deaf 5-year-old Paint gelding (B). Each tracing is the average of 500 sweeps following a stimulus of 100 db nHL auditory clicks. Tracings for the left and right ears are superimposed in A and duplicated and separated (left on the left, right on the right) in B. Identifiable waves (labelled I, III, V, in A) including cochlear microphonics (between click artifact and wave I) are not discernible in the deaf horse, suggesting bilateral cochlear or acoustic nerve degneration.

(Problem 6) (Marshall et al., 1981) and in calves with neomycin toxicity (Crowell et al., 1981).

Categories of Disease and Differential Diagnosis
*NOTE: Only those diseases marked * are discussed in this section.*

I. Congenital and Familial
    1. Ovine Ceroid Lipofuscinosis (Problem 1)
II. Physical
    1. Head Trauma (Problem 4)
III. Infectious, Inflammatory, Immune
    1. Bilateral Otitis-Media (Problem 6)
    2. Equine Protozoal Myeloencephalitis (Problem 10)
    3. Listeriosis (Problem 6)
V. Toxic
    *1. Aminoglycoside Toxicity
VI. Neoplastic
    *1. Acoustic Nerve Tumors
VII. Idiopathic
    *1. Idiopathic Deafness in the Horse

I. Toxic
    1. Aminoglycoside Toxicity
        These antibiotics are commonly used in large animals, but rarely cause clinical deafness; renal failure is more frequently found with overdosage. Neomycin given to calves at 2.25 and 4.5 mg/kg, BID, IM for 12 or 13 days resulted in clinical deafness, which was confirmed by ABR testing (Crowell et al., 1981). Rarely, might these antibiotics be expected to cause vestibular signs.
II. Neoplastic
    1. Acoustic Nerve Tumors
        Schwannomas of the acoustic nerve have been reported in cattle (Sullivan et al., 1985), but no cases of bilateral involvement and subsequent deafness have been reported in large animals.
III. Idiopathic
    1. Idiopathic Deafness in the Horse
        A Paint gelding was determined to be clinically deaf and had no demonstrable auditory brainstem responses (Fig. 11–1B). The horse always had a mellow temperament and the brown patches in the haircoat were blanched. The owner reported that other related horses also had faded haircoats, a quiet disposition, and were suspected of being deaf (Mayhew, 1987, unpublished observations). Although these cases may be an example of an inherited deafness associated with pigmentation defects, the possibility of acquired, possibly toxic, deafness is not ruled out.

REFERENCES

Crowell WA, Divers TJ, Byars TD. Neomycin toxicosis in calves. Am J Vet Res 1981; *42*:29–34.

Marshall AE, Byars TD, Whitlock RH, et al. Brainstem auditory-evoked response in the diagnosis of inner ear injury in the horse. J Am Vet Med Assoc 1981; *178*:282–286.

Marshall AE. Brainstem auditory-evoked response in the nonanesthetized horse and pony. Am J Vet Res 1985; *46*:1445–1450.

Rolf SL, Reed SM, Melnick W, et al. Auditory brainstem response testing in anesthetized horses. Am J Vet Res 1987; *48*:910–914.

Sullivan DJ, Anderson WA. Tumors of the bovine acoustic nerve—a report of two cases. Am J Vet Res 1958; *19*:848–852.

CHAPTER 12

Problem 8:
Opisthotonus, Tetanus, Myoclonus, Tetany, Tremor, and Other Localized Muscle Spasms and Movement Disorders

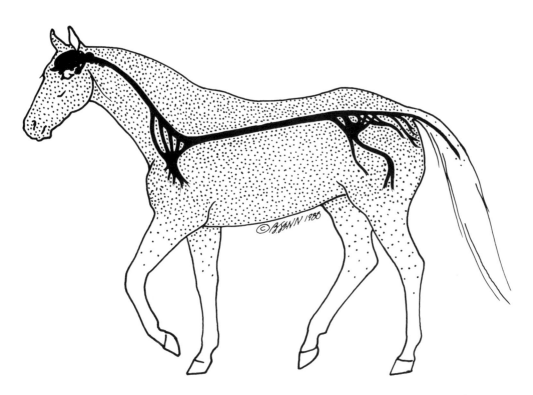

Locations of lesions resulting in opisthotonus, tetanus, tetany, tremor, localized muscle spasms, and movement disorders: diffuse and focal brain and spinal cord, nerve roots and peripheral nerves (blackened), and neuromuscular junctions and muscles (stippled).

The spectrum of disorders is divided into three clinical syndromes:

A. Opisthotonus, Tetanus, and Myoclonus
B. Tetany and Tremor
C. Other Localized Muscle Spasms and Movement Disorders

In fact, there is considerable overlap between these subdivisions. Thus, a case of *Clostridium tetani* intoxication may begin with mild muscle contractions and muscle tremor, proceed to tetany, then to tetanus, and finally to rigid opisthotonus with recumbency.

In many of these disorders, a strong correlation between the site of the lesions(s) (if any) and the clinical signs does not exist. In fact, several of them have no consistent lesion and many have diffuse lesions. Some characteristics of the various syndromes may be referrable to disturbances in cerebral function, in cerebellar function, in diffuse spinal cord function, or in neuromuscular function.

The motor system maintains a state of balance between muscle tone and muscle relaxation via the neuromuscular spindle and myotatic reflex arc. Fig. 12–1 shows that stimulation of 1a annulospiral afferent fibers, causing extrafusal muscle fibers to contract via alpha motor neurons, can occur in two main

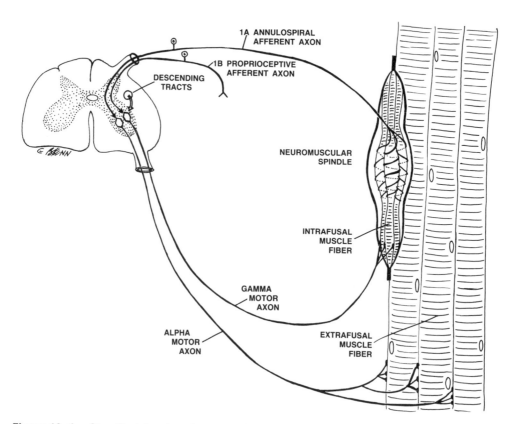

Figure 12–1. Simplified drawing of motor pathways, neuromuscular spindle, and myotatic reflex. (Adapted from de Lahunta, 1983.)

ways. Firstly, the influence of descending motor (UMN) pathways on gamma motor neurons can cause intrafusal muscle fibers in the neuromuscular spindle to contract, triggering the afferent axons. Secondly, a passive stretch of the intrafusal muscle fibers by gravity and posture, or by tendon reflex (proprioceptive input), can stimulate efferent gamma motor neurons and then 1a afferent axons. (For more detailed discussions see Palmer (1976) and de Lahunta (1976).) It is proposed that many of the syndromes resulting in abnormal muscular spasms and contractions discussed in this problem result from defective function of these motor system controls.

Problem 8A:

Opisthotonus and Tetanus

Opisthotonus ("backward tone") is a spasm of neck and limb muscles resulting in a dorsal and caudal extension of the neck and head with rigid extension of the limbs. Tetanus is a continuous (tonic) contraction of muscles without tremor. The most common cause of this syndrome is intoxication from *Clostridium tetani* neurotoxins. Head trauma, with rostral cerebellar damage, may rarely produce opisthotonus in a conscious large animal. Massive cerebral, and midbrain damage may result in opisthotonus, but the animal is severely depressed or in a coma (Problem 4). Many toxins may terminally cause similar posturing but they rarely do so without other more significant signs. Bacterial meningitis and other severe diffuse inflammatory diseases can mimic *Cl. tetani* intoxication (Problem 1).

Myoclonus describes shock-like, usually brief, intermittent contractions of muscle groups that may involve most of the body.

Severe congenital cerebellar disease, at least in calves and foals, may result in opisthotonus with recumbency (see Problem 9).

Categories of Disease and Differential Diagnosis
NOTE: Only those diseases marked * are discussed in this section.

    I. Congenital and Familial
        *1. Maple Syrup Urine Disease of Calves
        *2. Congenital Myoclonia (Neuraxial Edema) of Hereford Calves
        3. Citrullinemia (Problem 1)
        4. Hyperkalemic Periodic Paralysis of Horses (Problem 8B)
        5. Cerebellar Cortical Degeneration (Daft Lamb Disease) (Problem 9)
    II. Physical
        1. Head trauma (Problem 4)
    III. Infectious, Inflammatory, Immune
        1. Disseminated Meningoencephalitides (Problem 1)
    IV. Metabolic
        1. Hypomagnesemia and Hypocalcemia (Problem 8B)

V. Toxic
  *1. *Clostridium tetani* Neurotoxin
   2. Strychnine (Problem 2)
   3. Plant-Associated Tremor Syndromes (Problem 8B)
VI. Idiopathic
   1. Severe Australian Stringhalt (Problem 8C)

I. Congenital and Familial
  1. Maple Syrup Urine Disease of Calves
    Signalment. Newborn calves of the Horned and Polled Hereford breeds (and possibly other breeds) first show signs at a few days of age.
    History. Progressive dullness and opisthotonus is seen at 1 to 3 days with death by 1 week of age.
    Clinical Signs. Affected calves are depressed after having been bright, alert, and active at birth. This major finding helps differentiate this disease from other congenital and familial diseases of newborn calves (see Table 12–1). There are degrees of opisthotonus, and recumbency occurs quickly. Some calves are "floppy" when lifted, while others may show some extension of the hind limbs. Tremor and whole body tetany (rigidity) is not often seen. The urine may smell like burnt sugar (Baird et al., 1987), (Harper et al., 1986), (Healy et al., 1986).
    Assessment. It appears that this is another inborn error of amino acid metabolism (see Citrullinemia, Problem 1). Branched chain amino acids valine, isoleucine, and leucine accumulate in body fluids, presumably because of a deficiency in branched chain keto-acid decarboxylase (Harper et al., 1986).
    Vacuolation (status spongiosus) is severe in the white matter of the optic pathways, cerebellum, and cerebrum and in the grey matter of the brainstem and spinal cord (Baird et al., 1987).
    The disease, most likely, is inherited as an autosomal recessive factor, and is a model of maple syrup urine disease of man. Earlier reports of lethal syndromes in Hereford calves (Gregory et al., 1962) may be maple syrup urine disease.
    Prognosis. There is no treatment for this lethal disease.
  2. Congenital Myoclonia (Neuraxial Edema) of Hereford Calves
    Signalment. Newborn Horned Hereford, Polled Hereford, and Hereford cross calves are affected (Duffel, 1986), (Harper et al., 1986b).
    History. Often other cases have occurred in the herd. Inability to stand and hyperesthesia when handled are immediately evident signs. The gestational period is shortened to a mean of 274 days compared with 284 days for unaffected calves (Harper et al., 1986b).
    Clinical Signs. Affected calves are bright, alert, and remain recumbent from birth. Muscle tremor may be present, but whole body rigidity (which is intermittent) is prominent. Periods of tetanic muscle spasms of all four limbs and the neck and head are initiated by

Table 12–1. A Comparison of the Diseases Resulting in Tremor Syndromes and Myoclonia in Newborn Calves

Disease	Breed	Onset	Syndrome Characteristics	Major CNS Lesions	Problem No.
Maple syrup urine disease	Horned/Polled Hereford (Others)	Few days	Progressive opisthotonus; dullness; floppy when held up; extensor rigidity in hind limbs	Status spongiosus	8A
Congenital myoclonia (Neuraxial edema)	Horned/Polled Herefords and Crosses	Birth (in utero)	Shortened gestation; recumbent; stable; hyperesthesia; myoclonic extensor spasms; whole body rigidity; hip joint lesions	Neuraxial edema ± hypomyelination or no lesions	8A
Congenital tremor (Hypomyelinogenesis)	Holstein, Angus, Santa Gertrudis, Hereford Cross, Jersey, Shorthorn	Birth	Able to walk; stable; fine whole body tremor; sometimes cerebellar ataxia	Hypomyelinogenesis or no lesions	8B
Shaker calf syndrome	Horned Hereford	Birth	Walk with assistance; some progression; whole body trembling—shaking; fatigue; aphonia	Neurofibrillary degeneration	8B
Eggplant toxicity	Holstein, Others	Birth (and adult)	Tremor; cerebellar signs; recumbency	Poor myelin staining	8B

voluntary effort, by handling the calf, and especially by tapping the calf on the tip of the nose. After initiation of whole body muscular rigidity it takes 5 to 10 sec for the calf to relax, although it never achieves total relaxation. Muscle tremor ceases with rest. Amazingly, suckling does not initiate rigidity and there usually is no dystocia. Nystagmus or jerky eye movements may be seen.

Assessment. Degrees of vacuolation of the brain and spinal cord are frequently found at postmortem examination (Duffell, 1986). Such neuraxial edema may be prominent in white matter; this has been reported most often from California (Cordy et al., 1969) and the UK (Duffell, 1986). It also may be present in gray and white matter in affected Horned Hereford (Jolly, 1974) and Polled Hereford (Duffell, 1986) calves. Degrees of hypomyelinogenesis also have been reported (Duffell, 1986). In many cases, notably those reported from Australia, no consistent CNS lesions are found (Healy et al., 1986), (Harper et al., 1986b), (Donaldson et al., 1984). Other syndromes, such as "Doddler" calves (High et al., 1958), may represent this disease. Whether these discrepancies reflect phenotypic variations of one or more genetic disease(s), or a genetic disease and one or more acquired (in utero) disease(s), is unclear. At least the congenital myoclonia in Poll Hereford calves appears to be an autosomal recessive, inherited disorder (Harper et al., 1986b), (Donaldson et al., 1984).

The frequently found hip joint lesions (Donaldson et al., 1984) appear to be mechanical damage associated with the sustained, tetanic, muscle contractions.

Outcome. There is no treatment for this stable or progressive disorder. Affected calves should be destroyed and the sire and dam not used for breeding stock. Many muscle relaxant and anticonvulsant drugs have been tried with no success (Harper et al., 1986b).

II. Infectious, Inflammatory, Immune

1. Tetanus Due to *Clostridium tetani* Neurotoxin

Signalment. Young and adult horses often are affected, as are postpartum and neonatal ruminants (Fig. 12–2).

History. Often the disease involves neonatal animals with omphalitis, postpartum breeding animals, and all aged animals after injury or surgery. There is a sudden onset of a stiff gait, bloat, "funny-looking eyes," or recumbency.

Physical Examination. Retained placenta, wound, omphalitis, and surgical incision in all species, "nail prick" in horses, and bloat in ruminants all may be evident.

Neurologic Examination. The nostrils are flared, the nictitating membrane is prominent, the eyeballs retract readily with stimuli, and the nictitating membrane "flicks" when the head is tapped or in response to a hand clap. Erect ears, stiff jaw, opisthotonus, and an awkward stilted, hypometric gait with the tail-head elevated usually are present. Recumbency with profound opisthotonus is present in severe cases (Fig. 12–2).

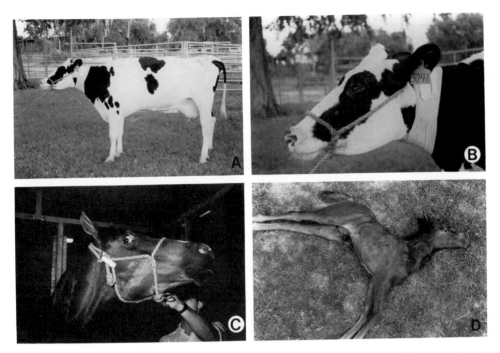

Figure 12–2. Tetanus due to *Clostridium tetani* in a cow (A, B), a horse (C), and a foal (D). Typical signs including a rigid stance, extended head posture, elevated tail-head, flared nostrils, drawn-back ears, and partly closed eyelids all are evident in the cow. Prominence of the nictitating membrane, particularly with tactile or auditory stimuli is clearly seen in the horse, along with a fixed facial expression. The cow and horse survived with treatment, but the foal, showing opisthotonus in recumbency, was euthanized because of the severity of its condition.

All signs are exaggerated with stimuli, especially a hand clap or head tap. Mild cases may only show a stiff gait.

Assessment. Hypertonia and hyperreflexia are the result of *Cl. tetani* neurotoxins interfering with interneurons in the CNS. These internuncial neurons often are inhibitory, therefore there is a lack of inhibition and consequent stimulation of lower motor neuron function. The organism grows in anaerobic sites to produce its toxins. Tetanus neurotoxin is bound to gangliosides in the CNS and the effect wears off as the neurotoxins are replaced. The characteristics of binding to gangliosides is similar to tetanus neurotoxin and for botulism toxin. Whether this is directly related to the molecular interference of synaptic function in each case is not yet clear (Mellanby, 1984).

Diagnosis. Colic, pleuritis, laminitis, meningitis, epilepsy, myopathy (e.g., white muscle disease), and fractured cervical vertebra can be important diseases to rule out from a clinical point of view. Demonstration of circulating neurotoxin and isolation of the organism from wounds to positively diagnose the disease can be extremely difficult.

Therapy. Treatment of tetanus in animal (Adams et al., 1979) is similar to treatment of tetanus in humans (Owen et al., 1959).

Keep the animal in a dark place, plug the ears with cotton, and do not disturb. Sedation (with chlorpromazine, diazepam, chloral hydrate, and pentobarbitone) and muscle relaxation (with glyceryl guaiacolate, methocarbamol, and xylazine combinations) are the basis of relieving the signs of tetanus (Adam et al., 1979). A balance between the amount of sedation and the degree of muscle relaxation is important. Drugs should be given to effect. Splenomegaly and anemia may occur with chronic phenothiazine usage in adult horses.

A moderate dose of homologous tetanus antitoxin (TAT) (e.g., 10,000 units TAT per horse) IV, or a high dose of heterologous TAT should bind residual circulating neurotoxin. All wounds should be debrided. Penicillin administration is advisable. Subarachnoid TAT might be indicated if treatment is begun in the early stages. This gives the clinician the opportunity to rule out meningitis by analyzing a sample of CSF. The dose of subarachnoid TAT probably should be 5 to 10,000 units for an adult horse, although up to 50,000 units have been recommended (Muylle et al., 1975). When using the higher volumes, one must be concerned about subarachnoid hemorrhage due to CSF pressure changes. Using subarachnoid TAT, one group (Muylle et al., 1975) reports a survival rate in horses of 77%, up from their expected 50% without using subarachnoid TAT. However, this was not a controlled trial and this form of therapy in human neonatal tetanus has not been proven to be particularly useful (Sedaghatian, 1979).

Prognosis. If the animal can still drink the prognosis is good with nursing care. If the animal is not recumbent the prognosis is fair to good (probably 75%). If the animal is recumbent the prognosis is poor for a small patient and bad for a large, adult patient. Recovery from tetanus does not protect against the disease, therefore patients still must be vaccinated. Vaccination of all other animals at risk is advised. Decubital lesions, fractured bones, and scoliosis can be lethal complications of the disease. Recovery without adequate muscle relaxant therapy appears to cause permanent, fibrous fixation and contracture of limbs.

Prevention. Use of homologous TAT or a booster tetanus toxoid is recommended at the time of occurrence of surgical and other wounds, at least in horses. A booster vaccination 2 to 4 weeks prior to parturition protects the dam and the offspring, assuming there is passive, colostral transfer of antibodies around this period. Unprotected newborn foals should receive 1 dose of TAT. Horses require at least 2 doses of aluminum-precipitated tetanus toxoid for protection (Liefman, 1981). Initiation of a vaccination program should begin by 12 weeks of age (Liu et al., 1982) and 3 doses of toxoid should be given in the first year to ensure protection. Although yearly revaccination is not necessary (Wintzer et al., 1975), booster vaccination at 1 to 5 year intervals or when a wound occurs, is necessary for guaranteed protection against the disease.

Tetanus toxoid and TAT can be administered at separate sites at one time to give immediate protection and to initiate a vaccination program (Liefman, 1980).

Problem 8B:

Tetany and Tremor

The state of tetany is characterized by repeated, violent, intermittent muscle spasms over the whole body, which frequently develop into a seizure. Tremor can be regarded as a milder form of tetany characterized by involuntary muscle contractions, which are frequently so mild that they are regarded as trembling or shivering. Thus, there is a gradation in severity of such involuntary muscle movements, from fasciculations, to shivering, to tremor, to tetany, to seizure.

Whole body tremor with no other neurologic signs is not common in large animals. Animals that are weak, especially as a result of conditions such as botulism ("shaker foals"), rhabdomyolysis, severe cervical spinal cord lesions, and even fractured pelvis or long bones, often tremble, particularly prior to becoming recumbent.

One foal suspected of suffering from a perinatal vascular accident (neonatal maladjustment syndrome—NMS) in the cervicothoracic spinal cord had limb and body tremor and severe spasms or tetany of one thoracic limb. It recovered with conservative therapy and nursing care, but had residual weakness and slight ataxia in the limb and muscle atrophy of the suprascapular and forearm musculature, indicating lower motor neuron involvement. One 18-month-old Quarterhorse is described with a "tic" or severe tremor, as well as paresis, localized to the right front limb (Beech, 1982).

In the early stages of diffuse, particularly bacterial, meningoencephalomyelitis prominent trembling or shivering may occur. Tetany and tremor can be caused by diffuse brain, cerebellar, and spinal cord diseases. Diseases involving myelin frequently result in asynchrony of electrical transmission and consequently in tremor syndromes. Also, alterations in normal synaptic transmission can cause tremor. For these reasons, many toxins can cause this syndrome.

Animals with several cerebellar diseases may present with prominent head tremor. Occasionally in these diseases, a truncal sway may also be thought of as a whole body tremor (Kidd et al., 1986).

Categories of Disease and Differential Diagnosis
*NOTE: Those diseases marked * are discussed in this section.*

I. Congenital and Familial
  *1. Congenital Tremor (Hypomyelinogenesis)
  *2. Shaker Calf Syndrome
  *3. Hyperkalemic Periodic Paralysis in Horses
  4. Maple Syrup Urine Disease of Calves (Problem 8A)
  5. Congenital Myoclonia (Neuraxial Edema) (Problem 8A)
  6. Citrullinemia (Problem 1)
  7. Ceroid Lipofuscinosis in Goats (Problem 1)
  8. Cerebellar Cortical Degeneration (Daft Lamb Disease) (Problem 9)
II. Infectious, Inflammatory, Immune
  1. Diffuse Meningoencephalomyelitides (Problem 1)
III. Metabolic
  *1. Hypocalcemia and Hypomagnesemia
IV. Toxic
  *1. Metaldehyde—Snail Bait (Problem 2)
  *2. Organophosphates (Problem 2)
  *3. Chlorinated Hydrocarbons (Problem 2)
  *4. Plant-Associated Tremor Syndromes
  *5. Eggplant
  6. Arsanilic Acid and 3-Nitro (Problems 2 and 10)
  7. Mild Tetanus (Problem 8A)
V. Idiopathic
  *1. Acquired Tremor Syndromes
  2. Grove Poisoning (Problem 2)

I. Congenital and Familial
  1. Congenital Tremor (Hypomyelinogenesis)
    Signalment. Newborn Piglets, lambs, and occasionally calves are affected. It is hereditary in Saddleback (U.K.) and Landrace pigs (Bradley et al., 1986) and in Jersey (Saunders et al., 1952), Shorthorn (Hulland, 1957), and Angus-Shorthorn (Young, 1962).
    History. At birth or shortly after, degrees of tremor of the limbs and the head is seen. Some affected animals appear more ataxic than others. Signs usually are not progressive and animals may improve, even to normal, over several weeks to months.
    Physical Examination. This is unremarkable unless the neonate is a "runt" or it cannot nurse, then cachexia will occur. Lambs have a hairy fleece and difficulty gaining weight (Psychick-Sheard et al., 1980). A grayness to the coat has been seen in Holstein calves in association with this syndrome.
    Neurologic Signs. These consist of a fine to jerky tremor, usually of the limbs, trunk, and head. The animal may have a basewide stance and a hypometric or rocking-horse gait. Such signs of cerebellar ataxia can be so severe that affected neonates cannot stand unassisted (Saunders, 1952). Ataxia is present, but usually without weakness. The tremor often can be enhanced with excitement and

movement and usually abates with rest and sleep. "Dancing pig disease" is a descriptive term in pigs, as is "Hairy shaker disease" in lambs and "Jittery calves" (Saunders. 1952).

Assessment. The syndrome of congential tremor (CT) consists of varying degrees of cerebellar and spinal cord white matter signs and lesions. However, sometimes no histologic abnormalities are present. The latter is classed as type B congenital tremor in pigs and has been studied best.

Table 12–2 summarizes the clinical, pathologic, and biochemical characteristics of these syndromes, which have been studied in detail in pigs (Bradley et al., 1986). Usually variations of cerebellar hypoplasia and cerebrospinal hypomyelinogenesis (type A congenital tremor in pigs) are found at necropsy. In pigs there are five divisions of CT type A: AI, caused by in utero infection with swine fever virus; AII, caused by another unidentified virus; AIII, a sex-linked form in Landrace pigs; AIV, an autosomal recessive form in Saddleback pigs; and AV, associated with exposure to organophosphates in utero. The last of these causes may be more frequent than initially thought (Bolske et al., 1978), (Knox et al., 1978). An unidentified virus, called congenital tremor virus, has been described in the USA (Gustafson et al., 1986) and may represent CT AII. It is possible that other viruses, such as pseudorabies virus, may occasionally be associated with CT in swine (Mare et al., 1974).

Border disease or Hairy shaker disease originally was identified in lambs from the Scottish-English border; it is a form of hypomyelinogenesis associated with in utero infection with a transmissible agent that shares some antigens with bovine virus diarrhea virus. Affected lambs have a hairy fleece.

This disease results when lambs are infected with the Border disease virus early in gestation. The virus in the lamb is persistent and the animal has no virus neutralizing antibody response. In comparison, it appears that infection with the virus later in gestation results in cerebral cavitation and cerebellar dysplasia (similar to presumed copper deficiency syndrome), no persistence of virus, and a high virus neutralizing antibody response. Infection in late gestation may result in irregular serologic responses and pathologic lesions, possibly dependent on the acquisition of immune competence by the lamb (Roeder et al., 1987).

Experimental evidence suggests that Border disease, virus-induced hypomyelination is associated with decreased circulating thyroid hormone concentrations due to insidious infection of the thyroid gland by the virus (Anderson et al., 1987).

Holstein-Friesian calves with congenital tremor and occasional tetanus, and degrees of incoordination, absent menace response (without blindness), and nystagmus, have been found to be persistently infected with bovine virus diarrhea virus in an outbreak in Holland (Binkhorst et al., 1983), (Straver et al., 1983). The signs varied in severity, but tended to improve and were associated with hypomyelination in the central nervous system.

Table 12–2. Diagnostic Characteristics of the Congenital Tremor Syndrome in Pigs

			Type*			
	AI	*AII*	*AIII*	*AIV*	*AV*	*B*
Cause	*Virus, Hog Cholera*	*Virus, Unknown*	*Genetic, Sex-linked Recessive*	*Genetic, Autosomal Recessive*	*Chemical, Trichlorfon*	*Unknown*
Field observations						
Proportion of litters affected	High	High	Low	Low	High	Variable
% piglets affected in litter	40%	80%	25%	25%	90%	Variable
Mortality	Medium-high	Low	High	High	High	Variable
Sex	Both	Both	Male	Both	Both	Any
Breed of dam	Any	Any	Landrace	Saddleback	Any	Any
Recurrence with rebreeding	No	No	Yes	Yes	Yes	?
Duration of outbreak	Months	Months	Indefinite	Indefinite	Variable	?
Laboratory observations						
Macroscopic						
Cerebellum:whole brain % (≤8% = abnormal)	↓↓	~ ~	~ ↓	~ ↓	↓↓	~ ~
Spinal cord size (weight)						
Microscopic (CNS)						
Myelin deficiency	+	+	+	+	+	?
Myelin aplasia (partial)	−	−	+	−	−	?
Oligodendrocytes swollen	+	+	−	−	−	?
Oligodendrocytes reduced	?	?	+	?	?	?
Neurochemistry (spinal cord)						
Total DNA	↓	~	↓	↓	↓	Variable
Whole lipid/g	↓	↓	↓	↓	↓	Variable
Cerebrosides/g	↓	↓	↓	↓	↓	Variable
Lipid hexose:phosphorous ratio	↓	↓	↓	↓	~	Variable
Cholesterol esters characteristic of demyelination	+	+	−	+	−	?
Serology						
Maternal antibodies to hog cholera	+	−	−	−	−	−

Note: + = present, − = absent; ~ = not significantly changed; ↓ = decreased; ? = unknown.

*Type: A = a form of congenital tremor with defined pathological characters and known etiology; B = a form of congenital tremor as yet inadequately characterized and/or of unknown etiology.

Reprinted by permission from: Bradley R, Done JT: Nervous and Muscular Systems. In: *Diseases of the Swine.* 6th Ed. Leman AD, Straw B, Glock RD, et al. eds. Ames: Iowa State University Press, 1986: Ch 4, p 73, Table 4.4.

Affected calves of many breeds have varying degrees of hypo-myelinogenesis and cerebellar hypoplasia (Cho et al., 1977). The same lesions were present in two captive Eland Antelope and two sibling Santa Gertrudis calves showing degrees of tremor and cerebellar dysmetria (Mayhew IG, Kollias GV, 1986, unpublished).

Diagnosis. Confirmation of the disease is by histology and by histochemistry of myelin lipids (see Table 12–2).

Prognosis. There is no treatment, but many animals recover with time. Considerations of genetic influences, infectious agents, and organophosphates should be made clear to the owner.

2. Shaker Calf Syndrome

Clinical Syndrome. This rare neurodegenerative disorder occurs in newborn Horned Hereford calves of both sexes. Calves are born normally, but cannot stand. In several hours they develop fine generalized tremor involving the head, body, and tail, which is exaggerated by spontaneous activity or handling the calves. With assistance, affected calves may stand and suck, but become fatigued easily. Progressive stiffness and ataxia is evident, particularly in the hind limbs. One calf survived for 3 months with continual tremor, hyperesthesia, and aphonia (Rousseaux et al., 1985).

Assessment. There is an excessive accumulation of neurofilamentous material in motor neurons in the central, peripheral, and autonomic nervous systems.

Outcome. The disease is inherited and is lethal. It may model some neurodegenerative motor neuron diseases affecting man.

3. Hyperkalemic Periodic Paralysis in Horses

Signalment. Young-adult (2 to 3 years), mostly male Quarterhorses have been reported to be affected (Cox, 1985). Although not many cases are reported, this may be a frequently occurring disease in families of Quarterhorses. Possibly, it occurs in other breeds.

History. The owner notices episodes of muscle trembling over the body or face that may lead to involuntary recumbency. Exercise and rest following exercise may precipitate episodes which can occur daily or monthly.

Clinical Syndrome. Between episodes, affected, well-muscled Quarterhorses appear essentially normal. The onset of a mild attack may begin with repeated yawning and intermittent flicking of the third eyelid (Cox, 1985), (Steiss et al., 1986), followed by fasciculations or muscle tremor (particularly involving the flank, shoulders and neck, and sometimes the face). During an episode the horse is alert, appears distracted and reluctant to move, and may stumble as if weak. A severe episode, perhaps following forced exercise (or KCl provocation), results in severe tremor and tetany of many muscles with recumbency and sweating. This is followed by a state of flaccidity, possibly with depressed spinal reflexes. Attempts to move result in further tremor and tetany, although the horse remains alert. Episodes last up to 15 minutes.

Although the disease does not appear to be fatal, one horse suspected of being affected was found dead in its stall and one affected horse had an episode triggered by anesthesia—a potentially fatal complication (Cox, 1985).

Diagnosis. The clinical syndrome is distinct. A KCl provocation test can be used with caution to make a diagnosis using 0.08 to 0.13 g KCl/kg BW by nasogastric tube (Spier et al., 1987), (Cox, 1985).

It is possible that a period of hypocalcemia (9.0 to 9.4 mg/dl) will occur immediately following an attack. Hemoconcentration also appears to occur.

Most often during a clinical or KCl-provoked attack, hyperkalemia (5.5 to 9.4 mEq/L) is detectable (Cox, 1985), (Spier et al., 1987). Electromyographic (EMG) examination reveals fibrillation potentials and myotonic discharges in most muscles (Spier et al., 1987), (Steiss, 1986). In one affected stallion, EMG examination of the same muscles, repeated while the horse was at rest and while anesthetized, revealed fluctuation in the severity of the abnormal EMG findings, which included fibrillation potentials, positive sharp waves, trains of positive waves, and bizarre high frequency discharges (Brewer BD, Mayhew IG, pers. observ.).

Assessment. This appears to be a familial and possibly inherited disease. Increased Na^+ and decreased K^+ concentrations detected within erythrocytes of affected horses (Spier et al., 1987) may relate to defective Na/K ATPase function at the cellular membrane level.

Treatment. Attacks of tremor and tetany appear to be short-lived, although treatment of horses during attacks with intravenous fluids containing Ca^{++}, HCO_3^-, glucose and acetazolamide may shorten an attack (Spier et al., 1987).

Prevention. Acetazolamide at 0.5 to 2.2 mg/kg, BID, orally and hydrochlorothiazide at 0.5 mg/kg, BID, orally appear to have lessened the frequency and severity of attacks.

II. Metabolic

1. **Hypocalcemia (milk fever) and Hypomagnesemia (also Problem 2)**

   Signalment. These metabolic derangements occur in periparturient cows, ewes, sows, and occasionally in mares; they also occur in pregnant or lactating animals and are stress-related. Transportation and starvation play a role in transit tetany in feedlot animals (Lucas et al., 1982). Hypomagnesemia (grass tetany) usually occurs in postpartum cattle on lush pastures, but also in bucket-fed calves.

   History. There is a sudden onset of tetany or tremor. In ruminants this proceeds rapidly to flaccid muscles and recumbency with hypocalcemia, and to hypertonicity and seizures with hypomagnesemia.

   Physical Examination. The lactating animal usually is producing a lot of milk. Weakness, ruminal atony, and a weak, slow heart beat, are characteristic in cows with milk fever.

   Neurologic Examination. Generally hypocalcemia results in tremor and weakness, whereas hypomagnesemia results in tetanic spasms, a pounding heart, and hyperresponsiveness. (Note some species differences.) Cattle have sluggish pupils and hyporeflexia in hypocalcemia and tetany with hypomagnesemia. Horses with low serum ionized calcium concentration show muscle tremor, a staggery, high-stepping gait, weakness, seizures, and synchronous diaphragmatic flutter ("thumps").

Assessment. Hypocalcemia (milk fever) in cattle is common in high-producing dairy cows in the first 3 days postcalving. Animals with high calcium diets prepartum are also predisposed to hypocalcemia. Hypocalcemia frequently is seen in ewes 6 weeks prepartum until lambing, usually associated with some stress factors. Cattle appear to be more susceptible to the hypocalcemic neuromuscular blockade, with subsequent hypotonia, that masks the tetany seen only in the early course of disease.

Hypomagnesemia (grass tetany) is seen in grazing cattle on lush pasture 1 to 3 months postpartum. Transit tetany in horses and lambs is perhaps related mostly to low blood calcium rather than magnesium concentrations (Pierson et al., 1975); although pure hypomagnesemia in foals and calves may be associated with tetany, seizures, and death (Haggard et al., 1978), (Harrington, 1974).

Diagnosis. Serum calcium and magnesium concentrations should be determined. Ideally, ionized calcium concentrations are of more significance than total serum calcium concentrations. Determination of cerebrospinal fluid magnesium concentration may be useful in the diagnosis of grass tetany in cattle, even up to 12 hours postmortem (Pauli et al., 1974).

Treatment. Intravenous and subcutaneous calcium or magnesium salts should be given to effect, with continual monitoring of cardiac function when IV therapy is instituted. Clinicians empirically often use Ca, Mg, PO_4, and glucose mixtures in treatment of these syndromes. Further calcium injections often are required in milk fever cows to prevent relapses.

Prevention. A relatively low calcium intake immediately prior to parturition, increasing calcium and magnesium intake during lactation, and avoidance of stress in pre- and postparturient dams, are factors that can reduce the incidence of these disorders.

Prognosis. Hypomagnesemic animals can die suddenly because of the excitement of therapy. Other cases often respond rapidly. Relapses can be prevented with appropriate management changes and magnesium supplementation.

IV. Toxic

1. Metaldehyde

Metaldehyde (snail bait) has caused tremor and tetany, usually leading to seizures and death in adult cattle and horses. Gastrointestinal lavage and general anesthesia are indicated treatments (see Problem 2).

2. Organophosphates

Also covered in Problems 1, 2, and 10, and in section I.1 (hypomyelinogenesis). The syndrome of acquired (postnatal) tremor associated with the use of these compounds probably results from a peripheral neuromuscular blockade or a nicotinic effect (Scheidt et al., 1987).

3. **Chlorinated Hydrocarbons**

Usually seizures (see Problem 2) occur with tremor.

4. **Plant-associated Tremor Syndromes**

Signalment. Sheep, cattle, and less often, horses are affected, usually when they are out at pasture.

History. Multiple animals usually are affected with ataxia, tremor, recumbency, and sometimes death. The number affected may fluctuate day to day. Outbreaks are seasonal and often occur later in the period of plant growth. Several syndromes are recognized and are associated with specific plants (see Table 12–3).

Neurologic Examination. Signs include a stiff, ataxic, sometimes hypermetric gait, with a prominent, although often fine, muscle tremor that worsens when animals are disturbed (Fig. 12–3). Usually the tremor involves the head and trunk. When forced to move, animals may fall to the ground with tetanic movements (possibly with convulsions), jerky eye movements, and paddling (Fig. 12–3). They may die, especially with phalaris toxicity, although with ryegrass staggers most recover if left undisturbed.

Assessment. The pathogenesis of these diseases probably involves bio- or mycotoxins (Seawright, 1982) (see Table 12–3). Dallis and paspallum staggers result from infestation of grass with the ergots of *Claviceps paspali,* which produce a neurotoxin (Buck et al., 1986). Phalaris (canary) grasses contain three tryptamine alkaloids that interfere with serotonic neurotransmitter release. Phalaris neurotoxicity may be altered by cobalt administration or topdressing of pastures, although this has not been substantiated. Accumulation of pigment in neurons, axonal degeneration, and fibrillary astrogliosis all have been found in sheep with Canary grass staggers (East et al., 1988). *Penicillium* sp molds that can produce tremorogenic indoles (penitrems) may account for some outbreaks of these syndromes. Cattle, sheep, pigs, and horses can be affected by a tremor syndrome similar to ryegrass staggers, which results from presumed

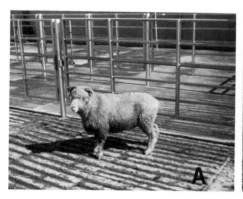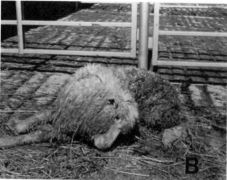

Figure 12–3. Two sheep grazing in a phalaris grass pasture showing degrees of a tremor that are typical of plant associated syndromes. The ram (A) had a slight head tremor and ataxia. With stimulation it would develop whole body tremor and became recumbent like the ewe (B), showing jerky, tetanic paddling movements.

Table 12–3. Several Acquired Tremor Syndromes Affecting Cattle, Sheep, and Horses Associated With Ingestion of Biologic Tremorogens

Syndrome	Associated Plants	Clinical Signs	Probable Source of Toxin	Pathogenesis	Neural Lesions	*Prognosis
Ryegrass staggers	Perenial ryegrass (*Lolium perenne*)	Ataxia, tremor, tetany	*Acremonium loliae* fungal endophytes	Lolitrem B (A,C) tremorogenic indoles	Secondary Purkinje cell degeneration	Excellent
Phalaris staggers	Canary grasses (*Phalaris* spp)	Tremor, tetany, seizures, cardiac arrhythmia, death	Phalaris grasses	Dimethyltryptamine alkaloids; monoamine oxidase inhibition	Neuronal pigmentation (indole melanins); axon degeneration, astrogliosis	Poor
Nervous form of ergotism	Dallis, Tobosa, Galleta grasses (*Paspallum* spp)	Ataxia, tremor, rarely convulsions	*Claviceps paspalli* (and other) ergot sclerotia	Ergot alkaloids or tremorogenic indoles	None	Good
Annual ryegrass toxicity	Annual or Wimmera ryegrass (*Lolium rigidum*)	Tremor, tetany, opisthotonus, convulsions	Bacterial galls (*Corynebacterium rathayi*) introduced by nematode (*Anguina agrostis*)	Corynetoxin glycolipids	Edema in cerebellar meninges	Fair
Aspergillus spp tremor syndrome	Sorghum beer residue (Others)	Tremor, ataxia, paralysis, death	*Aspergillus clavatus*	*Aspergillus* tremorogens	Degeneration of motor neurons	Bad
Miscellaneous plant-associated tremor syndromes	Bermuda grass (*Cynodon dactylon*), Rayless goldenrod (*Iscoma wrightii*), Coyotillo (*Karwinskia humboldtiana*), Mountain laurel, Mescalbeen (*Sophora* spp), (Others)	Trembling, ataxia, paralysis, death (others)	Plant or associated mycotoxin	Unknown	Variable: None to axonopathy to myopathy	Poor to bad

*Treatment includes removing animal from access to known or suspected toxin and catharsis. Diazepam and chlordiazepoxide, for control of tremor, and phenobarbital, as an anticonvulsant, may be tried when indicated.
Data from: Seawright, 1982; BL Smith, 1986; Buck et al., 1986; Bailey, 1986; Kellerman et al., 1976; Finnie et al., 1985; Berry et al., 1980; Norris et al., 1981; Munday et al., 1985.

ingestion of mycotoxins in stored feeds or while grazing. The best described of these is Penitrem A, a neurotoxin produced by *Penicillium cyclopium* (Seawright, 1982).

Currently it is believed that lolitrem B is the staggers toxin produced when the endophyte *Acremonium loliae* infests ryegrass (*Lolium perenne*) pastures (BL Smith 1986, pers. comm.), (Munday et al., 1985) or seed cleanings (Munday et al., 1985). Plants have been shown to be able to take up tremorogenic mycotoxins through intact roots and concentrate it in the growing shoots (Day et al., 1980). One mechanism, which has been studied, that may relate to the clinical signs in ryegrass staggers is neurotransmitter release (Mantle, 1983). It has been shown that cerebrocortical synaptosomes of affected sheep have the ability to spontaneously release excessive amounts of aspartic and glutamic acids, which are excitatory neurotransmitters.

Miscellaneous poisonous plants (see Table 12–3) can induce tremor syndromes either directly, or through, as yet unidentified, bio or mycotoxins (Bailey, 1986).

Diagnosis. The diagnosis is made clinically, ruling out other possibilities, and observing the affected animal's response to moving from the suspected pasture. Identification of some tremorogenic toxins is possible (Munday et al., 1985), (Kellerman et al., 1976), (Seawright, 1982).

In one outbreak of Canary grass staggers, CSF from affected sheep had slightly increased protein content and a mild mononuclear pleocytosis, with pigment granules present in some of the macrophages (East et al., 1988).

Treatment. Quickly and quietly remove the animals from the pasture or take away contaminated feed. Some sedation (with benzodiazepine drugs) (Norris et al., 1981) and nursing care may be required. Using cobalt (<28 mg/sheep/week orally, or topdress pastures) for phalaris staggers has been suggested. Cautious administration of cathartics seems appropriate.

Prognosis. Many animals recover, especially in some syndromes (Table 12–3).

5. Eggplant

Feeding eggplant (*Solanum melongena*) to cattle rarely has been associated with continual tremor and cerebellar signs in pregnant cows and their newborn calves. However, death can occur following recumbency and seizures. Histologically, evidence of disruption of myelin, with diffuse status spongiosis in cerebral and cerebellar white matter, is present in some cases.

V. Idiopathic

1. Acquired Tremor Syndromes

Acquired whole body tremor and tetany occurs in adult horses. It is not understood what mechanism is operative; mild cases of tetanus, meningitis, and mycotoxicosis cannot always be excluded from the diagnosis. Usually affected animals survive.

Landrace trembles is a disease of Landrace pigs that have tremor of the tail and ears, which is exacerbated by backing the animal. Occasionally the tremor involves more of the body, but is not incapacitating. Signs are most often seen at 4 to 6 months of age and regress over several weeks (Gedde-Dahl et al., 1970).

Problem 8C:

Other Localized Muscle Spasms and Movement Disorders

Spasticity usually refers to stiffness when a limb is positioned or moved, and it also indicates a state of continuous muscular hypertonia. If spasticity is caused by upper motor neuron disease, then it is accompanied by degrees of weakness; if there is spinal cord or caudal brainstem disease, usually ataxia occurs. The syndromes discussed herein do not, for the most part, relate to a focal CNS lesion. In man, lesions in areas of the extrapyramidal upper motor neuronal system, particularly in the basal nuclei, can cause intermittent writhing or flailing movements, referred to as athetosis or ballismus, respectively. Whether or not these occur in large animals is not clear, but specific upper motor neuron (functional) lesions may be suspected in some of the syndromes described below. More likely, several of these syndromes involve other components of the myotatic reflex, which control muscle tone (see Fig. 12–1).

On occasion, a large animal may show intermittent, usually irregular, muscle spasms of part of the neck or trunk or a limb. Some of these signs disappear and others remain constant. Partial damage to peripheral nerves or muscles or mild localized myelopathies usually are considered as causes, but this has not been proven (Fig. 12–6B).

Categories of Disease and Differential Diagnosis
*NOTE: Only those diseases marked * are discussed in this section.*

- I. Congenital and Familial
    - *1. Spastic Syndrome of Adult Cattle
    - *2. Spastic Paresis of Calves
    - 3. Hyperkalemic Periodic Paralysis (Problem 8B)
- II. Physical
    - *1. Fibrotic Myopathy
- III. Infectious, Inflammatory, Immune
    - 1. Focal Myeloencephalitides (Problems 1, 10)
- IV Toxic
    - 1. Mild Tetanus (Problem 8A)
    - 2. Lathyrism (see Stringhalt below)
    - 3. Delayed Organophosphate Toxicity in Swine (Problem 10)

VI. Nutritional
  *1. Pantothenic Acid Deficiency
VII. Idiopathic
  *1. Stringhalt, Lathyrism, Shivering
  *2. Hindlimb Spasticity in Piglets
  *3. Upward Fixation of the Patella

I. Congenital and Familial

  1. **Spastic Syndrome of Adult Cattle (Standings Disease, Barn Cramps, Crampiness, Stretches, Periodic Spasticity)**

  Signalment. Adult cattle, particularly 3- to 7-year-old Holstein and Guernsey bulls, at artificial breeding centers are affected (Roberts, 1965).

  History. There is an onset of progressive, periodic jerking and stiffness of the pelvic limbs and back, particularly noted when the animal stands up (Fig. 12–4).

  Clinical Signs. Periodic contraction of extensor muscles of the lumbar region and extensor and abductor muscles of the pelvic limbs, which may last many minutes, result in lordosis and in limb abduction and caudal extension (Fig. 12–4). Trembling of the hindlimbs, which may be violent, usually is seen. This motion has been likened to stringhalt, but is not a flexion movement of the hip, stifle, and hock. Signs usually are worse when the animal first stands up; they abate during recumbency. Movement is impossible during attacks (Palmer, 1976). Early on it is difficult to distinguish the syndrome from lumbosacral spondyloarthrosis, hip lesions, gonitis, upward patellar fixation, and excessively straight hindlimb conformation.

  Assessment. A familial tendency has been observed. Pedigree analysis of 892 bulls culled from artificial breeding establishments strongly indicates the disease was inherited as an autosomal dominant gene with incomplete penetrance (Sponenberg et al., 1985). A defect in the myotatic reflex arcs or postural reaction (upper motor neuron) pathways may be present. No significant neuromuscular pathologic findings are present (Wells et al., 1987).

  Treatment. Mephenesin (30 to 40 mg/kg, orally, for 2 to 3 days) may control severe signs for some weeks, but has not been consistently useful (Braun RK, pers comm). The syndrome persists for the animal's life and usually progresses.

  2. **Spastic Paresis of Calves (Elso Heel)**

  Signalment. This syndrome occurs frequently in calves 1 week to 12 months old, which usually are at pasture and suckling their dam. Many breeds are affected, particularly Holstein-Friesian, Angus, Ayrshire, and Shorthorn breeds in the USA and UK. Occasionally, a similar syndrome occurs in adult cattle (Bradley et al., 1980).

  Physical Examination. The calves have excessively straight hocks and an awkward, stiff, usually asymmetric pelvic limb gait. The forelimbs often are straight also (Fig. 12–5A).

  Neurologic Examination. The hocks are straight and the gastroc-

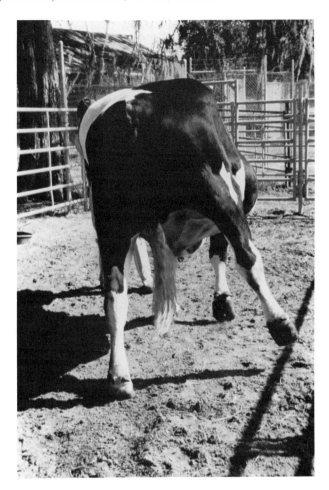

Figure 12–4. Spastic syndrome of adult cattle. This mature Holstein show steer demonstrates the typical motion of the hind limbs. Both limbs are rigidly extended and are abducted during protraction. The lumbar muscles also are contracted. Signs abate somewhat with movement.

nemius muscles have excessive tone. Usually both limbs are affected, but one more severely, causing it to be held extended behind the calf and to jerk forward without touching the ground at each step.

Assessment. Chemical (dilute epidural procaine) or surgical de-afferentation of the gastrocnemius muscle obviates spasticity, therefore the pathogenic mechanism underlying the syndrome is thought to be an overactive myotatic reflex (De Ley et al., 1977), (De Lay et al., 1979/1980). Some evidence that there is an imbalance of seroto-nergic vs dopaminergic neurotransmitter activity in spinal fluid has been presented (De Ley et al., 1975).

The syndrome appears to be familial and certain famous sires have been incriminated as genetic carriers. These include an East Friesland bull, Elso II (hence the name Elso heel) and a Dutch bull, Adema 197, both Frieslands. The evidence available suggests that if this syndrome is genetically controlled, it is of low heritability (Daw-

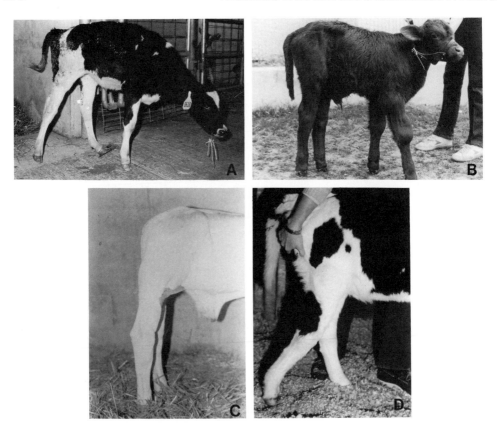

Figure 12–5. Spastic paresis of calves (Elso heel) and some conditions that must be differentiated from it. With typical spastic paresis (A) there are stiff, pendular movements of the hind limbs, often more severe in one limb. The forelimbs are usually straight also. Several conditions, including polyarthritis (B), congenital upward fixation of the patella (C), and laxity with overextension of the hock in Holstein calves (D), can result in stiff movement of the pelvic limbs and must be differentiated from spastic paresis.

son, 1975). The role of environmental factors, including micronutrients such as magnesium, has been raised (Leipold, 1982).

Diagnosis. This is based on the clinical syndrome. However, gonitis and generalized arthritis (Fig. 12–5B), upward patellar fixation (Fig. 12–5C), arthrogryposis, and congenital laxity and overextension of the hock joints in Holstein calves (Fig. 12–5D), frequently are confused with this syndrome and must be ruled out.

Therapy. Partial or total tibial neurectomy is esthetically pleasing, simple, and relatively effective. This is performed on the lateral aspect of the stifle between the two heads of the biceps femoris muscle (Bouckaert et al., 1966). Gastrocnemius tenotomy is not cosmetic, but it can be an effective salvage procedure. Lithium gluconate, 50 mg/kg/d, orally for 1 month has been claimed to be successful if begun early in the course of disease (Arnault, 1982).

Prognosis. This syndrome is assumed by many to be inherited but this has not been proven. If no therapy is undertaken, with time joint deformities in the back, stifle, and hip occur, progressing to recumbency.

II. Physical

1. Fibrotic Myopathy

Signalment. An abnormal slapping-type gait developing in one pelvic limb of a light-breed horse is regarded as typical for fibrotic myopathy.

History. It occurs most often in adult Quarterhorses, but has been observed as a congenital condition. A few cases follow single or repeated intramuscular injections in the caudal thigh musculature, or external injury to the limb (Turner et al., 1984), (Bramlage et al, 1985).

Examination. A firmess or scar, with or without mineralization, may be palpable in the semimembranosus, biceps femoris, or most often, in the semitendinosus muscle. The gait is characterized by sudden caudoventral movement of the foot near the end of the protraction phase with the hoof striking the ground with a variably increased force. No weakness or ataxia is present.

Assessment. It is assumed that a mechanical interruption by the scar tissue of normal muscle contraction results in the gait abnormality. However, a sensory neurologic defect disrupting gamma efferent function (myotatic reflex), similar to that occurring in stringhalt, may be operative. On occasion, horses with confirmed thoracolumbar spinal cord disease, most often caused by equine protozoal myeloencephalitis (see Problem 10), have demonstrated a prominent fibrotic myopathy-like gait, along with other signs of mild paraparesis and ataxia.

Treatment. Traditionally, surgical removal of affected muscle and scar tissue usually resulted in complete alleviation of the signs (Turner, 1984), (Turner et al., 1984). However, tenotomy of the tibial insertion of the semitendinosus tendon is far more cosmetic and probably results in a greater cure rate with fewer complications (Bramlage et al., 1985).

III. Nutritional

1. Pantothenic Acid Deficiency

Ataxia, with prominent high stepping or goose-stepping action of the pelvic limbs, appears to be related to pantothenic acid deficiency in swine. There is a degenerative polyneuropathy (Palmer, 1976). The complete syndrome warrants comparison with Australian Stringhalt.

IV. Idiopathic

1. Stringhalt, Lathyrism, and Shivering

Signalment. Adult horses of any breed are affected with Stringhalt and Lathyrism. Shivering occurs most often in draft breeds and is progressive.

History. Usually there is an abrupt onset of excessive flexion of one or both hind limbs (Fig. 12–6). The signs may progressively worsen (Australian stringhalt and lathyrism) and may occur in outbreaks (Australian stringhalt).

Clinical Syndromes. A stringhalt gait (Fig. 12–6A), with degrees

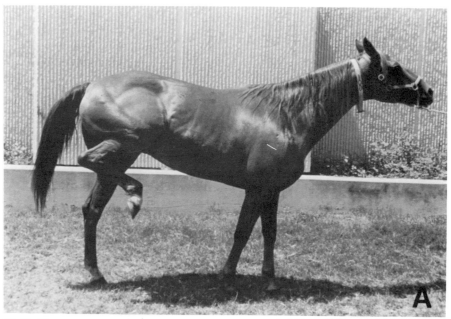

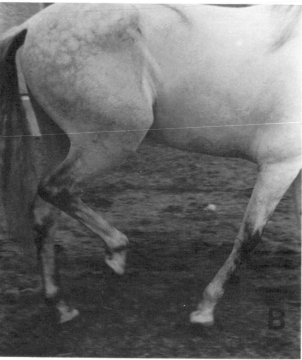

Figure 12–6. Stringhalt in the horse. The involuntary, hyperflexion of a pelvic limb, typical of stringhalt, is shown by this light bred mare (A). In this case the signs were bilateral, unassociated with injury to the limbs, and resolved over a period of several months, thereby resembling Australian stringhalt or lathyrism. The horse in B had spinal cord disease and demonstrated a stringhalt-like gait as well as some asymmetric ataxia and weakness. Treatment for protozoal myelitis was instituted and the signs improved.

of hyperflexion of one or both hind limbs during movements, is an ancient syndrome that frequently occurs as a sporadic syndrome in adult, light breed horses, probably worldwide (Cahill, 1985), (Pemberton et al., 1980). The syndrome is like that produced by tibial neurectomy, with unopposed hock flexion and digital extension (peroneal nerve) function predominant; the hoof may even strike the abdomen. Australian (epidemic) stringhalt refers to the syndrome that occurs often in outbreaks, with involvement (often profound) of both rear limbs and even the forelimbs and neck. With such severe signs, extensor and flexor muscle spasms occur and the horse can hardly move, and is considered to be in a state of tetanus (see Problem 8A). Atrophy, particularly involving the distal limb muscles, may be present in severe cases although, paradoxically, increased muscle tone is present. Intoxication with sweet pea plants (lathyrism) results in a clinically identical syndrome.

Shivering, with mild muscle tremor involving the hind quarters and tail and occurring with movement, especially backing, particularly affects draft breeds (also see Fig. 14–35).

Assessment. These syndromes could potentially be caused by a sensory neuropathy, a myopathy, or spinal cord disease. They also resemble some of the human, extrapyramidal, upper motor neuron disorders, but this site of lesion seems less tenable in horses. In all cases an alteration to the neuromuscular spindle and gamma efferent, and 1A and 1B afferent pathways, which controls muscle tone and contraction at the local spinal cord and peripheral nerve levels is likely (see Fig. 12–1). In lathyrism and Australian stringhalt distal nerve fiber degeneration in the sciatic nerve occurs (Cahill et al, 1986). Presumably, this first occurs in afferent fibers, with later involvement of α motor fibers, and subsequent neurogenic muscle atrophy in severe cases. Other long nerves, including the recurrent laryngeal nerves, may be affected; the lesions present in Australian stringhalt have been likened to those present in Roarers (see Problem 5H). Some isolated monomelic cases are associated with previous injury to the hock; these could represent an acquired resetting of the neuromuscular spindle trigger (Fig. 12–1).

Shivering is not currently well documented and one case described (Deen, 1984) bears resemblance to spastic syndrome of adult cattle and to complex, abnormal gaits seen with equine protozoal myeloencephalitis.

Diagnosis. This is based on the clinical syndrome and on ruling out other problems. Mild forms need to be differentiated from upward fixation of the patellar and other musculoskeletal lameness. Occasionally, equine protozoal myeloencephalitis and other spinal cord diseases (Problems 10, 11) result in a stringhalt-like gait (Fig. 12–6B).

Therapy. Horses should be removed from toxic plants or, if there are multiple cases, from the area. Mephenesin (Dixon et al., 1969) and several other muscle relaxant drugs do not appear to be useful in relieving the condition. Many cases of sporadic stringhalt and possibly all mild cases of epidemic stringhalt improve slowly with time (Cahill,

1985). Tenectomy of the lateral digital extensor tendon (Turner, 1984) often helps, even in cases of lathyrism; however, this does not cure severe cases. Unless evidence of hock trauma is present, it may be better to rest the horse for a while (months) before attempting surgery (Cahill, 1985).

2. Hindlimb Spasticity in Piglets

An outbreak of stiffness, interpreted as spasticity, was seen in all 61, 2-week-old piglets of 8 litters born during a 4 month period in a single piggery in South Africa (Newsholine et al., 1980). Neuronal chromatolysis and degeneration was detected and may be associated with the syndrome. The cause was not determined.

3. Upward Fixation of the Patella

Although this is a musculoskeletal disorder, it warrants consideration as a differential diagnosis for several of the above diseases.

This syndrome may be congenital (Fig. 12–5C) and also occurs in horses and cattle as an apparently acquired disorder. The patella and its medial patellar ligament become momentarily (mild) or permanently (severe) caught above the medial trochlear of the femur (Figs. 12–5C and 12–7). When the patella releases, the limb flexes

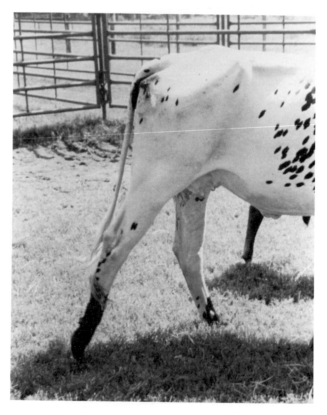

Figure 12–7 Upward fixation of the patella may be acquired (here) or may be congenital (Fig. 12–5C) in cattle and horses. The acquired condition can mimic stringhalt (and is referred to as such in cattle) because the hyperextended limb (as shown) may release rapidly to hyperflex to the position seen in Figure 12–6.

forward rapidly, resembling stringhalt; cattlemen in Florida refer to the acquired condition as stringhalt. More permanent fixation results in a syndrome almost identical to spastic paresis (Fig. 12–5), from which it is differentiated by there being no constant tension in the gastrocnemius tendon. Severe cases have disuse atrophy of the quarter. Medial patellar desmotomy (Turner, 1984) and improving general muscle conditioning and strength usually resolve the problem.

REFERENCES

Adams JM, Kenny JD, Rudolph AJ. Modern management of tetanus neonatorum. Ped 1979; *64*:472–477.

Anderson CA, Higgins RJ, Smith ME, et al. Border disease. Virus-induced decrease in thyroid hormone levels with associated hypomyelination. Lab Invest 1986; *57*:168–175.

Bailey ME. Principal poisonous plants in the southwestern United States. *Current Veterinary Therapy: Food Animal Practice,* 2nd Ed. Howard JL, ed. Philadelphia: WB Saunders, 1986. pp 412–416.

Baird JD, Wojcinski ZW, Wise AP, et al. Maple syrup urine disease in five Hereford calves in Ontario. Can Vet J 1987; *28*:505–511.

Beech J. Forelimb tic in a horse. J Am Vet Med Assoc 1982; *180*:258–260.

Berry PH, Howell JMcC, Cook RD, et al. Central nervous system changes in sheep and cattle affected with natural or experimental annual ryegrass toxicity. Aust Vet J 1980; *56*:402–403.

Binkhorst GJ, Journee DLH, Wouda W, et al. Neurological disorders, virus persistence and hypomyelination in calves due to intrauterine infections with bovine virus diarrhea virus. I. Clinical symptoms and morphological lesions. Vet Q 1983; *5*:145–155.

Bolske G, Kronevi T, Lindgren NO. Congenital tremor in pigs in Sweden. A case report. Nord Vet Med 1978; *30*:534–537.

Bouckaert JH, DeMoor A. Treatment of spastic paralysis in cattle: Improved de-nervation technique of the gastrocnemius muscle and post-operative course. Vet Rec 1966; *79*:226–229.

Bradley R, Wijeratne WVS. A locomotor disorder clinically similar to spastic paresis in an adult Friesian bull. Vet Pathol 1980; *17*:305–317.

Bradley R, Done JT. Nervous and Muscular Systems. In: *Diseases of Swine,* 6th Ed. Leman AD, Straw B, Glock RD, et al., eds. Ames: Iowa State University Press, 1986. pp 58–81.

Bramlage LR, Reed SM, Embertson RM. Semitendinosus tenotomy for treatment of fibrotic myopathy in the horse. J Am Vet Med Assoc 1985; *186*:565–567.

Buck WB, Cysewski SJ. Nervous form of ergotism. *Current Veterinary Therapy: Food Animal Practice,* 2nd Ed. Howard JL, ed. Philadelphia: WB Saunders, 1986. p 369.

Cahill JI, Goulden BE, Pearce HG. A review and some observations on stringhalt. NZ Vet J 1985; *33*:101–104.

Cahill JI, Goulden BE, Jolly RD. Stringhalt in horses: A distal axonopathy. Neuropathol Appl Neurobiol 1986; *12*:459–475.

Cho DY, Leipold HW. Congenital defects of the bovine central nervous system. Vet Bull 1977; *47*:489–504.

Cordy DR, Richards WPC, Stormant C. Hereditary neuraxial edema in Hereford calves. Vet Pathol 1969; *6*:487–501.

Cox JH. An episodic weakness in four horses associated with intermittent serum hyperkalemia and the similarity of the disease to hyperkalemic periodic paralysis in man. Proc 31st Annu Conf Am Assoc Equine Pract Nov/Dec 1985; 383–391.

Dawson PLL. The economic aspect of spastic paresis of the hind legs of Friesian cattle. Vet Rec 1975; *97*:432–433.

Day JB, Mantle PG. Tremorogenic forage and ryegrass staggers. Vet Rec 1980; *106*:463–464.

de Lahunta A. *Veterinary Neuroanatomy and Clinical Neurology.* 2nd Ed. Philadelphia: WB Saunders, 1976. pp 130–155.

De Ley G, De Moor A. Bovine spastic paralysis: Results of selective γ-efferent suppression with dilute procaine. Vet Sci Comm 1979/1980; *3*:289–298.

De Ley G, De Moor A. Bovine spastic paralysis: Cerebrospinal fluid concentrations of homovanillic acid and 5-hydroxyindoleacetic acid in normal and spastic calves. Am J Vet Res 1975; *36*:227–228.

De Ley G, De Moor A. Bovine spastic paralysis: Results of surgical desafferentation of the gastrocnemius muscle by means of spinal dorsal root resection. Am J Vet Res 1977; *38*:1899–1900.

Deen T. Shivering, a rare equine lameness. A case report. Equine Pract 1984; *6*:19–21.

Dixon RT, Stewart GA. Clinical and pharmacological observations in a case of equine stringhalt. Aust Vet J 1969; *45*:127–130.

Donaldson C, Mason RW. Hereditary neuraxial oedema in a Poll Hereford herd. Aust Vet J 1984; *61*:188–189.

Duffell SJ. Neuraxial oedema of Hereford calves with and without hypomyelinogenesis. Vet Rec 1986; *118*:95–98.

East NE, Higgins RJ. Canary grass (*Phalaris* sp) toxicosis in sheep in California. J Am Vet Med Assoc 1988; *192*:667–669.

Finnie JW, Jago MV. Experimental production of annual ryegrass toxicity with tunicamycin. Aust Vet J 1985; *62*:248–249.

Gedde-Dahl TW, Standal N. A note on a tremor condition in adolescent pigs. Anim Prod 1970; *12*:665–668.

Gregory KE, Arthaud VH, Koch RM, et al. Inheritance of a spastic lethal in cattle. J Hered 1962; *53*:130–132.

Gustafson DP, Bolin SR. Congenital tremors. In: *Diseases of Swine,* 6th Ed. Leman AD, Straw B, Glock RD, et al., eds. Ames: Iowa State University Press, 1986, pp 395–398.

Haggard DL, Whitehair CK, Langham RF. Tetany associated with magnesium deficiency in suckling beef calves. J Am Vet Med Assoc 1978; *172*:495–497.

Harper PAW, Healy PJ, Dennis JA. Maple syrup urine disease as a cause of spongiform encephalopathy in calves. Vet Rec 1986a; *119*:62–65.

Harper PAW, Healy PJ, Dennis JA. Inherited congenital myoclonus of polled Hereford calves (so-called neuraxial oedema): A clinical, pathological and biochemical study. Vet Rec 1986b; *119*:59–62.

Harrington DD. Pathologic features of magnesium deficiency in young horses fed purified rations. Am J Vet Res 1974; *35*:503–513.

Healy PJ, Harper PAW, Dennis JA. Diagnosis of neuraxial oedema in calves. Aust Vet J 1986; *63*:95–96.

High JW, Kincaid CM, Smith HJ. Doddler Cattle. An inherited congenital nervous disorder in Hereford calves. J Heredity 1958; *49*:250–252.

Hulland TJ. Cerebellar ataxia in calves. Can J Comp Med 1957; *21*:72–76.

Jolly RD. Congenital brain oedema of Hereford calves. J Pathol 1974; *114*:199–204.

Kellerman TS, Pienaar JG, Van Der Westhuizen GCA, et al. A highly fatal tremorgenic mycotoxicosis of cattle caused by *Aspergillus clavatus*. Onderstepoort J Vet Res 1976; *43*:147–154.

Kidd ARM, Done JT, Wrathall AE,. et al. A new genetically-determined congenital nervous disorder in pigs. Brit Vet J 1986; *142*:275–285.

Knox B, Askaa J, Basse A, et al. Congenital ataxia and tremor with cerebellar hypoplasia in piglets borne by sows treated with Neguvon® vet. (metrifonate, trichlorfon) during pregnancy. Nord Vet Med 1978; *30*:538–545.

Leipold HW. Review of Arnault S. *Study of Bovine Spastic Paresis.* Bovine Pract 1982; *3*:31–32.

Liefman CE. Combined active-passive immunisation of horses against tetanus. Aust Vet J 1980; *56*:119–122.

Liefman CE. Active immunisation of horses against tetanus including the booster dose and its application. Aust Vet J 1981; *57*:57–60.

Liu IKM, Brown SL, Kuo J, et al. Duration of maternally derived immunity to tetanus and response in newborn foals given tetanus antitoxin. Am J Vet Res 1982; *43*:2019–2022.

Lucas MJ, Huffman EM, Johnson LW. Clinical and clinicopathologic features of transport tetany of feedlot lambs. J Am Vet Med Assoc 1982; *18*:381–383.

Mantle PG. Amino acid neurotransmitter release from cerebrocortical synaptosomes of sheep with severe ryegrass staggers in New Zealand. Res Vet Sci 1983; *34*:373–375.

Maré CJ, Kluge JP. Pseudorabies virus and myoclonia congenita in pigs. J Am Vet Med Assoc 1974; *164*:309–310.

Mellanby J. Comparative activities of tetanus and botulinum toxins. Neuroscience 1984; *11*:29–34.

Munday BL, Monkhouse IM, Gallagher RT. Intoxication of horses by lolitrem B in ryegrass seed cleanings. Aust Vet J 1985; *62*:207.

Muylle E, Oyaert W, Ooms L, et al. Treatment of tetanus in the horse by injections of tetanus antitoxin into the subarachnoid space. J Am Vet Med Assoc 1975; *167*:47–48.

Newsholme SJ, Marshall LW. Unilateral hindleg spasticity: Outbreak of a specific clinical condition in suckling piglets. J S Afr Vet Assoc 1980; *51*:195–198.

Norris RT. Treatment of ovine annual ryegrass toxicity with chlordiazepoxide: A field evaluation. Aust Vet J 1981; *57*:302–303.

Owen LN, Leam G. The treatment of tetanus with particular reference to chlorpromazine. Vet Rec 1959; *71*:61–65.

Palmer AC. *Introduction to Animal Neurology.* 2nd Ed. Oxford: Blackwell Scientific Publications, 1976. pp 44–48, 166, 1984.

Pauli JV, Allsop TF. Plasma and cerebrospinal fluid magnesium, calcium and potassium concentrations in dairy cows with hypomagnesaemic tetany. NZ Vet J 1974; *22*:227–231.

Pemberton DH, Caple IW. Australian stringhalt in horses. Vet Ann 1980; *20*:167–171.

Physick-Sheard PW, Hopkins JB, O'Connor RD. A border disease-like syndrome in a southern Ontario sheep flock. Can Vet J 1980; *21*:53–60.

Pierson RE, Jensen R. Transport tetany in feedlot lambs. J Am Vet Med Assoc 1975; *166*:260–261.

Roberts SJ. Hereditary spastic diseases affecting cattle in New York State. Cornell Vet 1965; *55*:637–644.

Roeder PL, Jeffrey M, Drew TW. Variable nature of border disease on a single farm: The infection status of affected sheep. Res Vet Sci 1987; *43*:28–33.

Rousseaux CG, Klavano GG, Johnson ES, et al. "Shaker" calf syndrome: A newly recognized inherited neurodegenerative disorder of horned Hereford calves. Vet Pathol 1985; *22*:104–111.

Saunders LZ, Sweet JD, Martin SM, et al. Hereditary congenital ataxia in Jersey calves. Cornell Vet 1952; *42*:559–590.

Scheidt AB, Long GG, Knox K, et al. Toxicosis in newborn pigs associated with cutaneous application of an aerosol spray containing chlorpyrifos. J Am Vet Med Assoc 1987; *191*:1410–1412.

Seawright AA. *Animal Health in Australia. Chemical and Plant Poisons.* Vol 2. Canberra: Australian Government Publishing Service, 1982.

Sedaghatian MR. Intrathecal serotherapy in neonatal tetanus: A controlled trial. Arch Dis Child 1979; *54*:623–625.

Smith BL. Ryegrass staggers. Ruakura Animal Research Station, New Zealand, 1986; pers. comm.

Spier SJ, Carlson GP, Madigan JE. Potassium fluxes in horses with episodic weakness resembling hyperkalemic periodic paralysis. Vth Annu Am Coll Vet Int Med Forum, Abstract No 53, 1987; p 913.

Sponenberg DP, Vanvleck LD, McEntee K. The genetics of the spastic syndrome in dairy bulls. Vet Rec 1985; 92–94.

Steiss JE, Naylor JM. Episodic muscle tremors in a quarter horse: Resemblance to hyperkalemic periodic paralysis. Can Vet J 1986; *27*:332–335.

Straver PJ, Journee DLH, Binkhorst GJ. Neurological disorders, virus persistence and hypomyelination in calves due to intrauterine infections with bovine virus diarrhoea virus. II. Virology and epizootiology. Vet Q 1983; *5*:156–164.

Turner AS. Large Animal Orthopedics. In: *The Practice of Large Animal Surgery.* Jennings PB, ed. Vol 2. Philadelphia: WB Saunders, 1984, Ch 16, pp 937–949.

Turner AS, Trotter GW. Fibrotic myopathy in the horse. J Am Vet Med Assoc 1984; *184*:335–353.

Wells GAH, Hawkins SAC, O'Tool DT, et al. Spastic syndrome in a Holstein bull: A histologic study. Vet Pathol 1987; *24*:345–353.

Wintzer H-J, Körber H-D, Holland U. Zur tetanusprophylaxe beim Pferd. Berl Münch Tierärztl Wschr 1975; *88*:181–183.

Young S. Hypomyelinogenesis congenita (cerebellar ataxia) in Angus-Shorthorn calves. Cornell Vet 1962; *52*:84–93.

CHAPTER 13

Problem 9:
Incoordination of the Head and Limbs: Cerebellar Diseases

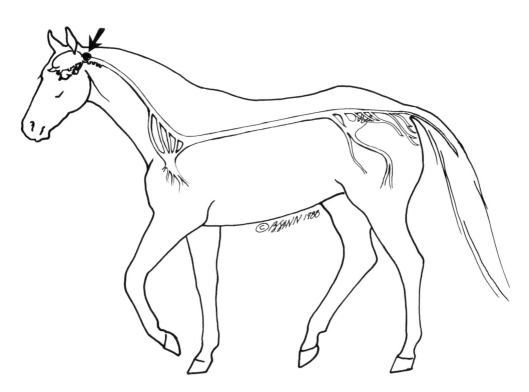

Locations of lesions resulting in incoordination of the head and limbs: diffuse and focal cerebellum (arrow).

Syndromes with combinations of ataxia, weakness, and dysmetria of the pelvic limbs, all four limbs, and sometimes of the head, and even rare cases of episodic weakness, have been referred to as wobblers, particularly in horses. The sites of lesions that result in such signs include the brainstem, cerebellum, cervical, thoracic, lumbar, and sacral spinal cord, spinal nerve roots, peripheral nerves, neuromuscular junctions, and muscles. Evidence of cranial nerve disorders should alert the examiner to vestibular disease (Problem 6) and other

227

brainstem and cranial nerve disorders (Problem 5). Diseases with additional signs such as widespread tremor, tetanus, and muscle spasms and those that particularly involve one limb or the tail and anus, are discussed in Problems 8, 11, and 12 respectively.

At the conclusion of a neurologic examination, the clinician should be able to identify cerebellar involvement. Although pure cerebellar diseases result in ataxia of the limbs, no weakness is evident. This distinguishes cerebellar disease from most of the other disorders discussed in Problem 10. The ataxic gait seen with cerebellar disease may be hypermetric (high stepping) ataxia, or hypometric (stiff legged) ataxia, or a combination of these signs (dysmetria). In addition, head signs are present. These include ataxia of the head and neck with wide, swinging, head excursions, jerky head bobbing, an intention tremor involving the head but not the body and limbs, and an abnormal menace response. With the latter finding the animal is able to see and to blink its eyelids, but does not blink in response to a menacing gesture directed toward each eye, although it may withdraw its head from the threatening gesture. This has been seen ipsilateral to unilateral cerebellar lesions. It is probable that the cerebellum positively influences the classic menace or eye preservation reflex. Thus, cerebellar lesions might suppress the reflex (see Chapter 2—Neurologic Examination).

Cerebellar syndromes often are seen in calves. In all large animals, these syndromes, when severe, frequently are diagnosed as cerebral disease, although a thorough neurologic examination usually is all that is required to separate these problems. Exacerbations of cerebellar signs, seen when severely affected animals are disturbed, can result in recumbency, thrashing, and opisthotonus—which can be called a "convulsion." This occurs especially in the familial and toxic cerebellar syndromes and most often in calves. In cats, it has been shown that cerebellar lesions alter the seizures resulting from convulsant drugs (Cook et al., 1952). Also, electroencephalograms taken from piglets (Kidd et al., 1986) and Arabian foals (Beatty et al., 1985) with cerebellar syndromes may be abnormal.

The floccular lobes of the lateral cerebellar hemispheres, the nodular lobe of the caudal vermis, and the pair of fastigial (medial) cerebellar nuclei all are interconnected with the vestibular nuclei within the medulla oblongata. Thus, severe, acquired cerebellar diseases sometimes include signs of vestibular derangement. Resulting vestibular syndromes can include paradoxical signs with leaning, turning, and head tilt—all away from the side of the lesion and the fast phase of any nystagmus toward the side of the lesion (also Problem 6).

Newborn animals frequently have a slightly hypermetric gait reminiscent of a cerebellar dysfunction (Fig. 13–1). In the context of congenital, cerebellar syndromes, clinical signs are present from birth or from when the neonatal animal is expected to ambulate well. Such syndromes may be inherited, but even if they are familial, there may be other environmental factors in utero that play a pathogenetic role.

The term cerebellar abiotrophy is used here to describe a clinical syndrome that is familial and that most often begins after the animal has had a normal gait for a period of time. Signs progress, and active degeneration of the cells of the cerebellum, usually Purkinje cells, may be demonstrated. Thus, the

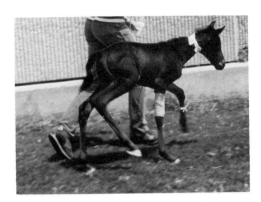

Figure 13–1. The gait of newly born large animals, particularly foals, often is hypermetric and similar in appearance to that seen with cerebellar dysfunction. Neonatal foals, such as the one shown, that are confined due to illness, have a prominently dysmetric gait when beginning to move around; this disappears within a few days to weeks.

clinical syndromes of the abiotrophies are taken to be familial and degenerative, but not usually congenital.

Congenital cerebellar disease may accompany the congenital tremor syndromes in Problem 8B, which includes in utero exposure to organophosphates (Knox et al., 1978), (Bölske et al., 1978). The Arnold-Chiari malformation and the Dandy Walker syndrome (agenesis of the caudal cerebellar vermis), have been related to cerebellar signs, although other signs resulting from hydrocephalus (see also Problem 1) and arthrogryposis (see Problem 10), and to agenesis of the corpus callosum, respectively, often predominate (Cho et al., 1977a), (Saunders et al., 1952), (Cudd et al., 1988).

Prominent cerebellar syndromes accompany the mannosidoses seen in calves and goats (see Problem 1). Angus calves with α-mannosidosis show progressive cerebellar ataxia, aggressiveness, and weight loss, whereas Anglo Nubian goats with β-mannosidosis are severely incapacitated early in life, with severe dysmetria and recumbency.

Acquired diseases that may involve the cerebellum, often resulting in asymmetric signs, include equine protozoal myeloencephalitis, migrating metazoan parasites (Fraser, 1966), nonsuppurative meningoencephalitis (van Bogaert et al., 1950), and injury.

Isolated cases of acute, diffuse cerebellar degeneration, which mimic abiotrophies, are seen in several breeds of cattle including Limousin (Oz et al., 1986) and Aberdeen Angus. They are most easily explained by an environmental toxic or infectious insult, but a genetic defect could be operative.

The relationship between site of lesions in the cerebellum and specific neurologic syndromes is discussed well by Holliday (1979/80). Interestingly, how incapacitating a particular cerebellar syndrome is, does not always relate to the severity of the gross and histologic lesions detected. Also, clearly evident lesions, detected unexpectedly at postmortem examination (Wheat et al., 1957), may or may not be clinically relevant.

If the cerebellum is small, cerebellar atrophy (formed then shrank), hypoplasia (did not form), or abiotrophy (postnatal degeneration) are the suspected causes. Determining the cerebellum to whole brain weight ratio (%)

confirms selective smallness of the cerebellum. A figure of less than 8% indicates selective smallness of the cerebellum (Mayhew, 1988), (Bölske et al., 1978), (Knox et al., 1978), (Dane, 1975), (Scott et al., 1973).

Categories of Disease and Differential Diagnosis
NOTE: Only those diseases marked * are discussed in this problem.

   I. Congenital and Familial
      *1. In Utero Viral Infections: Bovine Virus Diarrhea, Akabane, Aino, Bluetongue, Hog Cholera, Wesselbron Disease, and Rift Valley Fever Viruses
      *2. Cerebellar Abiotrophy
      *3. Familial Convulsions and Ataxia in Calves
      *4. Cerebellar Cortical Degeneration (Daft Lamb Disease)
      *5. Congenital Cerebellar Hypoplasia and Degeneration and Miscellaneous Malformations
      6. Mannosidosis (Problem 1)
  II. Physical (Problem 4)
      1. Head Trauma
 III. Infectious, Inflammatory, Immune (Problem 1)
      *1. Scrapie (Problems 1 and 13)
      *2. Louping Ill
      3. Otitis Media-Interna with Epidural Empyema (Problem 6)
      4. Verminous Encephalitis and Myelitis (Problems 1 and 10)
      5. Equine Protozoal Myeloencephalitis (Problem 10)
  IV. Toxic
      *1. Gomen Disease
      *2. Miscellaneous Cerebellar and Cerebellovestibular Disorders Associated with Toxic Plants (Problems 1, 2, 8B, 10)
      *3. In Utero Organophosphate Exposure
      *4. Chronic Methylmercurialism (Problem 10)
   V. *Neoplastic

   I. Congenital and Familial
      1. In Utero Viral Infections: Bovine Virus Diarrhea (BVD), Akabane, Aino, Bluetongue (BT), Hog Cholera (HC), Wesselbron Disease (WD), Rift Valley Fever (RVF) Viruses
        Signalment. Calves, less often lambs and piglets.
        Primary Complaint. Incoordination of limbs and head, recumbency or "seizures" are usually reported. Combinations of signs of hydranencephaly (somnolence, blindness) and arthrogryposis (congenital contractures) occur with some viruses more than others.
        History. Signs are first seen when affected animals try to ambulate: they may have difficulty getting clear of their fetal membranes. In an outbreak, abortions, mummified feti, birth of weak offspring, and neonatal ill thrift may occur. Usually the ataxia remains stable or the animal may compensate for the deficits.
        Physical Examination. Certain clinical findings often occur when

the syndrome is associated with a particular virus. Calves may have ophthalmic lesions with BVD (Scott et al., 1973), calves and lambs often have arthrogryposis (also Problem 10) with Akabane and Aino viruses (Konno et al., 1982a), (Coverdale, 1978), and piglets in particular may be stunted ("runts") by Hog Cholera.

Neurologic Examination. Of the viruses listed, BVD most consistently results in signs of cerebellar damage (Kahrs, 1970b), (Wilson et al., 1983). Signs of cerebellar disease are variable, but they are usually symmetric and vary from recumbency with opisthotonus and extensor rigidity of the limbs, to a mildly spastic (stiff, hypometric) or hypermetric ataxia and slight head tremor. Abnormal, jerky eye movements may be seen. Signs of cerebral disease can be caused by concomitant hydrocephalus, hydranencephalus, or porencephalic cysts. These cerebral lesions frequently occur with Akabane, Aino, BT, WD, and RVF in utero infections (Coetzer et al., 1979), (MacLachlan et al., 1985), (Konno et al., 1982a). Piglets exposed in utero to HC virus usually show tremor as well as ataxia; this also has occurred in calves exposed to BVD in utero (also Problem 8).

Assessment. These viruses, and possibly others, destroy portions of the developing brain (Konno et al, 1982b), (Brown et al., 1974), (MacLachlan et al., 1985), (Coetzer et al., 1979), (Brown et al., 1973). The external germinal layer of the bovine cerebellum is selectively destroyed by BVD virus if it gains access to the fetus at about 102 to 183 days gestation (Brown et al., 1933), (Kahrs et al., 1970b). Severe destruction of cerebral tissue may result in hydranencephaly (Fig. 13–2) (MacLachlan et al., 1985), (Konno et al., 1982b). Spinal cord ventral gray horn (LMN) and skeletal muscle lesions can explain the arthrogryposis (Konno et al., 1982b). Many times this syndrome occurs and there is no proof of the nature of the inciting in utero agent (Fig. 13–2).

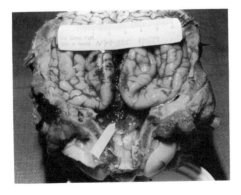

Figure 13–2. Severe cerebellar hypoplasia (indicated by white marker) and hydranencephaly (evident by the sunken occipital lobes between the marker and the rule) occur because of many in utero agents, particularly viruses. Only a small remnant of the cerebellum remains in this case, yet the affected calf could walk around unassisted with a severely dysmetric gait. As often is the case, no proof of a specific viral agent acting in utero could be determined.

The degree of cerebellar hypoplasia does not always relate to the severity of the clinical syndrome (Scott et al., 1973).

Diagnosis. A positive presuckle viral titer in serum and possibly in CSF is incriminating (Kahrs et al., 1970b), (Scott et al., 1973). Usually no virus can be detected in calves with cerebellar hypoplasia (MacLachlan et al., 1985), (Coetzer et al., 1979), although persistent BVD infection has been associated with congenital tremor (see Problem 8B) and cerebellar ataxia in calves (Straver et al., 1983). Confirmation of exposure of the dam to the virus during midgestation also is good circumstantial evidence (Kahrs et al., 1970a). If the ratio of cerebellum to total brain weight is less than 8% cerebellar hypoplasia is diagnosed (Scott et al., 1973).

Prognosis. There is no therapy, but the syndrome usually does not worsen. This is not a hereditary disease. Cattle with serum-neutralizing antibody titers to BVD resist challenge with pathogenic BVD virus at 150 days gestation and do not produce calves with cerebellar hypoplasia (Scott et al., 1973), (Brown et al., 1974). Therefore use of appropriate vaccine virus preparations may prevent these syndromes.

2. **Cerebellar Abiotrophy of Foals, Piglets, Calves, and Sheep**

Signalment. These clinical syndromes, for the most part, are not congenital. Affected animals have a normal gait for a period postnatally, then demonstrate a syndrome related to progressive cerebellar degeneration.

Arabian (Fig. 13–3a) and Arabian cross and Gotland pony foals of either gender are affected, usually between 1 and 6 months of age, rarely at birth (Björck et al., 1973), (Palmer et al., 1973), (Baird, et al., 1974). Oldenberg foals usually are 1 to 2 months old when the signs first occur (Koch et al., 1950). Affected Yorkshire piglets usually are 3–12 weeks old (de Lahunta, 1983), Holstein calves (Fig. 13–3B) usually are 3–8 months old (White et al., 1975), and Merino sheep are 3 to 6 years old (Harper et al., 1986) at the onset of signs. Isolated cases of acquired cerebellar syndromes occur in other breeds of large animals. Some of these may be inherited abiotrophies, but toxicities (below) must be strongly considered.

History. Usually a progressive gait abnormality with head tremor occurs. Progression of signs varies. In Yorkshire piglets and Oldenberg foals progression is abrupt, whereas in Arabian foals signs may progress insidiously. The incidence of disease has been recorded as 1.2% in Gotland ponies (Björck, 1973), but as high as 6 to 8% in families of Arabian horses (Sponseller, 1967).

Neurologic Examination. Signs are typical of diffuse, symmetric, cerebellar disease. A head bob, intention tremor, and deficient menace responses usually are present. A basewide stance and hypermetric or hypometric ataxia may be prominent; some affected animals show hypometric gait at a walk, which becomes hypermetric at faster gaits (Fig. 13–3). As with many neurologic diseases that result in abnormal gait in large animals, affected animals pace. No weakness occurs. Severely affected animals may use their noses to assist in posturing.

Assessment. The term abiotrophy is derived from Greek: a =

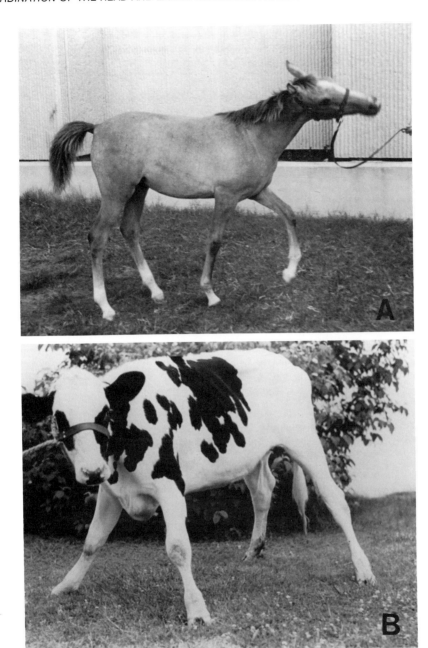

Figure 13–3. Cerebellar abiotrophy in an Arabian foal (A) and a Holstein calf (B). Ataxic movements of the head and neck (A), hypermetria (A), and a stiff, basewide stance (B) are evident in these syndromes of delayed, progressive cerebellar disease. The diseases are believed to be inherited.

absence; bios = life; trophy = nourishment. There is a presumed deficiency of a vital, trophic substance in cells (cerebellar neurons in this instance), which results in degeneration and depletion of Purkinje and granular cells. Ultimately, the cerebellum usually becomes small—less than 8% of total brain weight (Johnson et al., 1958), (Björck et al., 1973).

Histologically, evidence of degenerative Purkinje and granular cells and swollen Purkinje axons (torpedoes) may be prominent (de Lahunta, 1983). Because of great histologic variations in Holstein calves (Johnson et al., 1958), (White et al., 1975) and Yorkshire piglets (de Lahunta, 1983), more than one form of cerebellar abiotrophy may exist in these breeds.

An unusual finding of focal mineralization with mild gliosis in the rostral thalamus of affected Arabian foals (Beatty et al., 1985) may represent similar vulnerability of these thalamic neurons to the (inherent) insult affecting cerebellar neurons; it may also reflect trans-synaptic neuronal degeneration.

Diagnosis. Based on the signalment, history, and neurologic examination a presumptive diagnosis can be made. Several clinico-pathologic findings have been described in a group of six affected Arabian foals, which may assist in diagnosing cerebellar abiotrophy in that breed (Beatty et al., 1985). The CSF protein content was elevated to 204, 207,and 268 mg/dl in 3 of 6 foals. The CSF-CPK activity was elevated to 62 and 21 IU in 2 of 4 foals. The EEGs of all 6 were abnormal, showing prominent synchrony and abrupt frequency changes compared to unaffected horses.

Prognosis. This is grave. No treatment exists and because the signs are progressive most animals have to be euthanized, although some affected Merino sheep (Harper et al., 1986) and Gotland ponies (Björck et al., 1973) may survive for several years.

3. Familial Convulsions and Ataxia in Calves

Signalment. Aberdeen-Angus and Angus cross calves with this disorder are affected at birth or by a few months of age (Barlow et al., 1968). One 9-month Charolais calf was affected by a similar disorder (Cho et al., 1978).

History: One or several "convulsive" episodes usually occur in the first few days of life. Ataxia occurs in calves that survive several of these episodes (Fig. 13–4). Signs abate and by 12 to 15 months the convulsive episodes rarely occur; by 2 years survivors are clinically normal (Barlow, 1979). Up to 30% of the calves in a herd may be affected (Barlow, 1979).

Syndrome. This disorder is seen as waxing and waning signs of cerebellar disease. At times the extensor tone and opisthotonus is so strong the animal falls to the ground in an apparent convulsive episode, but with rest it becomes ambulatory again.

Assessment. The convulsive episodes may be true cerebral seizures, but more closely resemble exacerbations of cerebellar signs— or cerebellar fits (see page 228). Several factors that corroborate this statement are: the relationship to excitement and induced movement;

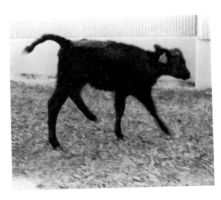

Figure 13–4. This Angus-Holstein cross calf suffered from the syndrome of familial convulsions and ataxia. Between convulsive-like episodes, from which it could be aroused, it demonstrated a variable, dysmetric, stilted gait (as shown) without being weak. This is typical of cerebellar ataxia. An affected herd-mate was euthanized and found to have subtle cerebellar lesions consistent with the disorder. This calf improved with time and was apparently normal by a year of age.

the ease with which the episode can be aborted (by positioning the calf upright and calming it); the absence of signs of autonomic involvement; the absence of depression and blindness, even after prolonged episodes lasting several hours; and the absence of abnormalities on EEG tracings (Barlow et al., 1968), (Barlow, 1979). Also, during these episodes, two affected Angus/Holstein cross-bred calves were found to be easy to attract and sucked on offered fingers.

There are fusiform, spheroidal, or argyrophilic swellings found on Purkinje cell axons (Barlow, 1981). Early in the disease, these may be difficult to detect. Unaffected parents of affected calves may have similar changes. Recovered calves have no lesions.

The disease may be inherited as an autosomal dominant gene with incomplete penetrance (Barlow, 1979).

Outcome. There is no specific treatment. Although affected calves may have to be destroyed, many survive and can be salvaged (Fig. 13–4). In the UK the disease has been controlled by gradual elimination of affected lines of Aberdeen-Angus cattle (Barlow, 1981).

4. Cerebellar Cortical Degeneration (Daft Lamb Disease—DLD)

Signalment. This rare disease, or group of diseases, occurred in many breeds of newborn lambs in the UK and Canada (van Bogaert et al., 1950).

Syndrome. Affected lambs with Daft Lamb Disease type A (DLD-A) have great difficulty rising and only some can walk (with wide-based, ataxic movement). They may wander, circle, and stagger. Head tremor and wide swinging head movements may be seen and most stand and sit with the head and neck hyperextended. Usually they are bright and can suckle. Most die if considerable nursing care is not offered.

Assessment. The clinical syndrome may be related to the neuropathologic lesions described in DLD-A (Van Bogaert, 1950). In this form cerebellar Purkinje cell degeneration and Bergmann glia proliferation occur. However, suggestions of weakness, patellar hyperreflexia, blindness, and deafness make only cerebellar disease unlikely. Also, in what is claimed to be an identical syndrome (DLD—B) patients have been described as having no cerebellar lesions (Terlecki et al., 1978). Indeed, the characteristic head and neck posture (stargazing) with the dorsum of the head often resting on the withers, but even decreased tone in the neck muscles, and wide swinging movements of the head—could represent bilateral vestibular disease (Terlecki et al., 1978). Further confounding information are the indications of skeletal fragility (Terlecki et al., 1978) and myopathy (Bradley et al., 1977), at least in DLD—B.

The disease has been likened to familial convulsions and ataxia in calves (Cho et al., 1978), and is thought to be inherited as an autosomal recessive trait (van Bogaert et al., 1950), (Terlecki et al., 1978). However, environmental factors have not fully been excluded from the pathogenesis of the syndromes.

Outcome. The outlook is grave; families in which the disease has occurred should not be used as breeding stock.

5. **Cerebellar Hypoplasia and Degeneration and Miscellaneous Malformations**

The first description of bovine hereditary cerebellar hypoplasia was in Hereford calves (Innes et al., 1940). Affected calves were recumbent and exhibited stiff thrashing movements of the limbs. Opisthotonus and tremor also were mentioned. The cerebellums were small in size and cell numbers in all layers were reduced. In Hereford calves that are usually recumbent from birth, at least one disease is believed to be the result of an autosomal recessive trait, which results in combinations of hydrocephalus, polymicrogyria, stenosis of the mesencephalic aqueduct, and severe cerebellar cortical maldevelopment. Cataracts and retinal dysplasia with detachment and myopathy also are seen. Signs are stable from birth and usually are accompanied by cerebral or other signs (Greene et al., 1974), (de Lahunta, 1983).

Inherited cerebellar hypoplasia in Shorthorn (Swan et al., 1982) and Illawarra Shorthorn and Shorthorn cross (O'Sullivan et al., 1975) calves occurred in Australia at an annual prevalence of 1% of newborns, but up to 8% on severely affected farms (Swan et al., 1982). Signs of spastic, widebased, ataxia and head tremor were seen at birth and remained stable. A marked sparsity of cells in the granular and Purkinje cell layers and thinning of the molecular layer were identified (O'Sullivan et al., 1975).

Ayrshire, Angus and unknown breeds of calves also have been suspected of having hereditary cerebellar hypoplasia. The mode of inheritance of most of these congenital cerebellar hypoplasia syndromes is thought to be autosomal recessive (Cho et al., 1977b).

A reproducible, congenital, cerebellar maldevelopment—presumed to be genetically determined—occurred as an outbreak in several litters of Wessex Saddleback X Large White piglets (Kidd et al., 1986). Piglets were unable to stand at first and showed perverse limb movements. With time they were able to walk with significant dysmetria, at which time body tremor was seen. Depletion of granular and Purkinje cells and the presence of Purkinje axonal swellings were present in the cerebellum of affected piglets.

Permanent recumbency, associated with severe cerebellar hypoplasia, has been seen in a 6-day-old thoroughbred colt (Oliver, 1975). Also, profound jerky and dysmetric (though strong) movements characterized a congenital syndrome in 2 Paso Fino foals, which were unable to sit sternal or stand, even after 1-month of nursing care in one foal. Wide floppy movements of the head and trembling eyeball movements also were present. Both foals had cerebellar hypoplasia (cerebellum <6% total brain) and depopulation and degeneration of cells in the granular and Purkinje layers.

Congenital agenesis of the caudal cerebellar vermis (central lobe) has been seen in a lamb (Pass et al., 1981), a kid (Verhaart, 1942), a calf (Cho et al., 1977b), and a thoroughbred foal that survived until weaning (Cudd TA et al., 1988). In the latter two cases, there was also agenesis of the corpus callosum. Signs in the lamb and foal, for the most part, represented cerebellar hypoplasia. All of these cases can be likened to the Dandy-Walker syndrome in children in which there often are other midline malformations (Tal et al., 1980).

A maldeveloped cerebellum is part of the Arnold-Chiari malformation seen in human infants and in calves of many breeds, but signs associated with other malformations—especially hydrocephalus and spina bifida—often overshadow signs of cerebellar disease (Cho et al., 1977a).

Several other congenital cerebellar syndromes are reported, in calves in particular, that most likely are associated with in utero viral infection (Allen, 1977), (Howell et al., 1966), or at least an environmental factor acting in utero (Greene, 1978), (Cho et al., 1977b). Exposure of sows to organophosphates (trichlorphon) on days 55 to 70 days of gestation is likely to result in cerebellar hypoplasia, which may be subclinical (Pope et al., 1986). These teratogenic factors are associated with congenital tremor and cerebellar ataxia in newborn animals (also Problem 8B).

II. Infectious, Inflammatory, Immune
  1. **Scrapie (also Problems 1 and 13)**
      Signalment. Scrapie is a transmissible disease of 2- to 5-year-old sheep (of particular breeds) and of goats; it has a prolonged incubation period of months to years (Palmer, 1976).

      Clinical Syndrome. The disease is characterized by cerebellar incoordination and pruritis, with eventual emaciation, seizures, recumbency, and death. A fine head tremor often is present. Pruritis usually is severe and even noxious stimuli applied to the skin appear to be misinterpreted—the animal moves toward the stimulus. The various names given to this disease are somewhat whimsical but apt: Gnubber Krankheit and Traber Krankheit (Germany), la tremblante (France), rubbers and goggles (England), and cuddy trot, yeuky pine, and scrapie (Scotland).

      Assessment. A spongiform encephalomyelopathy, with neuronal vacuolation and necrosis, and astrogliosis, involves particular neuronal groups in the brainstem and spinal cord. In particular, necrosis of Purkinje cells also is seen. The scrapie agent is resistant to environmental factors and persists in endemic areas. A genetic predisposition has been defined in certain breeds of sheep, and in families within one breed there can be a significant difference in susceptibility (Davies et al., 1985). In fact, it appears that the sheep's major histocompatibility locus (OLA) is associated with at least one gene that relates to susceptibility/resistance to scrapie; this may be used as a marker of genetic resistance (Millot et al., 1985). Finally, this disease, particularly adapted to mice, is a model disease for the contagious, spongiform, dementing diseases (Kuru and Creutzfeldt-Jakob disease), and possibly for Alzheimer's disease, in humans (Manuelidis, 1986).

   Outcome. The disease is fatal and no treatment exists. It is a notifiable disease.

2. Louping Ill

   This is a neurotropic encephalomyelitis of sheep transmitted by the tick *Ixodes ricinus,* which occurs in Europe. It also affects cattle, horses, and deer. Affected sheep bound or leap in a characteristic manner, are ataxic, and their heads flop from side to side. There is widespread destruction of neurons, including Purkinje cells (Palmer, 1976). Horses may show similar signs as well as severe weakness (Timoney et al., 1976).

III. Toxic

1. Gomen disease

   Adult horses, indigenous to, or brought in to one part of New Caledonia in the South Pacific may show progressive incoordination, debility, and death through misadventure (LeGonidec et al., 1981). There is widespread loss of Purkinje cells in the cerebellum, with pigment accumulation in neurons throughout the central nervous system (Hartley et al., 1982). The disease is thought to be an environmentally induced lipofuscinosis, and is likely to be caused by a toxic plant.

2. Miscellaneous Cerebellar Disorders Associated with Toxic Plants (also Problems 1, 8B, 10)

   Coyotillo (*Karwinskia humboldtiana*) produces cerebellar ataxia and progressive weakness in livestock, particularly goats, in southwestern USA (Charlton et al., 1970). Intoxication of cattle with *Solanum fastigiatum* in Brazil (Riet-Correa et al., 1983), *Solanum kwebense* in South Africa (Pienaar et al., 1976), and *Solanum dimidiatum* in the USA (Menzies et al., 1979) results in cerebellar degeneration. These diseases appear to be induced lysosomal storage diseases, possibly gangliosidoses. Mannosidosis is induced in animals by Darling Pea plants in Australia and by Locoweeds in the USA (also Problem 1). Cerebellar signs are prominent, along with aggression, seizures, and weight loss.

3. In Utero Organophosphate Exposure

   Newborn piglets and calves, exposed in utero to organophosphate compounds, have been found to have degrees of cerebellar hypoplasia and degrees of ataxia. Congenital tremor usually is prominent (see Problem 8B).

4. Chronic Methylmercurialism (also Problem 10)

Chronic methylmercury intoxication may induce neurologic syndromes that often are related to cerebral neuronal necrosis, which occurs in swine (Davies et al., 1976). Early signs of intoxication in calves include ataxia and swinging head movements and probably relate to degeneration of cerebellar granular cells (Herigstad et al., 1972). Prominent ataxia, dysmetria, hypermetria, and head nodding were seen in a horse with chronic methylmercurialism. Focal atrophy of granular cells in the cerebellum as well as more widespread neuronal and fiber necrosis were present (Seawright et al., 1978).

IV. Neoplastic

Neoplasia involving the central nervous system in large animals is rare. However, bovine lymphosarcoma and bovine medulloblastoma (a primitive neuroepithelial tumor) in adult and young animals, respectively, are two specific neoplasms that may result in purely cerebellar syndromes (also Problem 6).

REFERENCES

Allen JG. Congenital cerebellar hypoplasia in Jersey calves. Aust Vet J 1977; 53:173–175.

Baird JD, Mackenzie CD. Cerebellar hypoplasia and degeneration in part-Arab horses. Aust Vet J 1974; 50:25–28.

Barlow RM. Morphogenesis of cerebellar lesions in bovine familial convulsions and ataxia. Vet Pathol 1981; 18:151–162.

Barlow RM. Further observations on bovine familial convulsions and ataxia. Vet Rec 1979; 105:91–94.

Barlow RM, Linkater KA, Young GB. Familial convulsions and ataxia in Angus calves. Vet Rec 1968; 83:60–65.

Beatty MT, Leipold HW, Cash W, et al. Cerebellar disease in Arabian horses. Proc 31st Ann Meet AAEP 1985; 241–255.

Björck G, Everz KE, Hansen HJ et al. Congenital cerebellar ataxia in the Gotland pony breed. Zentralbl Veterinarmed 1973; 20:341–354.

Bölske G, Kronevi T, Lindgren NO. Congenital tremor in pigs in Sweden. A case report. Nord Vet Med 1978; 30:534–537.

Bradley R, Terlecki S. Muscle lesions in hereditary "Daft lamb" disease of Border Leicester sheep. J Pathol 177; 123:225–236.

Brown TT, de Lehunta A, Scott FW, et al. Virus induced congenital anomalies of the bovine fetus. Cornell Vet 1973; 63:561–578.

Brown TT, de Lahunta A, Bistner SI, et al. Pathogenetic studies of infection of the bovine fetus with bovine viral diarrhea virus. Vet Pathol 1974; 11:486–505.

Charlton KM, Pierce KR, Storts RW, et al. A neuropathy in goats caused by experimental coyotillo (Karwinskia humboldtiana) poisoning. Pathol Vet 1970; 7:435–447.

Cho DY, Leipold HW. Arnold-Chiari malformation and associated anomalies in calves. Acta neuropathol (Berl) 1977a; 39:129–133.

Cho DY, Leipold HW. Cerebellar cortical atrophy in a Charolais calf. Vet Pathol 1978; 15:264–266.

Cho DY, Leipold HW. Congenital defects of the bovine central nervous system. Vet Bull 1977b; 47:489–504.

Coetzer JAW, Theodoridis A, Herr S, et al. Wesselbron disease: A cause of congenital proencephaly and cerebellar hypoplasia in calves. Onderstepoort J Vet Res 1979; 46:165–169.

Cook WH, Stavraky GW. A cerebellar component of convulsive manifestations. Arch Neurol & Psychiatr 1952; 68:741–754.

Cudd TA, Mayhew IG, Cottrill CM. Agenesis of the corpus callosum and cerebellar vermian hypoplasia in a foal resembling the Dandy-Walker syndrome. Equine Vet J 1989; In press.

Cybinski DH, St. George TD. Congenital abnormalities in calves associated with Akabane virus and Aino virus. Aust Vet J 1978; 54:151–152.

Done JT. The congenital tremor syndrome in pigs. Vet Annual 1975; 98–102.

Davies DC, Kimberlin RH. Selection of Swaledale sheep of reduced susceptibility to experimental scrapie. Vet Rec 1985; *116*:211–214.

Davies TS, Nielsen SW, Kircher CH. The pathology of subacute methylmercurialism in swine. Cornell Vet 1976; *66*:32–55.

de Lahunta A. *Veterinary Neuroanatomy and Clinical Neurology,* 2nd Ed. Philadelphia: WB Saunders, 1983, pp 262–272.

Fraser H. Two dissimilar types of cerebellar disorder in the horse. Vet Record 1966; *78*:608–612.

Greene HJ, Leipold HW, Hibbs CM. Bovine congenital defects: variations of internal hydrocephalus. Cornell Vet 1974; *64*:596–616.

Greene HJ. Congenital hydranencephaly and cerebellar hypoplasia in calves. J Am Vet Med Assoc 1978; *173*:1008–1010.

Harper PAW, Duncan DW, Plant JW, et al. Cerebellar abiotrophy and segmental axonopathy: Two syndromes of progressive ataxia of Merino sheep. Am Vet J 1986; *63*:18–21.

Hartley WJ, Kuberski T, LeGonidec G, et al. The pathology of gomen disease: A cerebellar disorder of horses in New Caledonia. Vet Pathol 1982; *19*:399–405.

Herigstad RR, Whitehair CK, Beyer N, et al. Chronic methylmercury toxicosis in calves. J Am Vet Med Assoc 1972; *160*:173.

Holliday TA. Clinical signs of acute and chronic experimental lesions of the cerebellum. Vet Sci Comm 1979/1980; *3*:159–278.

Howell JMcC, Ritchie HE. Cerebellar malformations in two Ayrshire calves. Pathol Vet 1966; *3*:159–168.

Innes JRM, Russel DS, Wilsdon AJ. Familial cerebellar hypoplasia and degeneration in Hereford calves. J Pathol Bacteriol 1940; *50*:455–461.

Johnson KR, Fourt DL, Ross RH, et al. Hereditary congenital ataxia in Holstein-Friesian calves. J Dairy Sci 1958; *41*:1371–1375.

Kahrs RF, Scott FW, de Lahunta A. Congenital cerebellar hypoplasia and ocular defects in calves following bovine viral diarrhea-mucosal disease infection in pregnant cattle. J Am Vet Med Assoc 1970; *156*:1443–1450.

Kahrs RF, Scott FW, de Lahunta A. Bovine viral diarrhea-mucosal disease, abortion, and congenital cerebellar hypoplasia in a dairy herd. J Am Vet Med Assoc 1970a; *156*:851–857.

Kidd ARM, Done JT, Wrathall AE, et al. A new genetically-determined congenital nervous disorder in pigs. Br Vet J 1986; *142*:275–285.

Knox B, Askaa J, Basse A, et al. Congenital ataxia and tremor with cerebellar hypoplasia in piglets borne by sows treated with Neguvon® vet. (metrifonate, trichlorfon) during pregnancy. Nord Vet Med 1978; *30*:538–545.

Koch P, Fischer H. Die oldenburger fohlenataxie als erbkrankheit. Tierärztl Umschan 1950; *5*:317–320.

Konno S, Moriwaki M, Nakagawa M. Akabane disease in cattle: Congenital abnormalities caused by viral infection. Spontaneous disease. Vet Pathol 1982a; *19*:246–266.

Konno S, Nakagawa M. Akabane disease in cattle: Congenital abnormalities by viral infection. Experimental disease. Vet Pathol 1982b; *19*:267–279.

LeGonidec G, Kuberski T, Daynes P, et al. A neurologic disease of horses in New Caledonia. Aust Vet J 1981; *57*:194–195.

MacLachlan NJ, Osburn BI, Ghalib HW, et al. Bluetongue virus-induced encephalopathy in fetal cattle. Vet Pathol 1985; *22*:415–417.

Manuelidis L, Manuelidis EE. Recent developments of scrapie and Creutzfeldt-Jakob disease. Prog Med Virol 1986; *33*:78–98.

Mayhew IG. Neurological and neuropathological observations on the equine neonate. Equine Vet J 1988; Suppl *5*:28–33.

Menzies JS, Bridges CH, Murl Bailey Jr E. A neurologic disease of cattle associated with *Solanum dimidiatum.* Southwestern Vet 1979; *32*:45–49.

Millot P, Chatelain J, Cathala F. Sheep major histocompatibility complex OLA: Gene frequencies in two French breeds with scrapie. Immunogenetics 1985; *21*:117–123.

Oliver RE. Cerebellar hypoplasia in a Thoroughbred foal. NZ Vet J 1975; *23*:15.

O'Sullivan BM, McPhee CP. Cerebellar hypoplasia of genetic origin in calves. Aust Vet J 1975; *51*:469–471.

Oz HH, Nicholson SS, Al-Bagdadi, et al. Cerebellar disease in an adult cow. Can Vet J 1986; *27*:13–16.

Palmer AC, Blakemore WF, Cook WR, et al. Cerebellar hypoplasia and degeneration in the young Arab horse. Clinical and neuropathological features. Vet Rec 1973; 62–66.

Palmer AC. *Introduction to Animal Neurology,* 2nd Ed. Oxford: Blackwell Scientific Publications, 1976. pp 175–178.

Pass DA, McCHowell J, Thompson RR. Cerebellar malformation in two dogs and a sheep. Vet Pathol 1981; *18*:405–507.

Pienaar JG, Kellerman TS, Basson PA, et al. Maldronksiekete in cattle: A neuronopathy caused by *Solanum kwebense*. Onderstepoort J Vet Res 1976; *43*:67–74.

Pope AM, Heavner JE, Guarnieri A, et al. Trichlorfon-induced congenital cerebellar hypoplasia in neonatal pigs. J Am Vet Med Assoc 1986; *189*:781–783.

Riet-Correa F, Mendex MDC, Schild AL, et al. Intoxication by *Solanum fastigiatum* var. *Fastigiatum* as a cause of cerebellar degeneration in cattle. Cornell Vet 1983; *73*:240–256.

Saunders LZ, Sweet JD, Martin SM, et al. Hereditary congenital ataxia in Jersey calves. Cornell Vet 1952; *42*:559–591.

Scott FW, Kahrs RF, de Lahunta A, et al. Virus induced congenital anomalies of the bovine fetus. I. Cerebellar degeneration (hypoplasia), ocular lesions and fetal mummification following experimental infection with bovine viral diarrhea-mucosal disease virus. Cornell Vet 1973; *63*:535–560.

Seawright AA, Roberts MC, Costigan P. Chronic methylmercurialism in a horse. Vet Hum Toxicol 1978; *20*:6–9.

Sponseller ML. Equine cerebellar hypoplasia and degeneration. Proc AAEP 1967; 123–126.

Straver PJ, Journee DLH, Binkhorst GJ. Neurological disorders, virus persistence and hypomyelination in calves due to intrauterine infections with bovine virus diarrhoea virus. II. Virology and epizootiology. Vet Q 1983; *5*:156–164.

Swan RA, Taylor EG. Cerebellar hypoplasia in beef Shorthorn cattle. Aust Vet J 1982; *59*:95–96.

Tal Y, Freigang B, Dunn HG, et al. Dandy-Walker syndrome: Analysis of 21 cases. Develop Med Child Neurol 1980; *22*:189–201.

Terlecki S, Richardson C, Bradley R, et al. A congenital disease of lambs clinically similar to "inherited cerebellar cortical atrophy" (Daft lamb disease). Br Vet J 1978; *134*:299– 307.

Timoney PJ, Donnelly JC, Clements LO, et al. Encephalitis caused by Louping ill virus in a group of horses in Ireland. Equine Vet J 1976; *8*:113–117.

van Bogaert L, Innes JRM. Cerebellar disorders in lambs. A study in animal neuropathology with some comments on ovine neuroanatomy. Arch Pathol 1950; *50*:36–62.

Verhaart WJC. Partial agenesis of the cerebellum and medulla and total agenesis of the corpus-callosum in a goat. J Comp Neurol 1942; *77*:49–60.

Wheat JD, Kennedy PC. Cerebellar hypoplasia and its sequela in a horse. J Am Vet Med Assoc 1957; *131*:291–293.

White ME, Whitlock RH, de Lahunta A. A cerebellar abiotrophy of calves. Cornell Vet 1975; 476–491.

Wilson TM, de Lahunta A, Confer L. Cerebellar degeneration in dairy calves: Clinical, pathologic, and serologic features of an epizootic caused by bovine viral diarrhea virus. J Am Vet Med Assoc 1983; *183*:544–547.

CHAPTER 14

Problem 10:
Tetraparesis, Paraparesis and Ataxia of the Limbs, and Episodic Weakness

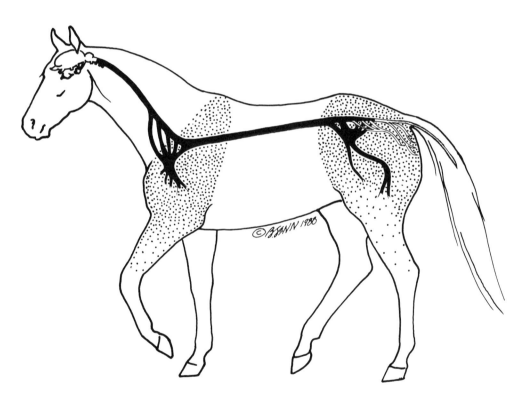

Locations of lesions resulting in tetraparesis, paraparesis, and ataxia of the limbs and episodic weakness: spinal cord, nerve roots and peripheral ganglia, plexuses and nerves of the limbs (blackened), and neuromuscular junctions and muscles of the limbs (stippled).

If following the neurologic evaluation, cerebellar involvement can be ruled out in a particular case showing ataxia and weakness of the limbs (wobbler), then the clinician must attempt to differentiate between the remaining disorders producing degrees of tetraparesis, paraparesis, and episodic weakness to arrive at a diagnosis.

The diseases causing degrees of this general syndrome can (on a clinical basis and particularly with ancillary aids) be divided into those primarily producing spinal cord lesions (A), those producing neuromuscular lesions (B), and those producing episodic weakness (C). These diseases are grouped this way in this problem.

Several diseases and syndromes have not been included in this text because of their parochial or rare nature or because of their uncertain clinical and neurological significance. However, the interested reader can refer to these examples: degenerative disk disease (Foss et al., 1983), (Rooney, 1969), ovine cervical vertebral stenosis (Palmer et al., 1981), bovine "knuckler" syndrome (Howard, 1971), congenital ataxia in artificially bred calves (McClintock et al., 1974), a rigid lamb syndrome in Dorper lambs in Rhodesia (Rudert et al., 1978), a suspected inherited neuromuscular disease in Dorset Down sheep in New Zealand (Thornton et al., 1985), kangaroo gait in ewes (Barlow et al., 1986), (Duffell et al., 1986), bovine paralysis in Zebu cattle in Cuba (Torano et al., 1975), spider syndrome in Suffolk sheep (Rook et al., 1986), segmental axonopathy (Murrurindi disease) in Australian sheep (Harper et al., 1986), and snakebite (Blood et al., 1983).

Problem 10A.

Spinal Cord Diseases

Spinal cord disease is common in large animals. A horse showing variations of this syndrome is called a "wobbler," although some people equate wobbler with cervical vertebral malformation.

With a mild or even moderate cervical spinal cord lesion in an adult cow or horse, signs of ataxia and weakness may be evident in the pelvic limbs only, especially if the patient is uncooperative. In this situation it is safest to conclude that the patient (with no head signs) has a lesion between C_1 and S_3. On the other hand, close scrutinization of the gait, posture, and postural reactions in the limbs, along with a search for localizing findings, often is productive. As a general rule, large patients that "dog-sit" for several minutes most likely have a lesion caudal to T_2. By being able to accurately define the site of the lesion(s), the clinician can reduce the number of possible diseases and thus can better direct the ancillary testing that is available.

Degrees of paraparesis often are seen in large animals. Frequently it is difficult to determine whether the thoracic limbs are involved. In such cases, a close scrutinization of the gait and a search for localizing findings often is productive. It is helpful to perform spinal reflexes and postural reactions on all small patients (<200 lb). Modified hopping with one forelimb held up is a useful postural reaction to test, even in large, adult animals—particularly horses. It is more difficult to test classical spinal reflexes and postural reactions in adult cattle, horses, and swine. Thus, the clinician relies on a critical evaluation of gait and posture, and additional spinal reflexes and responses performed during the neurologic examination to assist in localizing the lesion(s). Grading any gait abnormalities, testing local cervical, cervicofacial, and cutaneous trunci (panniculus) reflexes, and performing the laryngeal adductor response test are of considerable help in this regard for horses. All these tests are discussed in the neurologic examination section (Chapter 2).

In relating a spinal cord segment to a particular vertebra, it should be remembered that there are 8 cervical segments and only seven cervical vertebrae. Also, cows, sheep, goats, and horses (mostly) have six lumbar vertebrae, pigs have seven, and donkeys have five. The spinal cord usually ends at S_{1-2} but in pigs it ends at S_3.

It behoves the large animal clinician to complete a thorough neurologic workup as early as possible in the course of all neurologic syndromes. This is particularly so as more is known about various spinal cord diseases and more advanced medical and surgical therapeutic regimens become available. Ancillary aids, such as neuroradiology, electrodiagnostic techniques, and spinal fluid analysis can be of tremendous help in developing a plan for treatment early in the course of disease, before permanent neurologic signs and the consequent hopeless outlook for return of function arise. A CSF sample is best taken at the lumbosacral space (see Figs. 3–2 and 3–3) from patients with this problem because the fluid sampled is likely to be closest to the lesion. If this is unsuccessful it is worth trying at L_{5-6}, especially in lambs, kids, and calves, and at L_{6-7} in piglets.

Because of the considerable concern for life-threatening complications, and the high prevalence of equine protozoal myeloencephalitis (at least in horses coming from the eastern USA), many clinicians use glucocorticoids sparingly in treatment of wobblers and tetraplegic horses. Caring for a heavy, recumbent, adult animal is frustrating, time-consuming, and fraught with complications.

Categories of Disease and Differential Diagnosis
*NOTE: Only those diseases marked * are discussed in this problem.*

I. Congenital and Familial
   *1. Cervical Vertebral Malformation/Malarticulation
   *2. Occipitoatlantoaxial Malformations
   *3. Miscellaneous Vertebral and Spinal Cord Malformations
   *4. Neuroaxonal Dystrophy
   *5. Progressive Ataxia of Charolais Cattle
   *6. Bovine Progressive Degenerative Myeloencephalopathy
   *7. Arthrogryposis
   *8. Progressive Spinal Myelinopathy in Beef Cattle
   *9. Lysosomal Storage Diseases (also Problem 1)
   10. Equine Degenerative Myeloencephalopathy (section V.1 below)
II. Physical
   *1. Spinal Cord and Vertebral Trauma
   *2. Acquired Torticollis or "Wry-Neck"
III. Infectious, Inflammatory, Immune
   *1. Equine Herpesvirus-1 Myeloencephalitis
   *2. Caprine Arthritis—Encephalomyelitis

    *3. Visna-Maedi and Ovine Progressive Pneumonia
    *4. Vertebral Osteomyelitis and Discospondylitis
    *5. Equine Protozoal Myeloencephalitis
    *6. Verminous Myelitis (Problem 1)
     7. Louping Ill (Problem 9)
     8. Other Inflammatory Meningoencephalomyelitides (Problem 1)
IV. Toxic
    *1. Selenium
    *2. Delayed Organophosphate
    *3. Arsanilic Acid and 3-Nitro (also Problem 2)
    *4. Organomercury (also Problem 9)
    *5. Cystitis and Ataxia Associated with Sorghum Ingestion
    *6. Miscellaneous Toxic Plants (also VII.2 below and Problems 8B and 9)
     7. Bracken Fern (see Thiamin Deficiency—V.2 below)
     8. *Clostridium Tetani* Neurotoxin (Problem 8A)
V. Nutritional
    *1. Equine Degenerative Myeloencephalopathy
    *2. Bracken Fern and Horsetail-Induced Thiamin Deficiency
    *3. Enzootic Ataxia—Swayback—Copper Deficiency
     4. Pathothenic Acid Deficiency (Problem 8C)
VI. *Neoplastic
VII. Idiopathic
    *1. Premature Synosteosis of Thoracolumbar Vertebrae in Angus Calves
    *2. Poliomyelomalacia of Sheep, Goats, and Calves
    *3. Postanesthetic Hemorrhagic Myelopathy
    *4. Vascular Malformations
    *5. Thoracolumbar Spondylosis Deformans and Osteoarthrosis (Also 8, below)
    *6. Neurofibrillary Degenerations
    *7. Embolic Myelopathy
     8. Vague Neuromuscular Lameness and Back Problems (Problem 10B)
     9. Grove Poisoning (Problem 2)
    10. Enzootic Ataxia of Red Deer (see Swayback—V.3 above)
    11. Stringhalt (Problem 8C)

I. Congenital and Familial
1. Cervical Vertebral Malformation/Malarticulation

Signalment. Cervical vertebral malformation/malarticulation (CVM) is a common cause of "wobbles" in horses, worldwide (Mayhew et al., 1978), (Alitalo et al., 1983), (Yamagiwa et al., 1980), (Whitwell et al., 1987), (Reed et al., 1981), (Gerber et al, 1980). It affects any age and breed of horse, especially thoroughbreds a few months to 4-years-of-age.

Primary Complaint. Progressive ataxia (incoordination) of the pelvic limbs or all four limbs is observed. Occasionally there is an acute onset of tetraplegia, especially if external trauma plays a major role, and particularly with C_{2-3} and C_{3-4}, malarticulation with fixation in flexion.

History. Usually there is a slow onset of increasing clumsiness. Trauma may make the signs worse, but usually signs are evident before the horse falls. Signs frequently fluctuate.

Physical Examination. Sometimes a C_{2-3} or C_{3-4} flexion-fixation (kyphosis) can be seen and palpated. Affected horses tend to be large for their age and breed. Enlarged long bone physes frequently are a concurrent finding in younger patients.

Neurologic Examination. With a typical, mildly to moderately affected horse ataxia with circumduction of the limbs is present (wobbles). Sometimes ataxia is so pronounced in the pelvic limbs that the thoracic limbs may appear to be unaffected until they are critically evaluated. Weakness is evident by toe dragging (flexor weakness) and by the ease in which the horse is pulled to one side while walking (extensor weakness). Ataxia with hypometria (spasticity, stiffness) often is evident in the thoracic limbs, especially while walking the horse on a slope and with the head elevated.

The slap test is often, but not always, abnormal. Perhaps as frequently, asymmetry or hyporeflexia of cervical responses occur.

More severe lesions can produce paresis to paralysis with the same signs as any focal cervical lesion. Pelvic limbs are almost always more severely affected and typically are one grade worse than the thoracic limbs. However, in chronic cases with signs present for one or more years, there may be significant signs in the pelvic limbs with no detectable signs in the thoracic limbs.

Neck pain is infrequent, but may be present because of compression of intervertebral nerves or possibly because of intervertebral arthropathy. This usually occurs in older horses (4 to 8 years) with prominent arthropathy at C_6-T_1.

Assessment. Essentially, neurologic signs result from progressive spinal cord compression. Several or all of the following vertebral or surrounding structural changes may be operative (Mayhew et al., 1978a), (Whitwell et al., 1987), (Rantanen et al., 1981). See Figures 14–1, 14–2, 14–6, 14–7, 14–8, 14–9.

i. Vertebral malformation with stenosis of the vertebral canal. This may be absolute (static) or dynamic (occurring more on flexion or extension). The resulting spinal cord compression almost always is dorsoventral (saggital plane) rather than lateral (horizontal plane). Maximal narrowing often occurs at the caudal orifice of C_2 to C_5 and is associated with enlarged epiphyses (see v below). Maximal narrowing also occurs at the cranial orifice of C_5 to T_1 and is associated with "wedging" (see vii below). Vertebral canal stenosis can be regarded as the sine qua non of CVM. In the final analysis, there is not enough room for the spinal cord within the confines of the vertebral canal.

ii. Vertebral malformation with abnormal formation of, and alterations to, the articular processes. Cartilage degeneration and os-

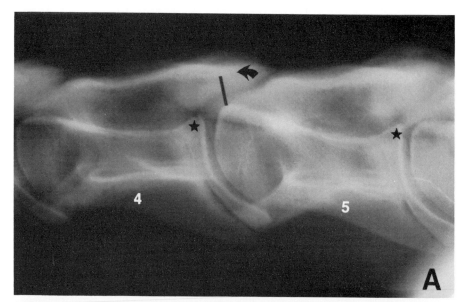

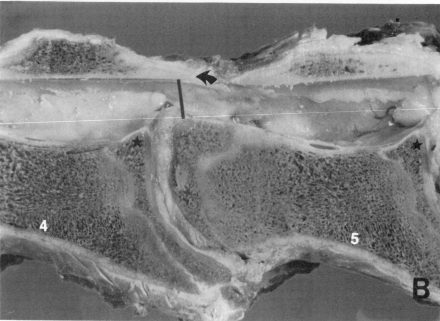

Figure 14–1. Left lateral views of the cervical radiographs (A) and median-sectioned 4th and 5th cervical vertebrae (B) of a yearling thoroughbred filly with CVM. Many of the radiographic characteristics of CVM are evident including: stenosis of the vertebral canal, which is most evident at the C_{4-5} site (black bar); angular deviation of C_5 on C_4; enlarged caudal epiphyses (stars), and caudal extension of the dorsal aspect of the vertebral arch (small arrows).

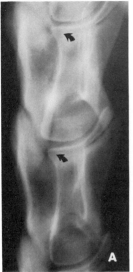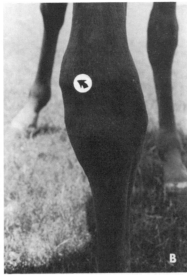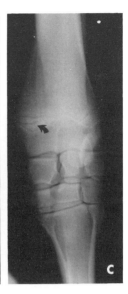

Figure 14–2. The morphologic characteristics of CVM, particularly the enlarged growing epiphyses (arrows) and associated angular deviation shown on a left lateral radiograph rotated 90° (A), bear considerable resemblance to the enlarged epiphyses and angular deformities (arrows) seen in the carpus (B) and on carpal radiographs (C) of a rapidly growing yearling horse.

teoarthrosis (osteochondrosis) occurs, sometimes intruding into the vertebral canal.

iii. Vertebral malformation with subluxation of the vertebrae on flexion (C_2 to C_5) or extension (C_5 to T_1) of the neck. In most cases this is more correctly referred to as the degree of angular fixation of vertebrae.

iv. Proliferation of soft tissues with impingement on the spinal cord. This can include formation of epidural and periarticular (synovial) cysts that compress the cord, usually at C_6 to T_1 (Fisher et al., 1981).

v. Enlarged vertebral epiphyseal growth regions. This is equivalent to the "physitis" in long bones of rapidly growing horses and certainly is part of the canal narrowing.

vi. Caudal extension of the dorsal aspect of the vertebral arch over the cranial aspect of the next caudal vertebral body. This allows dynamic stenosis when flexion and even normal movement occurs between vertebrae C_2 to C_5.

vii. Cranial and ventral extension of the craniodorsal edge of the vertebral arch ("wedging") allowing dynamic stenosis to occur during extension of vertebrae C_6 to T_1.

viii. External trauma plays a variable and often important role.

The overall assessment is that horses with CVM have various manifestations of osteochondrosis with rapidly growing epiphyseal growth plates and physeal enlargements, along with effects of external forces applied to these sites (see Fig. 14–2). Assessment of a group of horses with CVM in the UK did not support the theory that the disease has a genetic basis (Falco et al., 1976). However, a breeding trial using horses with CVM that had had corrective surgery resulted in offspring with a higher frequency of developmental orthopedic diseases than expected, but this did not include CVM (Wagner et al., 1985a). I believe that some degree of familial predisposition almost certainly occurs. A high or even excessive intake of protein and energy almost certainly is necessary for expression of the disease; CVM is not seen in malnourished or wild equidae. The role of micronutrients, especially copper and zinc, in all the developmental orthopedic diseases of horses is a topical subject, but is of unknown significance at this stage (Knight et al., 1985), (Knight et al., 1987).

These bone and joint changes result in chronic bone and soft tissue impingement on the spinal cord, resulting in necrosis in the white matter, and some focal loss of neurons. With time, secondary Wallerian-like, neuronal fiber degeneration in ascending white matter tracts cranial to the focal lesion and in descending white matter tracts caudal to the lesion occurs. This pattern of fiber degeneration can assist the neuropathologist in detecting a focal lesion in a wobbler and determining if the lesion is of a compressive nature (Fig. 14–3A).

Diagnostic Aids. Needle electromyography infrequently reveals mild focal changes consistent with denervation in cervical paravertebral muscles (Mayhew et al., 1978a).

Plain radiographs show stenosis of the vertebral canal, which is often exaggerated by flexion or extension of the vertebrae, and osteoarthrosis of the articular processes (Rantanen et al., 1981), (Whitwell et al., 1987). Plain radiographs are best exposed with the horse in a relaxed, standing position to obtain best alignment of vertebral bodies. Particularly in big horses under anesthesia, degrees of cervical torticollis result, which are difficult to correct.

To assist in deciding whether a myelogram is indicated, it is helpful to make several measurements from cervical radiographs (Fig. 14–4), particularly of the minimal sagittal diameter (MSD) within each vertebra (Mayhew et al., 1978a). Values approaching or lower than those for the control population (Table 14–1) strongly indicate that compression could be occurring. Significant angular deformities and severe osteoarthrosis occurring alone also are indications to proceed with contrast myelography. Many normal variations and inconsequential findings must be realized in interpreting cervical radiographs (Whitwell et al., 1987), (Rendano et al., 1978). See Figure 14–5. The frequent finding (possibly in 5% of thoroughbreds) of transpositioned ventral processes of C_6 to C_5 and more often to C_7 on one or both sides must be considered when vertebrae are being identified on radiographs (Whitwell et al., 1987).

Using the figures for MSDs (Table 14–1) and incorporating them with semiquantitative grading of the contributing structural changes (i through viii above) evident from plain cervical radiographs, a score

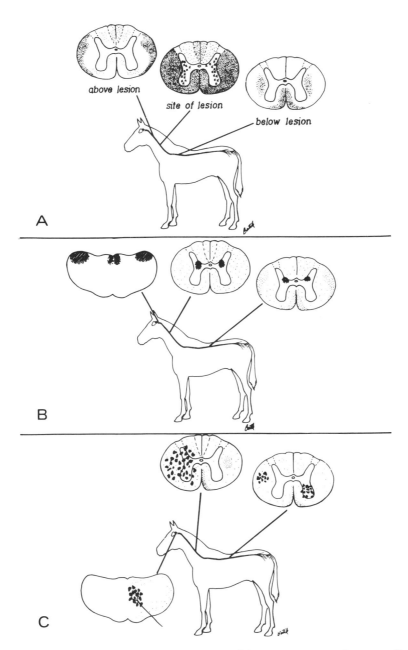

Figure 14–3. Diagrams of the lesions seen in some of the most common diseases affecting the spinal cord of horses resulting in wobblers in North America. Darkened areas indicate sites of the various lesions. A. Cervical vertebral malformation (and trauma). There is a focal, cervical, pressure-induced lesion affecting gray and especially white matter. Secondary white matter fiber degeneration is present in ascending pathways above and descending pathways below the lesion. B. Equine degenerative myeloencephalopathy with no focal lesion. Degeneration of ascending and descending white matter tracts throughout the spinal cord, particularly in the superficial lateral (ascending) and ventromedial (descending) pathways of the thoracic segments. Selective gray matter degeneration (neuroaxonal dystrophy) in caudal medullary, cranial cervical, and thoracic regions. C. Equine protozoal myeloencephalitis. Asymmetric, multifocal, nonsuppurative inflammatory lesions affecting gray and white matter in the brain and particularly the spinal cord. (From Mayhew IG, de Lahunta A, Whitlock RH, et al. Spinal cord disease in the horse. Cornell Vet 1978; *68* (suppl 6):110–111.)

Table 14–1. Minimum Values of Equine Cervical Vertebral Plain Radiographic and Myelographic Measurements*

| Body Weight | Minimum Sagittal Diameter (MSD) (mm) | | | | | |
	C_2	C_3	C_4	C_5	C_6	C_7
Under 320 kg	20.8	18.1	16.7	17.3	18.3	19.8
Over 320 kg	21.1	18.5	17.7	18.7	19.0	22.2
	Minimum Flexion Diameter (MFD) (mm)					
	C_2-C_3	C_3-C_4	C_4-C_5	C_5-C_6	C_6-C_7	
Under 320 kg	19.3	13.4	13.2	16.1	21.6	
Over 320 kg	22.8	15.6	14.8	17.9	28.5	
	Minimum Flexed Dural Sagittal Diameter (MDD) (mm)					
	C_2-C_3	C_3-C_4	C_4-C_5	C_5-C_6	C_6-C_7	
Under 320 kg	11.3	9.0	9.9	11.9	17.3	
Over 320 kg	12.9	10.5	10.8	11.4	17.6	

*Values represent the 2.5 percentile figures for the population. Adapted from Mayhew IG, Whitlock RH, and de Lahunta A: Spinal cord disease in the horse: Electromyographic and radiographic studies. Cornell Vet 1978; *68* (Suppl 6):44–70.

for the status of individual foals with respect to the likelihood of development of CVM has been developed (Mayhew IG, Donawick WJ, Galligan DT, Green S, 1987, unpublished data). Using this CVM score we have been able to predict the onset of signs of spinal cord disease in the nine foals that were graded with a CVM score above all others.

Myelography is necessary to demonstrate impingement on the spinal cord by a stenotic vertebral canal, by flexion or extension movement (dynamic stenosis), or by periarticular soft tissue or cyst (Figs. 14–5, 14–6, 14–7). Considerable care must be taken to not compromise the spinal cord with excessive manipulation of the neck under general anesthesia. With strong flexion, the dorsal and ventral contrast myelographic columns can be totally obliterated in normal foals (Fig. 14–5). Lateral compression of the spinal cord by medially displaced and proliferated articular processes, which usually show osteochondrosis and associated exuberant soft tissue, is not frequent. Dorsoventral views are necessary to confirm this form of compression, although a general blanching of the contrast column and even a widening of the spinal cord shadow may be evident on lateral views (Fig. 14–8).

Prior to deciding on surgical decompression or vertebral fusion, myelographic evidence of spinal cord compression is mandatory. Positive contrast myelography under general anesthesia is not an innocuous procedure in the horse (Beech, 1979), (Nyland et al., 1980). A hemorrhagic, aseptic, neutrophilic meningitis occurs 6 to 48 hours following the procedure, which can be associated with complicated recoveries (Beech, 1979) and often with fever (Nyland et al., 1980). Newer nonionic, water-soluble agents, such as iopamidol (May et al., 1986) and iohexol, appear to be better tolerated and to give better contrast than metrizamide. Standing myelography in the conscious horse (Foley et al., 1986) must not be undertaken.

Prominent spinal cord compression can readily be determined with myelography (Fig. 14–6; 14–7); however, often subjective evidence of contrast-column compromise exists, which is of question-

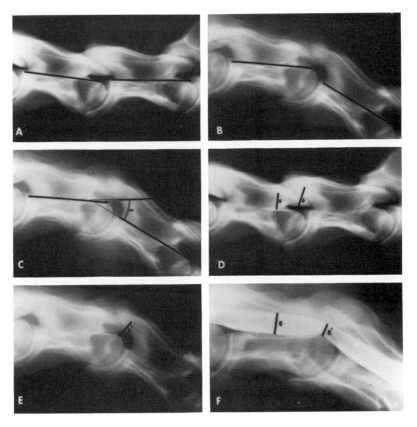

Figure 14–4. Methods for determining various measurements from radiographs that can be helpful in the diagnosis of CVM, particularly to help decide whether or not a myelogram should be performed. The flexion angle (FA, α) between adjacent vertebrae, the minimum sagittal diameter of the vertebral foramen (MSD, a), the minimum sagittal diameter between adjacent vertebrae in a neutral position (b) and in a flexed position (MFD, b'), the dural sagittal diameter within each vertebral foramen (c), and the minimum dural sagittal diameter during flexion of the cervical vertebral column (c'). A: Lines indicate extent of the floor of the vertebral foramina of adjacent cervical vertebrae in neutral position. B: Like A, with vertebral column in flexed position. C: Overlaying vertebra on left side in B, on the same vertebra in A, allows measurements of the FA (α). D: MSD taken within vertebral foramen at smallest measurement (a). The intervertebral sagittal canal diameter, measured in a neutral position (b), is not usually helpful (see b' in E). E: MFD taken from the dorsal rim of the caudal orifice of one vertebral foramen, to the closest point (on the cranial epiphysis) of the body of the next caudal vertebra, b'. F: The minimum dural sagittal diameter during flexion, c'. Intraforamenal dural sagittal diameter (c) is not usually utilized. (From Mayhew IG, de Lahunta A, Whitlock RH, et al. Spinal cord disease in the horse. Cornell Vet 1978; *68* (suppl 6):46.)

able significance (see Fig. 14–5) because of the lack of definitive, objective criteria (Mayhew et al., 1978a), (Rantanen et al., 1981), (Beech, 1979), (May et al., 1986). If a question ever exists concerning the presence of a myelographic cervical spinal cord compression in a horse, then I strongly recommend using Table 14–1 as an objective guide (adapted from Mayhew et al., 1978a). Using these figures (2.5 percentile) for the minimal vertebral canal measurements, and more particularly the minimal flexed dural diameters, the presence or

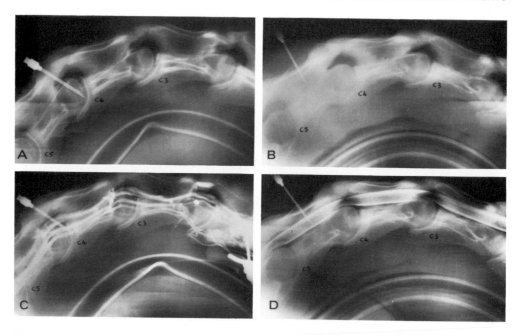

Figure 14–5. Plain (upper) and contrast (lower) radiographs of the flexed cervical vertebrae of two normal horses (left and right). Note hypodermic needle used as marker in skin. A and B: The cervical vertebral canals are wide. There is considerable flexion at each C_{3-4} space, and a tendency for each cranial epiphysis to rise dorsal to each caudal epiphysis. C: Venogram of A with intramedullary trocar in C_2. The two dorsal dye columns outline the cervical, ventral, internal, vertebral plexus running along the floor of the vertebral canal. At C_{3-4} and C_{4-5} there is a greater than 50% reduction in the diameter of this plexus. The two ventral dye columns outline the vertebral veins, and anastomoses are between these veins and the vertebral plexus. Residual dye remains in the body of C_2. (The technique for performing cervical vertebral venography is described in Mayhew et al. 1978a.) D: Myelogram of B showing the normal "blanching" of the total dye column and obliteration of the ventral dye column at each intervertebral site. In this control case there is also a greater than 50% reduction in the thickness of the dorsal dye column at C_{3-4} and C_{4-5}. (From Mayhew IG, de Lahunta W, Whitlock RH, et al. Spinal cord disease in the horse. Cornell Vet 1978; *68* (suppl; 6):58–59.)

absence of pathologic narrowing of the vertebral canal and consequent spinal cord compression then can be stated with 97.5% accuracy.

Cerebrospinal fluid analysis generally is normal in cases of CVM, but a slight increase in protein content and occasionally xanthochromia and macrophages showing erythrophagocytosis can be present.

Therapy. Use of glucocorticosteroids and other anti-inflammatory drugs provide transient neurologic relief, but do not solve the problem. Thus the process continues to progress. Rest, neck braces, and correction of faulty nutrition has helped stop the progress of the disease; radiographic as well as clinical improvement has occurred. By analysis of feeding programs and institution of a strict, well-balanced, novel diet (based on minimal though adequate growth), along with exercise restriction, we have observed six foals show clinical signs of CVM with high radiographic CVM scores over

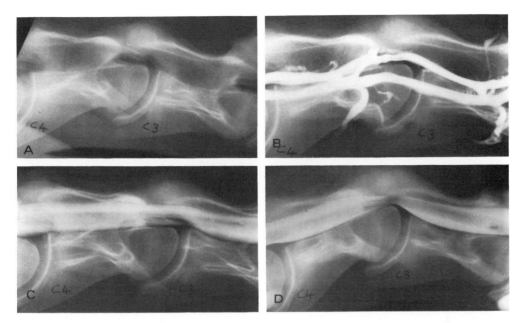

Figure 14–6. Plain and contrast radiographs of C_3 and C_4 from a horse with CVM. A: Stenosis occurred at the caudal orifice of the vertebral foramen of C_3 (14 mm) and at the intervertebral ($C_{3–4}$) portion of the canal above the cranial epiphysis of C_4, even in this partly flexed view. B: The two dye columns of the vertebral plexus are superimposed, but considerable narrowing of each can be seen above the cranial epiphysis of C_4 in this venogram. C: In this partly flexed myelogram, the ventral dye column is already obliterated. D: Massive compromise of the total contrast column (6.5 mm) is evident in this fully flexed myelogram. There is even further narrowing of the intervertebral flexion diameter to 8 mm compared with A. (From Mayhew IG, de Lahunta A, Whitlock RH, et al. Spinal cord disease in the horse. Cornell Vet 1978; *68* (suppl 6):60–61.)

a period of 2 years. All six foals have improved to show no clinical signs and their CVM scores have improved to be no different from those of unaffected siblings (Donawick WJ, Galligan DT, Mayhew IG, 1987, unpublished observations).

Surgical techniques have been developed for various aspects of the disorder (Wagner et al., 1979), (Wagner et al., 1981), (Wagner et al., 1985b), (Wagner, 1987), (DeBowes et al., 1984), (Nixon et al., 1983), (Nixon et al., 1985), (Nixon et al., 1983a;b), (Stashak et al., 1984), (Grant et al., 1985a). Dorsal laminectomy, especially between C_6 and T_1 is indicated for absolute stenosis associated with osteoarthrosis and proliferated soft tissue. Postoperative complications are frequent with this surgery (Nixon et al., 1983a;b). A modified Cloward technique, using ventral fusion with a bone plug or a stainless steel basket, is useful in selected horses. This procedure has been successful in early cases involving one site between C_2 and C_6. Also, cases with absolute stenosis and enlarged articular processes (usually C_5 to T_1) have radiographically and clinically improved with intervertebral fusion surgery, and this may well be the best procedure to consider in all cases of CVM. Myelographic confirmation is a mandatory prerequisite for surgical intervention. It is of note that

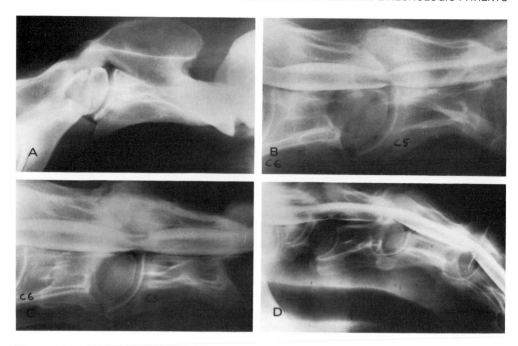

Figure 14–7. Plain and contrast radiographs from three cases of CVM (A, B, and C) and one of EPM + (D). A: Stenosis of the caudal part of the vertebral foramen of C₂ (15 mm) and the cranial part of the vertebral foramen of C₃ (15 mm), with an abnormal angle (kyphotic) between C₂ and C₃ seen in a radiograph taken with the neck in a neutral position. B: Stenosis of the cranial orifice of the vertebral foramen of C₆ (14 mm), with severe compromise of the total dye column. Narrowing of the dorsal dye column at the cranial orifice of the vertebral foramen of C₇ is shown at the extreme left of this radiograph. This is seen in the majority of control (and other) horses and is exaggerated by further neck extension. Neutral neck position. C: Massive arthrosis of the C₅₋₆ intervertebral articulations are visible. These are asymmetrically compressing the dural dye column from each side, resulting in two borders to the dorsal dye column. Using these two borders, the resulting measured sagittal diameters are 20 mm and 11 mm respectively. Neutral neck position. D: A significant narrowing of the dorsal, and particularly the ventral dye columns, and a blanching of the total dural dye column can be seen at the level of C₆ (center) and C₇ (left). At postmortem examination the cord was found to be swollen from C₅ to C₈ because of protozoal myelitis. Note the needle used as a skin marker (right). Flexed neck position. (From Mayhew IG, de Lahunta A, Whitlock RH, et al. Spinal cord disease in the horse. Cornell Vet 1978; *68* (suppl 6):62–63.)

these surgical procedures have not been widely accepted outside the USA.

Prognosis. The outlook is fair if the proper surgical technique is performed early. No controlled trials have been performed; however, some surgeons believe a 40 to 60% prognosis for return to full performance can be given in selected acute cases (Nixon et al., 1985), (Grant et al., 1985b). On the other hand, poor results were reported for 16 horses that underwent surgical repair of CVM (Beech, 1985). There may be degrees of multiple intervertebral site involvement, and in these cases the prognosis is poor.

Some cases showing mild to moderate signs have improved with conservative therapy of dietary correction and restriction, and rest (see Therapy above). The disease probably is as heritable as osteo-

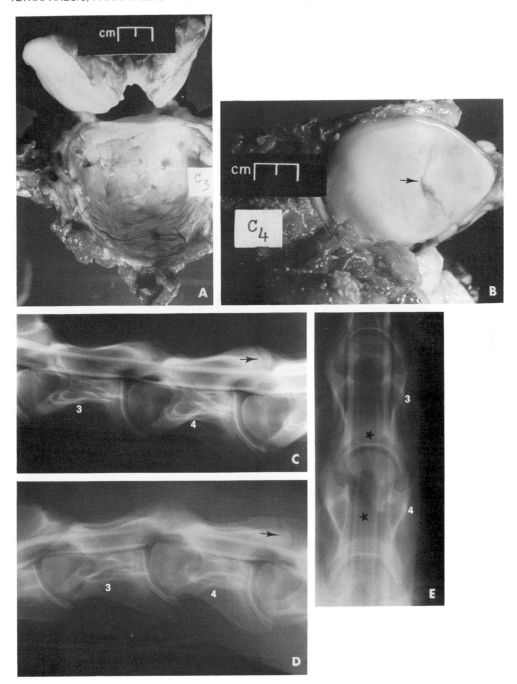

Figure 14–8. Lateral compression of the spinal cord alone occurs infrequently in CVM cases. Medially displaced caudal articular processes of C_3 can be seen in this example (A). Osteochondral lesions, including fissures, were present at several articulations and are indicated by arrows in B, C, and D. No dorsoventral compression was demonstrated on a myelogram with the neck in a neutral position (C). However, obliteration of both dorsal and ventral contrast columns occurred with flexion (D). Notably, blanching of the complete contrast column is associated with a widening of the shadow of the spinal cord (C). At the levels of mid-C_3 and mid-C_4 the cord measures 11 mm high, whereas at the C_{3-4} interspace it measures 12.5 mm. These factors indicate either a swollen spinal cord or lateral compression. The latter was confirmed on a ventrodorsal radiograph (E). The myelographic contrast column measures 25 mm at the level of the upper star (C_3), 24 mm at the level of the lower star (C_4), and 20 mm at the mid-point between them.

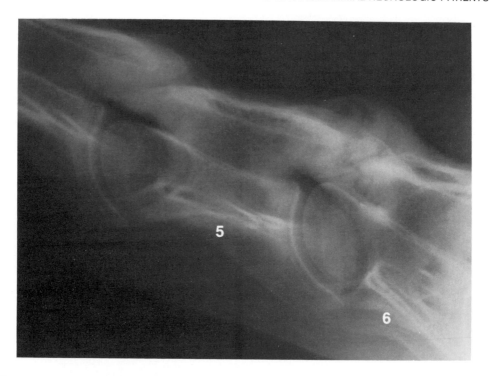

Figure 14–9. Severe degenerative joint disease with fissures present, shown here at the C_{5-6} articulations, can cause spinal cord compression. At this chronic stage of disease it is impossible to determine whether osteochondral disease (CVM), or trauma, or both, are the primary initiating factor(s).

chondrosis is, and certainly is multifactorial in its etiopathogenesis. Manipulation of diet, exercise, and growth rate, and maintenance of injury-free rearing, breaking, and training practices, may allow us to reduce the expression of this debilitating disease of horses. The ultimate goal must be to prevent this important disease of performance horses.

2. Occipitoatlantoaxial Malformations (OAAM)

Signalment. These disorders are uncommon in large animals. Arabian foals, newborn to several months of age, have been diagnosed as having OAAM perhaps more often than other groups of large animals (Whitwell, 1978), (Watson et al., 1983), (Mayhew et al., 1978b). Isolated cases occur in young horses of other breeds (Wilson et al., 1985). Calves, particularly of the Holstein breed (White et al., 1978), (Watson et al., 1985), and sheep (Watson et al., 1983) have been found with similar malformations.

History. Affected animals can be born dead, be ataxic at birth, or show progressive ataxia (wobbles) as yearling animals (Mayhew et al., 1978b), (White et al., 1978), (Boyd et al., 1987). Occasionally no neurologic signs are present, just restricted movement of the neck (Watson et al., 1983).

Physical Examination. An extended neck posture often is seen. A malformed atlas and axis can be palpated. Reduced flexion at the atlanto-occipital junction and a clicking sound as the animal moves its head or when the head is manipulated may be detected. Scoliosis may be present.

Neurological Examination. Sometimes no neurologic abnormality is present. Usually there are varying degrees of tetraparesis and ataxia leading to tetraplegia.

Assessment. Various developmental anomalies of the occiput, atlas, and axis are present, including atlanto-occipital fusion, hypoplasia of the dens, and additional bony pieces. The disease is probably inherited in Arabian horses (Watson et al., 1983), (Mayhew et al., 1978b).

Diagnosis. The clinical syndromes are distinctive, but the disease must be confirmed with radiography (Fig. 14–10). In an Arabian foal, OAAM should not be confused with CVM and cerebellar abiotrophy. Chronic, healed atlanto-occipital injury can mimic the clinical and radiographic signs of OAAM (Wilson et al., 1985).

Treatment. No therapy is indicated in Arabian horses because

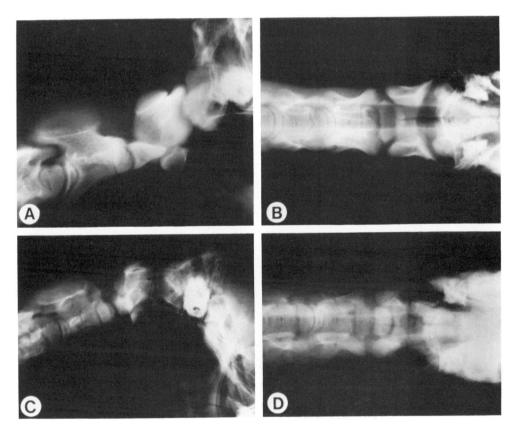

Figure 14–10. Craniovertebral radiographs of a normal 4-day-old foal (A and B) and of a 2-day-old Arabian foal with OAAM (C and D). In conjunction with atlanto-occipital fusion there is occipitalization of the hypoplastic atlas, and atlantalization of the axis with a hypoplastic dens and broad transverse processes. (From Mayhew IG, Watson AG, Heissan JA. Congenital occipitoatlantoaxial malformation in the horse. Equine Vet J 1978; *10*:4, fig. 1.)

it is most likely inherited. Therefore, the same family lines should
not be bred.

3. **Miscellaneous Congenital Vertebral and Spinal Cord Malformations**

Cases of block vertebrae, spina bifida, cavitated vertebrae, and
myelodysplasia are rarely seen in calves (Cho et al., 1977b), lambs
(Saperstein et al., 1975), (Hartley et al., 1962), piglets (Done, 1968),
and foals (Cho et al., 1977a). See Figures 14–11 and 14–12. Characteristically affected calves (Wasserman, 1986), (Henninger et al.,
1983) and foals (Cho et al., 1977a) have been noted to have bilaterally
synchronous, voluntary (bunny-hopping) and reflex movements of
the pelvic limbs (Fig. 14–11c). A bunny-hopping gait without bilaterally-active reflexes can, however, be associated with several
musculoskeletal lesions, including osteochondrosis and lumbar myopathy.

Congenital kyphosis, scoliosis, and torticollis often are associated with cases of arthrogryposis, including the contracted foal and
twisted calf syndromes (see section I.6). Toxins acting in utero can

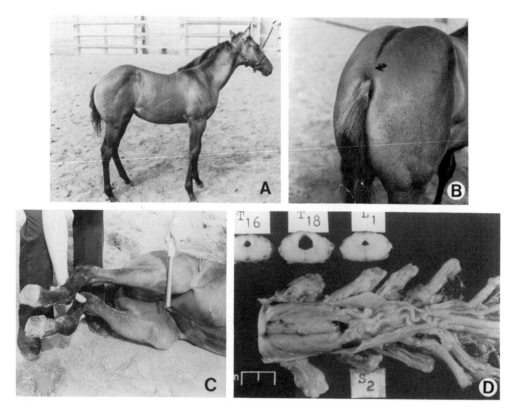

Figure 14–11. This weanling, dun Quarterhorse filly (A), was born with an incomplete dorsal
midline stripe (arrow), a depressed coccygeal vertebra, and a slightly wry tail (B). The filly had
a bunnyhopping gait and bilaterally active flexor and patellar reflexes in the pelvic limbs (C),
typical of myelodysplasia. The malformation in this case was hypoplasia of the coccygeal segments and hydromyelia of T_{16} through L_1 (D).

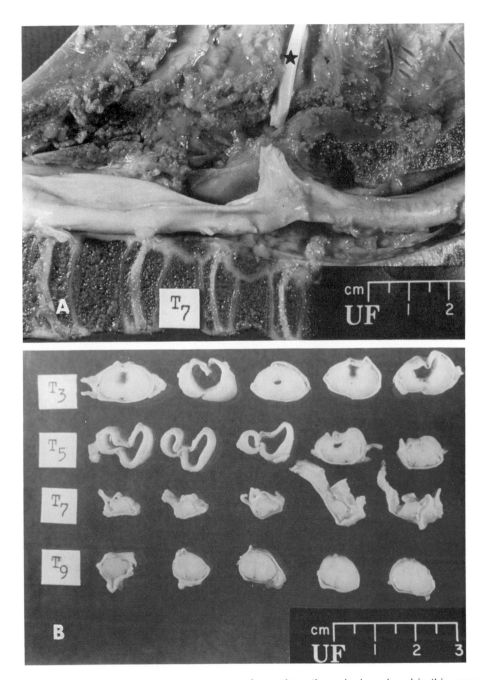

Figure 14–12. Myelodysplasia can occur anywhere along the spinal cord and in this case a newly born thoroughbred foal had meningomyelocele at T_8 (star in A), complex, severe hydromyelia, and spinal cord dysplasia from T_3 through T_{10} (B). Bilaterally active reflexes were present in the pelvic limbs and there was thoracic torticollis. (Courtesy of EM Santschi, Ocala, FL.)

effect skeletal and probably nervous system malformations (Leipold, 1973a), (Keller et al., 1981).

4. **Neuroaxonal Dystrophy**

A progressive ataxia and paraparesis progressing to tetraparesis and ataxia affects 1- to 6-month-old Suffolk lambs in the USA (Cordy et al., 1967). It is associated with accumulations of spheroids (dystrophic, swollen axons) in certain brainstem and spinal cord gray matter nuclei. It is familial and probably inherited.

A proportion of 6- to 18-month-old animals in certain families of Romney and probably other breeds of sheep in Australia (Hartley WJ, 1984, pers. comm.) and New Zealand (Hartley et al., 1962), (Thompson J, 1984, pers. comm.) have a similar syndrome of progressive ataxia, sometimes leading to recumbency. Similar widespread neuroaxonal dystrophy is present, along with neuronal fiber degeneration in the spinal cord white matter. The lesions warrant comparison with those seen in equine degenerative myeloencephalopathy (see section I.6). However, the vitamin E status of affected families has not been evaluated.

5. **Progressive Ataxia of Charolais Cattle**

Charolais cattle in the UK and in North America have been affected with this disease (Palmer et al., 1975), (Cordy, 1986). They usually are 6 to 24 months at the onset of signs and both sexes are affected. There is progressive ataxia leading to recumbency in 1 to 2 years. Affected cattle may urinate in frequent short spurts and they show ataxia and paraparesis. There are histologic lesions involving white matter in the brain and spinal cord with demyelination and production of eosinophilic plaques (Blakemore et al., 1974). Defective oligodendroglia can be detected ultrastructurally and the plaques appear to represent redundant, proliferated, oligodendroglial processes at paranodal sites (Palmer et al., 1975), (Cordy, 1986). The disease is probably inherited.

6. **Bovine Progressive Degenerative Myeloencephalopathy ("weaver") of Brown Swiss Cattle**

Affected Brown Swiss calves of either sex are 5 to 8 months old at onset of paraparesis, ataxia, and dysmetria (Stuart et al., 1983), (Leipold et al., 1973b). There is Wallerian-like neuronal fiber degeneration seen diffusely in the spinal cord, with swollen axons (spheroids) present in spinal white matter, in some brainstem nuclei, and in the cerebellar granular layer (Stuart et al., 1985). The disease is seen throughout the USA (Stuart et al., 1985) and Europe (Braun et al., 1987). A familial pattern to the disease is seen, and it is suspected to be inherited. Brown Swiss breeders identify relatives of affected cattle in the US stud books with the aim of eliminating the trait.

A similar clinicopathologic syndrome has been seen in members of a closed herd of Watusi cattle.

7. **Arthrogryposis (congenital articular rigidity, crooked calf syndrome, contracted foal syndrome)**

Signalment. This is a common syndrome in calves, but is less

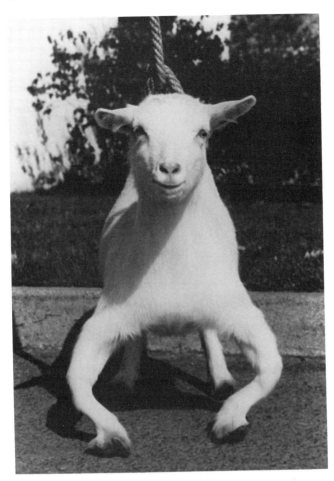

Figure 14–13. Arthrogryposis in a young goat showing mild but typical thoracic limb contractures.

so in foals, piglets, lambs and kids (Fig. 14–13 and 14–14). Newborn animals are seen to be affected when they attempt to stand and walk. In horses, the contracted foal syndrome is frequently seen in certain breeds, such as the thoroughbred in the US and small draft breeds in Europe (Vandeplassche et al., 1984). The crooked calf syndrome is common in beef calves in Western Europe (Van Huffel et al., 1987). In the western United States and Alaska it may occur at a frequency of 40% on some farms and is most common in calves from first calf heifers (Abbott et al., 1986).

History. Newborn animals have degrees of limb flexion- and extension-rigidity, with inability to stand plantigrade at birth (Fig. 14–14); sometimes the vertebral column and calvarium is similarly affected.

Examination. There are varying degrees of angular fixation of limb joints with restricted ranges of motion, muscle atrophy, and vertebral deviations such as kyphoscoliosis. Most often flexion fixation, valgus deformity of the thoracic limbs, and extension rigidity

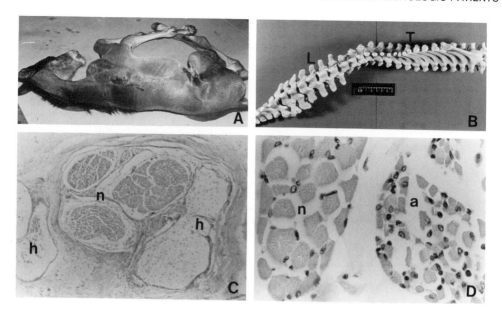

Figure 14–14. This neonatal thoroughbred "contracted foal" (A) has fixation contractures of the limbs in the position shown and thoracolumbar (TL) torticollis which is seen in this dorsal view of the vertebral column (B).

Asymmetric, partial depopulation of TL motor neurons was associated with many TL ventral nerve roots having normal (n) and hypoplastic or empty (h) fascicles (C), as well as with intervertebral multifidus muscles having normal (n) and atrophic (a) muscle fibers. This would account for the vertebral malformation.

of the pelvic limbs occurs. Cerebral signs, such as severe depression and blindness (hydranencephaly) and cerebellar signs may be present; these are most common in cattle and sheep. Charolais calves usually have a cleft palate, and severely affected foals have abdominal herniation or visceral eventration (Rooney, 1966), (Boyd, 1976).

Assessment. The term arthrogryposis means curved or sickle-shaped joints. This is secondary to anything that causes reduced movement of the fetus in utero, such as lower motor neuron (LMN) defects (Mayhew, 1984). See figure 14–14.

Even though it can occur with palatoschisis, arthrogryposis is not usually hereditary. In Charolais and Hereford cattle arthrogryposis occurs with palatoschisis and is probably inherited (Van Huffel et al., 1987), (Greene, 1979). Outbreaks of arthrogryposis and hydranencephaly in calves have occurred in several countries (Australia, Japan, Israel) with Akabane and other arboviruses (see Hydranencephaly, Problem 1).

The inherited forms of arthrogryposis, such as in Charolais cattle, are not common. Affected Charolais calves may have hypotonic (floppy) muscles, and although a neurogenic defect is suspected, the abnormal joints may be normal, lax, restricted, or fixed (Russell et al., 1985).

Akabane and other arboviruses affect fetal neurons, especially those in the spinal cord, as well as muscle cells. Thus, some lower motor neurons are absent and joints have limited mobility with subsequent angular fixations (Konno et al., 1982). Coxsackievirus A2 injected into chick embryos can result in myositis and arthrogryposis (Drachman et al., 1976). Thus, other viruses may be expected to cause the disease in other species.

Tobacco, sweet pea, locoweed, lupine, poison hemlock, and jimsonweed ingestion have been shown to produce the syndrome in pigs and cattle (Leipold et al., 1973), (Panter et al., 1985), (Keeler et al., 1981), (Van Huffel et al., 1987), (Greene, 1979). Ingestion of *Sorghum* spp grasses by pregnant cows and mares has been associated with the disease in offspring (Prichard et al., 1967), (Seaman et al., 1981).

Up to 40% of beef calves in some herds in the Western United States are affected. This is associated with ingestion of lupines by pregnant cows on day 40 to 70 of gestation; the principle toxin appears to be the quinolizidine alkaloid, anagyrine, which is present in certain species of lupines (Abbott et al., 1986). The syndrome of crooked calf disease, and the similar, frequently occurring calf arthrogryposis seen in Europe (Van Huffel, et al., 1987) are both particularly characterized by forelimb involvement.

The cause of the disease in many cases, including all cases of contracted foals, is not known. In addition to the factors already discussed, it is valid to consider several alternatives to the pathogenesis of arthrogryposis. These include: exposure to organophosphates (Rousseaux et al., 1985), anthelmintics (Drudge et al., 1983), hyperthermia (Edwards, 1978), and fetal overcrowding or fetal-maternal disproportion (Vandeplassche et al., 1984), (Vandeplassche et al., 1987).

The possibility that some cases of congenital contracted tendons in foals represent mild degrees of arthrogryposis is an interesting hypothesis (Gunn, 1976). Such a syndrome has been related to ingestion of locoweeds by pregnant mares (McIlwraith et al., 1982) and to states of hypothyroidism in affected foals (McLaughlin et al., 1986).

Treatment. Manipulation, splinting, and surgery is successful in even severely affected human patients, but the likelihood of becoming an athlete is remote. This would probably hold true with horses also. Combinations of capsulotomy, tenotomy, and desmotomy have been extremely successful (>80%) in salvaging crooked calves in Europe (Van Huffel et al., 1987). To date, only the distinct syndromes in Charolais and probably Hereford cattle have been shown to be inherited (Greene, 1979).

8. Progressive Spinal Myelinopathy in Beef Cattle

Pelvic limb ataxia and paraparesis beginning at birth, and usually progressing to severe tetraparesis, has been primarily seen in beef cattle of the Murray Gray breed in Western Australia (Richards et al., 1986). The syndrome is associated with fiber degeneration and probably a degree of demyelination in spinal cord white matter and is often severe in peripheral, subpial zones. Also, neuronal chromatolysis occurs in several gray matter nuclear regions of the brainstem and spinal cord. Lesions are reminiscent of enzootic ataxia of red deer and swayback in sheep. The exact etiology is not known, but the role of heredity, nutrient deficiencies, and environmental toxins have been discussed.

A similar disease is reported in two Murray Gray cattle in New Zealand (Belton et al., 1987)

9. Lysosomal Storage Diseases (also Problem 1)

Most of the rare, inherited, and toxin-induced lysosomal storage diseases result in evidence of progressive brain dysfunction and degrees of weight loss. However some of these, including globoid cell leukodystrophy in Polled Dorset sheep (Pritchard et al., 1980) and glycogenosis type II (Pompe's disease) in Corriedale sheep (Manketelow et al., 1975) and in Beef Shorthorn and Brahman cattle (Healy et al., 1987), (O'Sullivan et al., 1981), (Howell et al., 1981), may have progressive paraparesis and ataxia.

II. Physical

1. Spinal Cord and Vertebral Trauma

Trauma is the cause of spinal cord disease (in cases of wobbles and acute recumbency) that most frequently is suspected in clinical large animal practice.

Signalment. This involves animals of all ages and breeds, particularly those that are easily frightened and those that can attain high speeds. Pathologic fractures are seen in malnourished young stock.

History. Usually there is a sudden onset of reluctance to move, ataxia, or recumbency. Signs usually are peracute and nonprogressive, often with improvement. With hemorrhage, instability, and callus formation, signs can progress days or months following injury. Falls during performance, rearing and falling over backwards, breeding injury, and thunderstorms, may be significant historical factors.

Examination. The physical examination may be modified so the clinician first attends to life threatening problems and does not move the patient excessively—an unstable fracture may exist. Neurologic signs are not always present with vertebral damage, and syndromes are variable, with or without evidence of head trauma.

Probably C_1-T_2 is the most frequent area affected, especially the occipitoatlantoaxial region. Degrees of tetraparesis or recumbency result (Mayhew et al., 1982) (Figs. 14–15; 14–16; 14–17). Trauma to T_3-L_6 results in degrees of paraparesis leading to recumbency; the animal may dog-sit.

Of clinical significance is the fact that T-L vertebral injury resulting only in acute, mild ataxia and paraparesis (as opposed to paraplegia) is extremely rare in adult large animals. Considerable force is required to damage T-L vertebrae in these patients and most often, if the spinal cord is compressed at all, the vertebral fracture is unstable. Thus, the patient becomes paraplegic and recumbent.

Sacral fractures result in degrees of urinary and fecal incontinence, gait abnormalities in the pelvic limbs, and subsequent muscle

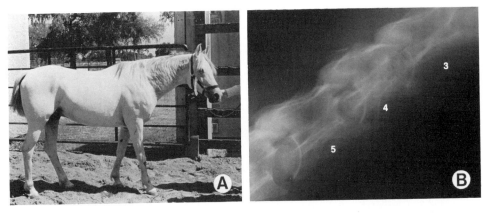

Figure 14–15. This Arabian stallion (A) injured its neck and became recumbent. Within several hours it could just rise and walk. Radiographs of the neck (B) revealed a compression fracture of C_4. The horse was treated aggressively with glucocorticosteroids and dimethyl sulfoxide and made a remarkable recovery (A). Eventually it became a successful stud horse.

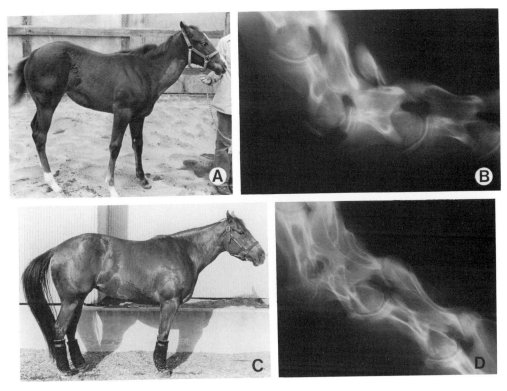

Figure 14–16. Remarkable fusion and remodelling can occur spontaneously following vertebral fractures. This Quarterhorse filly fractured C_4 and C_5 at 4-months-of-age and was severely ataxic and paretic (A and B). With stall rest and intensive anti-inflammatory therapy she made a complete neurologic recovery (C) and fusion and significant remodelling of C_4 and C_5 occurred (D).

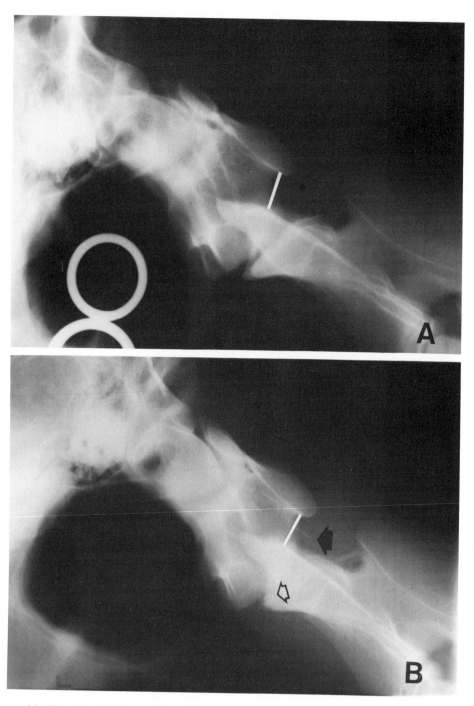

Figure 14–17. Injury to the occipitoatlantoaxial region occurs commonly in horses, and radiographs of the region can sometimes be difficult to interpret. A yearling foal injured its neck and became acutely ataxic, would not flex or extend its head, and resisted palpation of the cranial neck. Radiographs of the region were not remarkable (A). However, atlantoaxial subluxation was diagnosed because the dens was elevated from the body of the atlas and the vertebral canal diameter at C_{1-2} (white bar) measured 23 mm. An average measurement, taken from radiographs of normal weanling and yearling foals with the head in a neutral position, was 28.7 ± 2.0 mm (N = 16, min 26, max 34). Five weeks later the ataxia and neck pain had improved. The C_{1-2} measurement still was 23 mm (white bar in B). Evidence of previous trauma in the form of mineralization (filled arrow), (probably epidural) and remodelling of the ventral aspect of the dens (open arrow) was then evident.

atrophy. With sacrococcygeal involvement hypalgesia, hypotonia, and hyporeflexia of the perineum, tail, and anus occurs (see Problem 12).

Diffuse or localized sweating, the result of epinephrine release and sympathetic denervation (decentralization) respectively, often is present in horses severely affected by spinal cord injury.

Animals may be frantic as a result of pain and their inability to stand. Spinal shock (areflexia caudal to lesion) and Schiff-Sherrington signs (extensor hypertonus in otherwise normal thoracic limbs with a cranial thoracic lesion) are infrequently encountered and are short lived in large animals (Chiapetta et al., 1985), (Mason, 1971).

Initial Management. (Also see notes on head trauma in Problem 3.) For restraint, it may be necessary to utilize sedation (diazepam 0.05 to 0.1 mg/kg or xylazine 0.5 to 1 mg/kg) or to use low doses of general anesthetic agents to contain a thrashing patient suspected of suffering from spinal cord trauma.

If signs are mild, it may be best to do nothing but enforce rest. If neurologic signs of spinal cord compression are moderate or severe, most large animals probably should be given 0.1 to 0.25 mg/kg dexamethasone IV, BID to QID for 48 hours—unless immediate surgery is considered. Also, 1.0 g/kg, 10% dimethylsulfoxide in D5W, IV, appears to have been useful in relieving signs of traumatically induced spinal cord disease. Phenylbutazone and flunixin are likely to be beneficial, at least in horses. Furosemide and mannitol have not been dramatically helpful, especially in light of the profound dehydration resulting and the urinary bladder distention created—particularly in recumbent adult horses.

The use of thyrotropin-releasing hormone and naloxone in spinal cord trauma patients still is experimental, however, some promising results have been obtained (Faden et al., 1983).

Antibiotics probably are not required for vertebral fractures or spinal cord trauma, but may be necessary to treat concurrent skin lesions, cystitis, and pneumonitis—especially in recumbent patients.

In the final analysis, if a dramatic improvement occurs in the specific neurologic deficits of a patient with spinal cord trauma following a particular treatment, that treatment was probably indicated and consideration should be given to repeating it.

Initial Prognosis. At this stage of evaluation an initial prognosis frequently is requested. The outlook is guarded for all recumbent patients. However, much may be gained and little lost if final judgment is withheld for one to several hours, provided the patient is not suffering. Considering the acute phase of experimental spinal cord trauma, the functional loss is far more profound than that expected from the morphologic changes that can be seen in the spinal cord. Consequently, if further damage is prevented, return of functional integrity can be remarkable, even in control animals receiving no therapy and in clinical equine patients (Figs. 14–15,

14–16). Above all, time and good nursing care are paramount to a successful outcome.

Diagnosis. Radiography is an indispensable diagnostic aid (Figs. 14–15, 14–16, 14–17), particularly if external or internal fixation is considered. Radiography also is useful in detecting chronic osteoarthropathy, which is present in some cases of CVM, especially at C_6-T_1 (see Fig. 14–9). In these cases external injury precipitates spinal cord compresssion (Whitwell et al., 1987).

If increased intracranial pressure is suspected in a patient that may have sustained an injury, it is unwise to collect CSF from the atlanto-occipital site because of the risk of caudal herniation of the cerebrum and cerebellum. However, collection of CSF from animals that have suffered spinal cord trauma but that show no head signs is safe, particularly from the lumbosacral site. Analysis of CSF is sometimes of great assistance in ruling out other causes of peracute spinal cord disease, such as viral, verminous, and protozoal myeloencephalitis. Firm evidence of subarachnoid hemorrhage, however, may not always be found on analysis of CSF in spinal cord trauma cases. In fact, the results of CSF analysis in such animals often are normal.

Electromyography can be valuable in helping localize the site of subacute or chronic spinal cord trauma and can help to direct radiographic attention. Evidence of denervation of muscles only appears 1 to 3 weeks or probably longer after damage to the ventral gray matter or nerve roots. Prominent multifocal or diffuse denervation potentials found by electromyography on a patient with spinal cord disease would be strong evidence for a multifocal mechanism likely to be one other than injury.

Hematologic, chemical, serologic, and other tests can be useful in the differential diagnosis of spinal cord trauma cases. However, a hematologic stress pattern, unconjugated hyperbilirubinemia, uremia, and chemical and enzymatic evidence of soft tissue and possibly bone damage, may be expected in recumbent heavy animals.

External and Internal Fixation. Techniques for external fixation using newer, lightweight casting materials can be useful, especially in smaller patients such as foals, goats, and calves (Schneider, 1981), (Stashak et al., 1984). However, some horses fight such casts, necessitating their removal.

Selection of patients is vital to successful surgical intervention. Surgery probably is indicated if the patient's neurologic condition deteriorates after appropriate medical therapy, and if decompression of the spinal cord with stabilization of vertebral body luxations is feasible. Surgical texts are available describing these techniques (Stashak et al., 1984), (Wagner, 1987). Particularly in small patients, which are far easier to manage pre- and postoperatively, several of the surgical techniques of decompression and internal fixation devised for small animals (and modified for large animals) are worth attempting (Stashak et al., 1984), (Owen et al., 1978), (Guffy et al.,

1969), (Crawshaw et al., 1982), (Sorjonen et al., 1983), (Slone et al., 1979), (McCoy et al., 1984).

Prognosis. The prognosis for patients, particularly horses, suffering from spinal cord trauma associated with luxations or fractures of the vertebral body, arch, or articular processes is guarded to poor for return to use. Healing of such fractures frequently results in some degree of vertebral malalignment, sometimes with lordosis, kyphosis, scoliosis, or torticollis (Figs. 14–15, 14–16). Even after apparent healing and resolution of neurologic signs, delayed callus formation and degenerative changes in adjacent articulations can result in permanent spinal cord compression.

No simple rules can be given for the management of patient suffering from spinal cord trauma, but two points are worthy of emphasis. First, thorough and repeated neurologic examinations help the clinician arrive at a prognosis and evaluate progress of the case. Second, no individual medical or surgical therapeutic regimen is more singularly beneficial in healing spinal cord injuries than time; time alone can be the most beneficial factor in determining the patient's outcome. Hasty decisions to euthanize animals should not be made, although the clinician should consider pain and suffering (Figs. 14–15, 14–16).

2. Acquired Torticollis or "Wry-Neck"

Signalment. Foals, ponies, goats, calves, and lambs most often are affected.

History. There is usually a sudden onset of cervical torticollis whether or not the animal has a history of trauma or signs of spinal cord compression (Fig. 14–18).

Physical Examination. In the acute stage of the disease, the twisted neck can be straightened, at least to a degree, but later this becomes impossible. Usually ataxia or weakness is not present.

Diagnosis. Radiographs often are not helpful because no bone lesions are detected.

Assessment. A few cases show evidence of cervical myopathy, which is based on examination of muscle biopsy and on serum CPK activity and selenium status (McKelvey et al., 1979). Most cases probably involve subluxations of vertebrae. A high frequency of wry-neck occurred over a few years in a dairy goat herd in Australia (Dickson et al., 1986), which might suggest a nutritional factor.

Progressive, acquired torticollis associated with apparent pain has been seen in dogs and man (Child et al., 1986) and in a suckling foal. These syndromes are associated with forms of myelodysplasia, such as hydromyelia and syringomyelia, that may be acquired (Child et al., 1986).

Treatment. With uncomplicated wry-neck, external bracing has worked well when done early in the course of the syndrome (Stashak et al., 1984) (see Fig. 14–18). General anesthesia may be needed to realign the neck and apply a cast. Vitamin E and selenium therapy should be considered.

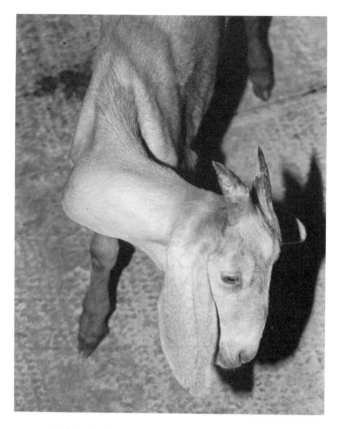

Figure 14–18. Acquired torticollis in a Nubian doe. No vertebral damage could be seen radiographically and the neck did straighten considerably with external cast support.

III. Infectious, Inflammatory, Immune

 1. Equine Herpesvirus 1 (Rhinopneumonitis) Myeloencephalitis

  Signalment. Usually adult horses of both sexes are affected, occasionally foals. Epizootics have most often been described in postfoaling mares (Jackson et al., 1977), (Charlton et al., 1976), (Greenwood et al., 1980), although outbreaks in adult horses in training have recently occurred with increasing frequency (Allen et al., 1986).

  The syndrome has been reported in almost all countries with a large equine population (Allen et al., 1986), (Carroll et al., 1985).

  Because of epizootics involving expensive breeding and performance horses, equine herpesvirus 1 (EHV1) myeloencephalitis is of major international importance. The disease has been suspected to occur in a captive zebra (*Equus burchelli*) (Montali et al., 1985).

  History. There is an acute onset of gait abnormality (ataxia) or acute recumbency. Signs generally are stable after 24 hours, though they may fluctuate somewhat. This disease often occurs in outbreaks and can be associated with abortions, respiratory infections, or fevers in the herd. Some horses may have fever (105° F) and a transient ataxia; pregnant mares, particularly, have a prodromal, distal limb edema. The disease has been seen after live virus EHV1 vaccination (Rhinoquin, now off the market) with 400 cases occurring out of 60,000 vaccinates (Liu et al., 1977), (Allen et al., 1986).

Physical Examination. Concurrent respiratory disease, fever, distal limb edema, and hypothermia have been reported, as has diarrhea in foals (Greenwood et al., 1980), (Crowhurst et al., 1981), (Pursell et al., 1979).

Neurologic Examination. Pelvic limb ataxia and paresis is usually symmetric but occasionally there is hemiparesis. Thoracic limbs can be involved. Frequently, urinary bladder paralysis with dribbling of urine, and sometimes repeated erections in males, occur. Sensory deficits over the trunk are rarely seen. Head signs, such as depression, diffuse face, jaw, tongue, and pharyngeal weakness, and signs of vestibular involvement occur less frequently (Greenwood et al., 1980), (Crowhurst et al., 1981), (Pursell et al., 1979), (Kohn et al., 1987), (Allen et al., 1986).

Assessment. The cause of the disease is the abortion-inducing strain of equine herpesvirus now called EHV1 (previously EHV1 type 1), as opposed to the primarily respiratory strain now called EHV4 (previously EHV1 type 2) (Allen et al., 1986). EHV1 is endotheliotropic, particularly for blood vessels in the CNS. Vasculitis of arterioles, with resulting ischemic necrosis of gray and particularly white matter in brain and especially spinal cord, is the underlying lesion explaining an acute (vascular) onset of neurologic signs (Little et al., 1976), (Charlton et al., 1976), (Platt et al., 1980), (Allen et al., 1986), (Jackson et al., 1977). Because of this, some authors refer to the disease as a myelopathy rather than a myelitis (de Lahunta, 1983), (Kohn et al., 1987). The pathogenesis is suspected to be an immune-mediated, Arthus-type reaction in vessels, particularly of the CNS. Apparently, reinfection (and possibly reactivation) with endotheliotropic EHV1 occurs and the virus is carried to the CNS in infected leukocytes. In the face of a particular titer of circulating anti-EHV1 antibodies, an immune-associated, Arthus-like, vasculitis ensues (Allen et al., 1986). Harvesting the virus from the CNS of affected horses has been difficult, perhaps because of its association with antibody (Allen et al., 1986), (Carroll et al., 1985), (Kohn et al., 1987), (Mumford et al., 1980). With specific, indirect antibody probes, virus antigen, IgG and complement all have been detected in arteriole walls within the CNS of clinical cases (Allen et al., 1986); however, a negative fluorescent antibody test for virus in the CNS does not exclude the diagnosis (Kohn et al., 1987). A trigeminal ganglionitis usually is present (Little et al., 1976).

Diagnosis. Cerebrospinal fluid, especially from the LS space, may have xanthochromia and elevated protein (100 to 300 mg/dl) content, but it has few cells (Kohn et al., 1987). Pre-existing EHV1 serum-neutralization titers do not appear to be protective and may in fact be necessary for the disease to occur. A fourfold rise in an affected EHV1 serum titer is good circumstantial evidence of EHV1 infection in affected individuals or in associative herd animals. Viral isolation from nasal swab, tracheal wash, and buffy coat cultures is also good evidence for the disease (Montali et al., 1985), (Kohn et al., 1987), (Allen et al., 1986).

Therapy. Probably it is best to use glucocorticosteroids in the acute phase of the disease: e.g., 0.1 to 0.25 mg/kg dexamethazone, IM, BID, for 3 days (Greenwood et al., 1980), (Kohn et al., 1987), (Mayhew et al., 1982). Good nursing care with catheterization of the urinary bladder if necessary, is most important for a successful outcome. EHV1 vaccination in the face of an outbreak is of unknown usefulness and conceivably may exacerbate an immune-mediated process. However, it may well be advisable to (re)vaccinate horses on a property where a case is suspected, if they can be regarded as unexposed (Allen et al., 1986). This is more important if EHV1 (and not EHV4 or EHV1 type 2) has been isolated (Allen et al., 1986).

Prognosis. Ambulatory horses usually improve over a few days to few months and return to neurologic normalcy. Even recumbent horses have recovered completely and raced successfully with careful nursing (Greenwood et al., 1980), (Little et al., 1976).

Prevention. Appropriate, repetitive administration of currently available EHV1 vaccines probably results in immunity to respiratory disease but not to infection (Allen et al., 1986). Thus, such animals may show EHV1 abortion or neurologic signs and may still be a menace as carriers of EHV1 (Allen et al., 1986), (Mumford, 1987), (Edington, et al., 1985). Exogenous glucocorticoids (Edington et al., 1985) and probably stress of shipping, breeding, foaling, weaning, and castration (Mumford, 1985), (Allen et al., 1986) can result in reactivation of EHV1 with virus shedding. Also, the disease can spread rapidly in an outbreak and be devastating. Therefore, it is prudent to isolate new arrivals to a property for 2 to 3 weeks, to not crowd animals undergoing weaning, vaccinating, deworming, and castration, and to be cognizant of the risk of using glucocorticoids, especially in late term mares (Mumford, 1985).

2. Caprine Arthritis—Encephalomyelitis (Viral Leukoencephalomyelitis of Goats)

Signalment. Typically the neurologic syndrome of caprine arthritis-encephalomyelitis (CAE) involves 1- to 4-month-old kid goats of many breeds, although it is now recognized in a wider age range (Cork, 1976), (Knight et al., 1982), (Cork et al., 1974), (Crawford et al., 1981), (Norman et al., 1983).

The disease varies in prevalence but probably occurs in all countries where goats are raised. Dairy breeds may be more frequently infected because of the practice of feeding pooled colostrum to dairy kids (Robinson et al., 1986).

History. Rapidly or slowly progressive ataxia, weakness and stiffness of the pelvic limbs followed by involvement of the thoracic limbs occurs. Often there is more than one kid affected over a period of time. A history of animals recently introduced to the herd, and adult goats with joint distensions, cachexia and a hard udder may be offered by the owner (Knight et al., 1982), (Robinson et al., 1986).

Physical Examination. This may detect chronic arthritis, interstitial pneumonitis, a hard udder, and weight loss (Knight et al., 1982), (Robinson et al., 1986). Infrequently, fever of 104–106° F occurs (Norman et al., 1983).

Neurologic Examination. Degrees of slightly asymmetric, paraparesis to paraplegia are initially encountered. This usually progresses to tetraplegia with hyperactive reflexes, although hypotonia and hyporeflexia (suggesting gray matter (LMM) involvement) may be present (Norman et al., 1983). Evidence of multifocal disease is helpful in making a presumptive diagnosis. Signs of cerebellar, cranial nerve, and brainstem involvement may be detected in up to 50% of cases (Norman et al., 1983).

Assessment. The etiologic, transmissible agent is a lentivirus (slow virus) of the family Retroviridae, which has only slight antigenic differences from ovine progressive pneumonia virus and visna-maedi virus in sheep (Knight et al., 1982), (Robinson et al., 1986), (Ellis et al., 1983). Perinatal, horizontal spread results from contact and particularly from colostrum and milk. The dam of affected kids often is young and primiparous. Often an area or farm has a high rate of infection (90%) but a low rate of clinical disease (10%). Young, infected kids may develop CNS signs, but arthritis usually is recognized in goats over 1 year old (Ellis et al., 1983).

Severe, granulomatous, pervascular myelitis (especially involving white matter) occurs. The virus also produces a nonsuppurative polyarthritis and probably a proliferative pneumonitis. Adult goats have been detected with histopathologic lesions of polyarthritis, pneumonitis, and varying degrees of encephalomyelitis; the latter is usually subclinical. This lentivirus infects monocyte-macrophage cells, which produce a unique interferon which seems to curtail viral replication and enhance expression of specific histocompatible antigens—perhaps augmenting the host's lymphoproliferative response (Zink et al., 1987).

Diagnosis. A CSF mononuclear pleocytosis and elevated protein content should be sought; it is present in about half the cases (Norman et al., 1983). Needle EMG studies may show mild, multifocal, gray matter (LMN) disease. Serum agar gel immunodiffusion (AGID) and enzyme-linked immunosorbent assay (ELISA) tests are helpful in confirming the presence of infection in a herd. However, a negative serum test result may not be diagnostic because such animals have been found to harbor virus and pathologic lesions (Norman et al., 1983), (Robinson et al., 1986), and only 42% of clinically affected goats may be seropositive (Grewal, 1986). Many flocks will have animals that show a positive AGID test, in which there may be no evidence of active disease in young stock but arthritis in older animals. Neonatal infection thus may result in apparent protection, CNS disease, arthritis, probably pneumonitis, or more often, nothing. Copper deficiency (see V.3 below) may complicate the diagnosis.

Therapy. There is no therapy, although anti-inflammatory drugs may delay progression of the disease.

Prognosis. Usually the neurologic syndrome is permanent and crippling and most often is fatal (Norman et al., 1983).

Control. The kids can be removed from their dams at birth to prevent infection via colostrum and milk. Kids then must be fed pasteurized milk from goats tested free of the disease, cows milk, or milk replacer. They need to be serotested several times until at least 90 days of age before joining other virus-free herd mates. A closed herd policy or introduction of seronegative animals that are quarantined for 90 days and tested negative also is required. Such schemes of colostrum deprivation and repeated neurologic testing, with removal of seropositive animals, form the basis of control and eradication programs (Robinson et al., 1986), (Knight et al., 1983), (Adams et al., 1983).

3. **Visna-Maedi and Ovine Progressive Pneumonia (OPP)**

Signalment. Adult sheep, usually over two years of age, are affected with the rare nervous form of this disease: ovine progressive meningoencephalitis or visna (Ellis et al., 1983), (Petursson et al., 1978).

History. Affected adult sheep or flock mates may show progressive respiratory difficulties and weight loss, with ataxia and stumbling progressing to recumbency.

Physical Examination. Sheep are cachectic, afebrile, and often have interstitial pneumonia, rarely arthritis (Ellis et al., 1983), (Zink et al., 1987).

Neurologic Examination. Degrees of ataxia, para- and tetraparesis are found.

Assessment. The causative lentiviruses of visna-maedi and OPP are almost identical and have only slight antigenic differences from CAE (Ellis et al., 1983), (Zink et al., 1987). Maedi (dyspnea) and visna (wasting) were described in Iceland in the 1930s, but have since been eradicated. Although OPP occurs in North America and Western Europe, neurologic signs associated with meningoencephalomyelitis are rare (Sheffield et al., 1980), (Cutlip et al., 1979), (Petursson et al., 1978), (Ellis et al., 1983). As with CAE, mononuclear cells become persistently infected with the retrovirus in the face of circulating and spinal fluid antibodies (Petursson et al., 1978), and invoke a chronic, prominent, mononuclear inflammation in lung, meninges, brain, spinal cord, mammary gland, and joints (Sheffield et al., 1980), (Cutlip et al., 1979), (Petursson et al., 1978).

Diagnosis. A specific circulating antibody appears within 4 months of infection, at which time the virus can be isolated from buffy coat and CSF mononuclear cells. Prominent (100 to 500 per μL) mononuclear pleocytosis occurs in CSF early in the disease course (Petursson et al., 1978).

Treatment. There is no treatment and affected sheep will die. The severity of CNS lesions can be significantly reduced with immunosuppression, but persistent virus shedding remains. (Petursson et al., 1978).

Control. Control measures based on artificial rearing, repeated serologic testing, and culling (as for CAE) are feasible but not practical.

4. Vertebral Osteomyelitis and Discospondylitis

Signalment. Usually this is a bacterial disease and is seen most frequently in neonates of all species (Stashak et al., 1984). Fungal osteomyelitis of vertebrae is rare in large animals (Markel et al., 1986).

Clinical Complaint. Neck or back pain, paresis, and ill thrift occur in various combinations (Markel et al., 1986), (Sherman et al., 1986), (Adams et al., 1985), (Stashak et al., 1984).

History. Often there is an acute onset of pain or stiffness, with or without progressive paresis.

Physical Examination. Diarrhea, polyarthritis, localized sepsis, docking abscesses, or intrathoracic or abdominal abscesses often are coexisting problems.

Neurologic Examination. Sometimes focal spinal cord compression is evident, but frequently only localizing signs of heat, pain, and swelling along the vertebral column are present. Areas of hyperreflexia, hyporeflexia, and patches of sweating (horse) also can occur.

Assessment. Osteomyelitis, vertebral arthritis, and discospondylitis occur at variable sites in the vertebral column, especially C_{1-2}, C_{6-7}, and lumbar vertebrae. Sometimes there is direct extension from external wounds, such as paravertebral injection abscesses, and from intrathoracic abscesses (Fig. 14–19). In ruminants the lesion usually develops from intervertebral (dorsal) joint sepsis with local extension (Dodd et al., 1964). Such a lesion is best termed an epidural empyema (Chaldek et al., 1976).

Many different organisms have been isolated, particularly *Streptococcus* spp, *Salmonella* sp, *Actinobacillus equuli, Eikenella corrodens,* and *Rhodococcus equi* (Fig. 14–19) in foals, and *Brucella abortus* and *Mycobacterium tuberculosis* in adult horses (Stashak et al., 1984), (Richardson, 1986), (Adams et al., 1985), (Markel et al., 1986), (Kelley et al., 1972). Organisms associated with this disease in ruminants include *Pasturella* sp, *Spherophorus* sp, *Corynebacterium* sp, and *Staphylococcus* sp (Sherman et al., 1986), (Dodd et al., 1964), (Finly, 1975). In swine with discospondylitis the organisms recovered have included *Cornebacterium pyogenes, Staphylococcus* sp, *Erysipelothrix insidiosa,* and *Streptococcus* sp (Doige, 1982), (Finly, 1975), (Dodd et al., 1964), (Doige, 1980).

Diagnosis. Needle electromyographic examination and radiographs are helpful in localizing the site and defining the nature of the disease, respectively (Stashak et al., 1984), (Whitwell et al., 1987), (Markel et al., 1986), (Adams et al., 1985). Cerebrospinal fluid analysis may be normal or it may show evidence of compression with xanthochromia, a mild increase in mononuclear cells, and an elevated protein content (Smith et al., 1984), (Sherman et al., 1986), (Adams et al., 1985), (Markel et al., 1986). Occasionally neutrophils are present, but rarely can the organism be cultured from CSF (Sherman et al., 1986), (Markel et al., 1986). Direct aspiration and anerobic

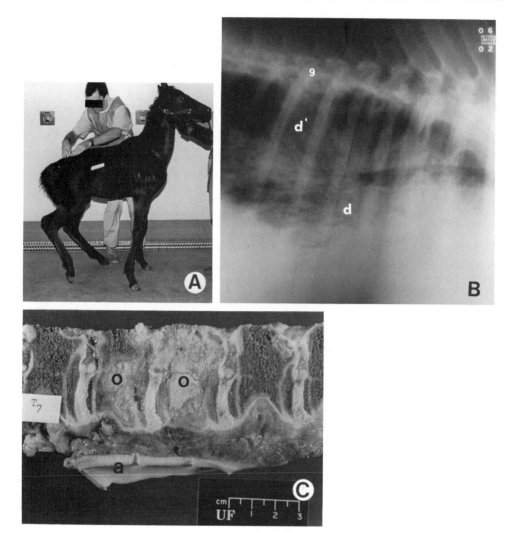

Figure 14–19. This 3-month-old filly was being treated for pneumonia and suddenly developed paraparesis (A). Partial sensory loss and a localized pain response indicated that there was a mid-thoracic spinal cord lesion. Thoracic radiographs (B) revealed patchy pulmonary densities (d), one of which (d′) projected up to the ninth thoracic vertebra (9). At postmortem examination *R. equi* pneumonia with abscessation was found. One abscess had spread around the aorta (a) to result in osteomyelitis (o) of T_8 and T_9 and an epidural empyema (C).

and aerobic culture from the lesion in the vertebrae has been useful in identifying the organisms and directing antimicrobial therapy. A tuberculin test, *Brucella* titer, and blood and urine cultures are indicated in adult horses.

Recently, nuclear scintigraphy (Markel et al., 1986), ultrasound (Richardson, 1986), and infrared thermography have been used to help identify the site of vertebral osteomyelitis.

Treatment. This is mainly prolonged antimicrobial therapy, preferably based on culture results (Richardson, 1986), (Adams et al., 1985), (Markel et al., 1986). Surgical drainage of osteomyelitis and spinal cord decompression should be considered; it has been successful in treating some cases (Richardson, 1986), (Palmer et al., 1963), (Smith et al., 1984). The prognosis is guarded, but can be good if prolonged therapy is possible and spinal cord compression is not severe.

5. Equine Protozoal Myeloencephalitis

Background. Equine protozoal myeloencephalitis (EPM) involves invasion of the equine central nervous system (CNS) by an as yet unidentified sporozoan parasite. It is a frequent cause of many syndromes of CNS dysfunction in horses in eastern North America (Mayhew et al., 1978). Also, from a clinical viewpoint, it is probably the most frequently diagnosed protozoal disease of horses in this part of the world.

The disease EPM is likely to be identical to focal myelitis-encephalitis described in Kentucky and Pennsylvania during the 1960s (McGrath, 1962), (Prickett, 1968), (Rooney et al., 1970). It is also probably identical to *Toxoplasma*-like encephalomyelitis subsequently reported from several eastern states (Beech et al., 1974), (Cusick et al., 1974), (Dubey, 1974), (Dubey et al., 1974).

More recently, identical protozoan parasites have been observed in CNS lesions in horses living in California (Dorr et al., 1984), (Madigan et al., 1987), Saskatchewan, Canada (Clark et al., 1981), and Brasil (Lombardo de Barros, L., 1985, pers. comm.; Macruz R, 1980, pers. comm.). In São Pâulo, Brasil the clinical syndrome was complicated by ophthalmitis, abortion, and irritability. Concurrent *Toxoplasma gondii* infection, evidenced by high Sabin-Feldman dye tests and indirect fluorescent antibody tests, likely occurred (Ishizuka et al., 1975), (Macruz et al., 1975). Horses that originated in Eastern USA, but resided in England, also have had clinical syndromes and histologic lesions containing protozoa identical to EPM organisms (Whitwell KE, 1984, pers. comm.). There may be more than one protozoal organism that can invade the equine CNS; however, EPM certainly is an emerging protozoan disease of horses with international significance.

Signalment. Young to adult, lightbred horses are most often affected with EPM, particularly standardbred and thoroughbred horses on breeding and training establishments. Horses of all common light breeds in North America and from 2 months to over 20 years of age have been affected. One 10-year old pony has been reported to have EPM (Dubey et al., 1986).

History. Clinically, variable syndromes reflect involvement of almost any part of the equine CNS; the lesions represent typically multifocal, necrotic, nonsuppurative myeloencephalitis. All aspects of the syndromes are extremely variable because of the variation in the site of CNS involvement and the extent and progression of the lesion. Historically, a mild lameness occurs, which frequently defies localization, or there may be an acute onset of ataxia, head tilt, weakness of one or more limbs, or recumbency. Lesions, as evidenced by the associated clinical signs, may be fulminant in hours to days or may remain quiescent for periods of months to years with or without therapy.

Physical Examination. This may reveal muscle atrophy, sweating, decubitus, constipation, urinary incontinence, or other problems related to the CNS lesions. No consistent involvement of other body systems has been reported.

Neurologic Examination. Almost any neurologic syndrome of horses can be produced by EPM. Extremely selective focal lesions may involve one nucleus or tract in the CNS. Thus, unilateral facial paralysis, hemiatrophy of the tongue, unilateral hypermetria, radial paralysis, or unilateral quadriceps (Fig. 14–20) or gluteal (Fig. 14–21) muscle atrophy may be present with no other signs of CNS involvement. More frequently, syndromes of brainstem or spinal cord disease, with asymmetric ataxia and tetra- or paraparesis, occur. Variable localizing findings of cranial nerve dysfunction and hyporeflexia, hypotonia, muscle atrophy, hypalgesia, and sweating of the neck, limbs, trunk, tail, and anus can be detected. On the other hand, many horses with EPM are first seen as wobblers with degrees of symmetric weakness, ataxia, and hypometria in the thoracic and/ or the pelvic limbs—indicating cervical spinal cord involvement. The unusual syndrome of moving with the thoracic limbs extended forward and the head held low (reflecting a caudal cervical gray

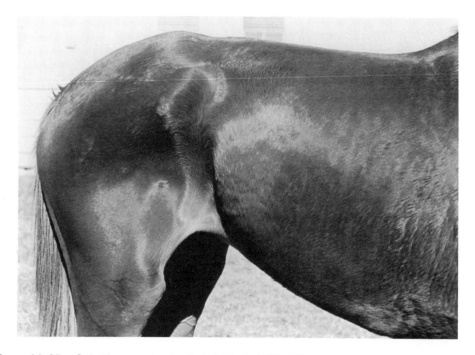

Figure 14–20.   Selective muscle atrophy is typical of EPM. This horse developed right quadriceps muscle atrophy with no initial change in gait. Extensor weakness and pelvic limb ataxia ensued and the horse was euthanized. Protozoal organisms were present in a nonsuppurative lesion at L_4.

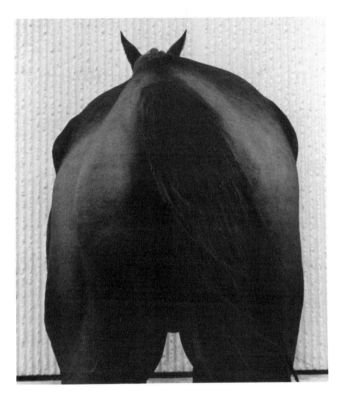

Figure 14–21. Unilateral (middle) gluteal muscle atrophy in lightbreed, mature horses from eastern North America most often is caused by EPM.

matter lesion and thoracic limb weakness) has most consistently been the result of EPM (Fig. 14–22).

Differential Diagnosis. Other diseases to be considered with cases of EPM vary considerably, but for the most part depend on the anatomic location of the lesion(s) (Fig. 14–3C). Diffuse cerebral involvement, although not frequently seen, can mimic equine viral encephalomyelitides, moldy corn poisoning, and hepatoencephalopathy. With acute brainstem involvement, particularly involving vestibular dysfunction, head trauma and verminous migrations need to be considered. Cervical vertebral trauma, cervical vertebral malformation, vertebral osteomyelitis, various verminous myelitides, equine herpesvirus-1 myelitis, and equine degenerative myeloencephalopathy, should be considered in the diagnosis of cases having just spinal cord involvement. Interestingly, with selective CNS involvement, the disease can mimic several other selective CNS and even peripheral nerve and muscle syndromes. These include tetanus, *Sorghum* sp intoxication, lathyrism, stringhalt, fibrotic myopathy, neuritis of the cauda equina, and peripheral nerve trauma.

Based on 210 cases of neurologic disorders in the horse, a presumptive clinical diagnosis and a definitive pathologic diagnosis were made; the accuracy of diagnosis of EPM was between 81 to

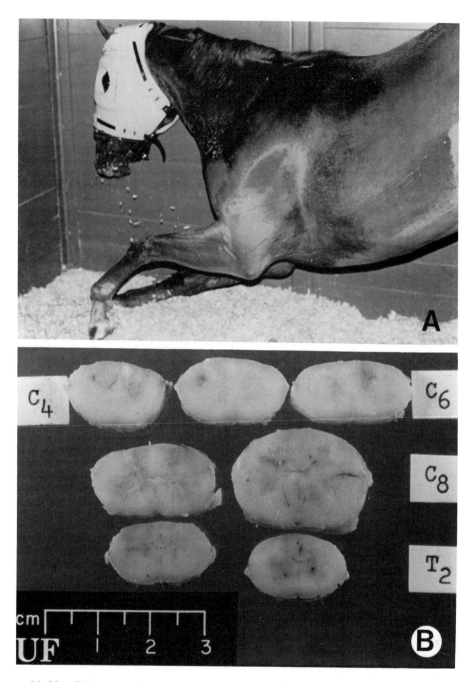

Figure 14–22. This unusual syndrome of selective thoracic limb extensor weakness with little change in pelvic limb gait (A) has been seen frequently with EPM. The lesion is at C_8-T_2 (B).

95%—depending on the accuracy parameter used (Mayhew, unpublished data, 1988).

Assessment. Typically one or more focal areas of pink, brown, or yellow discoloration are seen, as well as softening, with swelling of the tissue, in the brainstem or spinal cord (Fig. 14–22B). Histologically, necrosis and inflammation occurs in these areas, with macrophages, lymphocytes, eosinophils, and sometimes multinucleate cells and plasma cells also present. With severe necrosis focal hemorrhage and neutrophil infiltration occurs. Nucleated merozoites (1 to 4 μm long) individually, or in groups, without a well-defined cyst wall, can be seen within or near these lesions (Beech et al., 1974), (Dubey et al., 1974), (Mayhew et al., 1978a). The extent and the severity of the myeloencephalomeningitis accompanying EPM vary considerably. Sporozoan organisms may be seen in about half the cases in which typical lesions are present (Mayhew et al., 1978a), (Simpson et al., 1980).

Nature of the Protozoan Parasite. Ultrastructurally, the putative cause of EPM is a sporozoan with an apical complex that appears to divide by endopolyogeny (Clark et al., 1981), (Mayhew et al., 1978a), (Simpson et al, 1980). Further positive identification of this agent is lacking and indeed the possibility that there is more than one protozoan parasite causing EPM is not to be discounted.

As stated above, serologic evidence as well as ultrastructure characteristics suggest it is not *Toxoplasma gondii.* A group of horses with EPM showed some serologic evidence of exposure to *Sarcocystis cruzi*-like antigens (Mayhew et al., 1978a), although an attempt to infect horses with *S. cruzi* sporocysts failed (Mayhew et al., 1981). With some ultrastructural similarities to *Sarcocystis* spp and perhaps serologic cross reactivity to *S. cruzi* (Mayhew et al., 1978), it is reasonable to suppose that the EPM agent is at least related to *Sarcocystis.*

The possibility that the EPM agent is *Klossiella equi* has been expressed (Brown et al., 1977), although there was no difference in the frequency of the presence of *K. equi* in the kidneys of 10 horses that had EPM and 10 horses that did not have EPM (Mayhew et al., 1981). Merozoites have been detected in leukocytes within CNS vessels. Thus, like many coccidian parasites, there may be a parasitemia with secondary infection of the CNS. Any other route of infection of the CNS would be unusual for a protozoan parasite.

Diagnostic Aids. A specific antemortem diagnostic test for EPM does not exist. For the most part, ancillary aids are used to rule out other diseases from the differential diagnosis. Radiographs of the skull, vertebral column, and limbs assist in diagnosing many traumatic, developmental, and inflammatory bone diseases associated with neurologic syndromes. Results of hematologic, serum chemistry, serologic, and toxicity testing are necessary to evaluate for many diseases included in the differential diagnosis. Of some significance is the fact that no form of immunodeficiency or immunosuppression has so far been related to the disease at the time of clinical evaluation.

Electromyography can help localize lower motor neuron (gray matter) involvement. With multifocal sites of denervation potential, the likelihood of EPM—as opposed to many usually unifocal or diffuse disorders—becomes more probable.

Analysis of cerebrospinal fluid (CSF) is usually normal, but it can reveal a mild, moderate, or even profound (rarely) nonsuppurative inflammatory response with necrosis. Thus, some degree of xanthochromia, with large and small mononuclear cell pleocytosis, may be present. The CSF analysis is usually abnormal when taken from a site close to a large, acute lesion and usually normal when there are small, quiescent lesions present. Only rarely are eosinophils (Traver et al., 1978) or neutrophils present.

If or when the putative coccidian agent is identified and purified, serologic testing should become an invaluable diagnostic tool for EPM. Presently available serologic data would suggest that the organism is not *Sarcocystis cruzi, Toxoplasma gondii* (Beech, 1974), (Beech et al., 1974), (Dubey et al., 1974), (Mayhew et al., 1978a), or many of the common *Sarcocystis* spp affecting domestic animals in North America (Fayer et al., 1986).

Therapy. Based on clinical experience EPM appears to be a treatable disease. The basis of therapy is antifolate drugs, such as pyrimethamine and a sulfonamide given for a prolonged period. A common regimen used is pyrimethamine at 0.5 mg/kg, orally followed by 0.1 to 0.25 mg/kg, SID, orally and trimethoprim/sulfadiazine at 15 to 20 mg (total dose)/kg, BID, orally. Both should be given for 4 to 12 weeks. The folic acid inhibiting effect of these drugs should be monitored by observing for cytopenia and particularly neutropenia and thrombocytopenia. Vitamin B-complex can be given in view of the antimicrobial effect on gastrointestinal flora, although the antidote for toxicity of these drugs is folinic acid, and dosages of up to 40 mg/day/horse may be required. Reduction in dosages of the antifolate drugs has alleviated early signs of leukopenia.

If the disease is profound or acute then anti-inflammatory drugs usually are used. Phenylbutazone (5 mg/kg/daily, orally), dimethylsulfoxide DMSO (1 g/kg/daily, IV, 10% in D5W, for 1 to 5 days), and even glucocorticosteroids (0.05 to 0.2 mg/kg dexamethazone, IM, up to QID, for 1 to 5 days), have all been used. Side effects, such as laminitis with glucocorticosteroid therapy, must be taken into consideration. In addition, pyrimethamine and DMSO are not licensed for use in the horse. The intensity and duration of therapy frequently depend upon empirical evaluation of the severity and progressive nature of the lesion(s), and thus whether inflammation and edema are significantly contributing to the clinical signs. Prolonged use of glucocorticosteroids, alone, appears to be associated with the progression of EPM over periods of weeks, as does *Toxoplasma* encephalitis in immunosuppressed humans and animals

(Brewer, 1984), (Handler et al., 1983). Nevertheless, it is worthwhile to consider short-term use of such drugs to reduce inflammation during antiprotozoal therapy and before multiplication of coccidian zoites becomes rampant—a process that probably takes several weeks.

Certainly, hundreds of horses suspected of having EPM have been treated. However, with survival no definitive diagnosis is possible; thus accurate cure rates cannot be given. On the other hand, it is rare to see protozoa in typical EPM lesions of horses that have undergone necropsy after being treated with adequate antiprotozoal therapy for more than 48 hours. In a study of 73 horses with a definitive pathologic diagnosis of EPM, 41 had received appropriate antiprotozoal therapy for 1 day to 12 weeks and 32 had not received such therapy. In only 2 of those treated (5%) were organisms found histologically, whereas in 19 of those not treated (59%) organisms were found (Mayhew, unpublished data, 1988).

Prognosis. The disease probably is not transmittable from horse to horse, although clusters of cases are seen on single establishments over periods of months to several years. Untreated, the disease appears to be progressive, although therapy does appear to be able to arrest or to slow down progression of the lesion(s). There is no definitive antimortem diagnostic test, so it is not known what the horse has if it survives. With intensive therapy, progress of the disease often can be halted, but residual deficits may be unacceptable; therefore, the prognosis is usually guarded.

Prevention. Because the life cycle is not known, no specific recommendations can be made regarding prevention of either the disease or of the possibility of a reinfection or reexacerbation. Indeed, some horses that have recovered well from a syndrome suspected to be caused by EPM have returned to a similar environment and have had new and different signs of EPM. When they were destroyed, both chronic and peracute histologic lesions of EPM, consistent with the successive syndromes, were discovered. Because of these experiences, regimens of prophylaxis have been suggested in some cases. One such regimen might be 1 mg/kg pyrimethamine and 20 mg/kg trimethoprim-sulfadiazine orally, once every 7 to 14 days.

6. Verminous Myelitis (also Problem 1)

Signalment. This occurs in animals of any age, especially in young goats and lambs, adult cattle, swine, and horses. Affected animals are not necessarily severely parasitized.

History. Most often there is a peracute onset of an asymmetric gait abnormality, which progresses rapidly. However, stable periods of days to weeks can occur. Application of a systemic organophosphate anthelmintic a few hours to few days before the onset of signs may be significant in affected cattle.

Physical Examination. Usually this is noncontributory. Warble (*Hypoderma* sp) larvae may be evident on the backs of affected (and unaffected) cattle and horses.

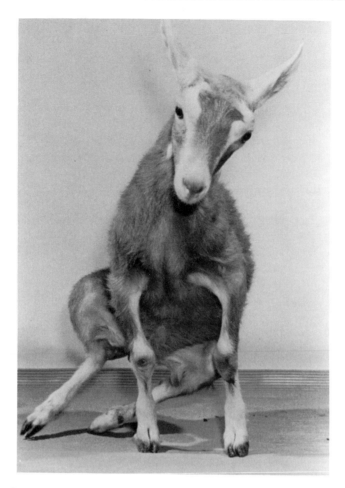

Figure 14–23. Several *Parelaphostrongylus tenuis* larvae migrating through the spinal cord to the brain stem resulted in progressive, asymmetric paraparesis, paraplegia, then tetraparesis and left vestibular signs in this young Toggenburg doe.

Neurologic Examination. Asymmetric mono-, para-, or tetra-paresis or paralysis occurs. Multifocal signs (*Parelaphostrongylus tenuis*) occur in kids and lambs, and occasionally in horses. Both upper (spastic) and lower (flaccid) motor neuron paralysis can occur. Also, head signs, especially asymmetric cranial nerve signs, and occasionally signs of cerebral disease, may be evident (Fig. 14–23).

Assessment. In goats and sheep, and several other wild and domesticated ruminant species, *P. tenuis,* the meningeal worm of white-tailed deer, often invades the spinal cord, brainstem, and cerebellum and often more than one parasite is present (Mayhew et al., 1976), (Alden et al., 1975), (Krogdahl et al., 1987), (Stackhouse, 1977).

In cattle usually a single *Hypoderma bovis* instar invades the spinal cord. Organophosphate therapy may cause death of epidural *H. bovis* instars and results in an acute necrosis and granulomatous inflammatory reaction (Andrews, 1981)—although this pathogenesis of acute ataxia has been questioned previously (Khan, 1969). Evidence of spinal cord involvement, mostly paraparesis or paraplegia in previously normal cattle, can thus occur hours to days following organophosphate treatment. Signs occurring days to weeks following use of such compounds are likely to be the result of delayed organophosphate intoxication (see section IV.2).

In swine, a single *Stephanurus dentatus* larva usually invades the lumbar spinal cord (Maxie, 1985).

With intrusion of *Strongylus vulgaris* larvae into the CNS of horses and donkeys an acute infarction, with or without subsequent parasite migration, usually occurs in the forebrain (Little et al., 1974) or thoracolumbar spinal cord (Vos et al., 1985), (Mayhew et al., 1984), (Little, 1972). Singular *Hypoderma* sp instars can enter through large natural foramina, such as the foramen magnum, the optic foramen, and occasionally intervertebral foramina (Hadlow et al., 1977). Multiple filarial parasites, such as *Setaria* spp, may invade the CNS, especially the spinal cord (Innes et al., 1955a), (Fraunfelder et al., 1980). Multiple, small, *Micronema (Halicephalobus) deletrix* usually cause diffuse acute encephalitis, sometimes associated with signs of renal disease (Rubin et al., 1974), (Blunden et al., 1987). Spiruroids like *Draschia megastoma* have invaded brain and possibly spinal cord tissue. One was quiescent for 6 weeks before re-migrating (Mayhew et al., 1982).

Various species of *Elaphostrongylus* can invade the vasculature of the head and produce blindness and other neurologic signs in various wild ruminants, such as elk, and reindeer, and possibly domestic ruminants (Adcock et al., 1969), (Kummeneje, 1974).

Diagnosis. Good diagnostic evidence of cerebrospinal nematodiasis and myiasis includes an eosinphilic or neutrophilic pleocytosis in CSF with varying numbers of macrophages and red blood cells. It would be possible to find some larval species such as *Parelophostrongylus tenuis* or *Micronema deletrix* in the CSF (Powers et al., 1977).

Therapy. Suggested anthelmintics (Mayhew et al., 1976), (Mayhew et al., 1982), (Shoho, 1954) for various hosts include: diethylcarbamazine (DEC), or levamisole or thiabendazole (TBZ) for goats and sheep; organophosphates (OP) for cattle; fenbendazole (FBZ) for swine; oxfendazole (OFZ), TBZ, FBZ, OP, DEC for horses (varies with sites of migration); ivermectin for all species.

Suggested doses of these anthelmintics are: TBZ 440 mg/kg; DEC 50 mg/kg; FBZ 60 mg/kg once, 50 mg/kg repeated in 2 to 3 days, or 7.5 mg/kg/daily for 5 days; OFZ 10 mg/kg; levamisole 14 mg/kg; routine systemic dose for OP.

Glucocorticosteroids are definitely helpful. Phenylbutazone obviates the systemic (lethal) effects of intravenous preparations of dead *Hypoderma bovis* in cattle (Eyre et al., 1981) and usually should be included in the therapy. Ivermectins might appear to be the drugs of choice at 200 µg/kg for horses; however, they can take up to 10 days to kill larvae.

Prognosis. Usually degrees of permanent deficit should be expected with this group of diseases, but some amazing recoveries have been seen when early, aggressive, anti-inflammatory and anthelmintic therapy has been undertaken. For prevention, avoid contact with natural hosts where appropriate and maintain routine anthelmintic programs.

IV. Toxic

1. Selenium Toxicity

Signalment. Neurologic signs due to selenium toxicity are usually seen in feeder pigs (Wilson et al., 1983).

Blind staggers occur in horses and cattle in the Southern Plain states and are associated with ingestion of selenium-accumulating plants (locoweeds). Signs of mania and ataxia predominate. Actually the disease is probably locoism—an induced mannosidosis (see Problem 1).

Clinical Syndrome. There is a sudden onset of ataxia and recumbency in several feeder pigs in a group. Some recumbent pigs can raise up on the thoracic or on the pelvic limbs. Flaccid areflexia, reflecting loss of lower motor neuronal function, occurs in the thoracic and/or the pelvic limbs (Fig. 14–24). Pigs still standing may show lameness with separation of the hoof at the coronary band (Wilson et al., 1988).

Assessment. An acute poliomyelomalacia, particularly in the ventral gray horns at the brachial and the lumbosacral intumescence,

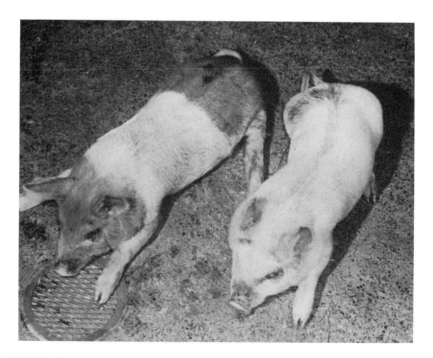

Figure 14–24. Selenium toxicity in swine results in an acute onset of para- or tetraplegia as shown, and is due to poliomyelomalacia involving the thoracic or lumbosacral intumescence. Severe depression of pelvic or thoracic spinal reflexes is characteristic of the syndrome.

occurs; it accounts for the flaccid paralysis (Harrison et al., 1983),(Casteel et al., 1985). Histologically, lesions can occur in several brainstem nuclei, including nucleus cuneatus, nucleus gracillis, facial nucleus, trigeminal motor nucleus, and reticular nuclei (Harrison et al., 1983), (Wilson et al., 1983), (Wilson et al., 1988). Clinical deficiencies of their function might be expected. Acutely, there are fibrinoid, degenerative, vascular changes, neuronal degeneration, and eosinophil infiltration. In chronic cases, significant necrosis of neurons and glia with microglial infiltration occurs, often resulting in microcavitation (Wilson et al., 1983), (Wilson et al., 1988).

Diagnosis. Results of spinal fluid analysis have revealed a mildly elevated (40 to 130 mg/dl) protein content (Harrison et al., 1983). Dramatic increases in cell counts would not be predicted.

Whole blood selenium concentrations in clinically (0.57 ± 0.06 μg/ml) and experimentally (3.7 ± 0.2 μg/ml) affected pigs have been higher than control (0.13 ± 0.01 μg/ml) values. Also, fresh liver selenium concentrations in clinically (3.8 ± 0.4 μg/g of liver) and experimentally (17.8 ± 2.3 μg/g of liver) affected pigs are far above control values (0.45 ± 0.01 μg/g of liver) and are the best diagnostic test available (Wilson et al., 1983).

Dietary selenium in excess of 20 μg/g of dry matter is sufficient to produce the syndrome (Casteel et al., 1985), (Harrison et al., 1983). Oral dosing of pigs with 1.4 to 4.2 mg/kg sodium selenite daily resulted in the syndrome between days 3 and 20 (Wilson et al., 1988).

A similar syndrome with sparing of neurons and more white matter damage has been produced experimentally with induced nicotinic acid deficiency (O'Sullivan et al., 1980). This mechanism should be given consideration if selenium deficiency can be ruled out in a particular outbreak.

Prognosis. Some mildly affected pigs can be salvaged and marketed once the toxic feed is removed (Casteel et al., 1985).

Prevention. Recommended, safe dietary selenium for growing swine is 0.24 ppm (Wilson et al., 1983).

2. Delayed Organophosphate Toxicity

Signalment. Young and adult sheep (especially Suffolk), cattle, and swine.

History. Most often an outbreak of acutely progressive ataxia and paraplegia occurs 1 week to several months after use of organophosphate (OP) spray or drench, or after accidental access to certain industrial organophosphates (Baker et al., 1970), (Williams et al., 1976), (Kruckenberg et al., 1973), (Wells, 1984). Some may die at the time of contact with signs of acute, anticholinesterase OP toxicity.

Neurologic Examination. Rapidly progressive, symmetric paraparesis and ataxia of the pelvic limbs occur; the animal becomes paraplegic and dog-sits (Fig. 14–25) and occasionally becomes tetraplegic (Williams et al., 1976), (Sanders et al., 1985), (Perdrizet et al., 1985), (Beck et al., 1977).

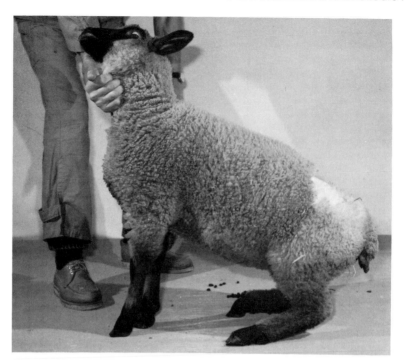

Figure 14–25. Acute ataxia and paraparesis occurred in a group of Suffolk lambs about 14 days after being drenched with an organophosphate anthelmintic (haloxon). Some lambs demonstrated acute organophosphate toxicity several hours after dosing, but the affected lambs were normal until the delayed neurologic signs appeared. Preservation of spinal reflexes helps distinguish this syndrome from enzootic ataxia (see V.3 below).

Pigs may initially have hypermetria and even a stringhalt-like gait in the pelvic limbs (Kruckenberg et al., 1973). Affected cattle have demonstrated dyspnea (Beck et al., 1977), presumably the result of laryngeal paralysis, which occurs in horses (also Problem 5).

Assessment. The potent neurotoxins triorthocresyl phosphate and triaryl phosphate can be found in industrial lubricants and wastes. Haloxon and possibly other OP anthelmintics and insecticides have been involved. The disease is not primarily related to suppression of blood cholinesterase activity, but may be associated with suppression of other neural esterases, effecting myelin and/or neuroaxonal metabolism. This results in symmetric fiber degeneration in the CNS and PNS (Barrett et al., 1985), (Perdrizet et al., 1985), (Sanders et al., 1985).

Certain breeds of animals (Suffolk sheep) have a familial predisposition to the disease, which is related to a particular pattern of identifiable esterase activity in the blood (Baker et al., 1970).

The lesions are thought to represent a distal (preterminal), central, and peripheral axonopathy (Perdrizet et al., 1985), (Sanders et al., 1985), (Barrett et al., 1985).

An acute onset of paresis or paralysis, several hours to a few days after systemic OP antiparasitic therapy in cattle, is likely to be the result of death of epidural *Hypoderma bovis* and subsequent necrotic myelitis rather than the direct effects of the OP compound (Andrews, 1981).

Diagnosis. Attempts should be made to identify the contaminant OP and remove it from the environment. Blood and tissue cholinesterase activity may be circumstantial evidence of intoxication. Blood cholinesterase activity in cattle can be difficult to interpret; a toxicology laboratory should be consulted.

Therapy. Nursing care is probably the only therapy. Perhaps 2-PAM and atropine can be used if acute systemic signs of OP toxicity coexist. Diphenhydramine hydrochloride (Benadryl) may be used to decrease the amount of atropine required to achieve a central anticholinergic (nicotinic) effect and to control the neuromuscular blockade effect (Clemmons et al., 1984); however, the dose for large animals is not known.

Prognosis. The outlook is poor if the animal is recumbent. A few mildly affected sheep have been salvaged, but considerable weight loss occurred (Williams et al., 1976).

Prevention. Because some lines of Suffolk sheep appear to be extremely sensitive, great care must be taken if exposing them to any OP compounds.

3. **Arsanilic Acid and 3-Nitro (also Problem 2)**

These relatively safe compounds are used as growth promoters and for the control of swine dysentery. Overdose has resulted in a wide spectrum of syndromes, including seizures (also Problem 2), peripheral blindness, tremor, and ataxia (Rice et al., 1980), (Harding et al., 1968), (Keenan, 1973). The precise clinical syndrome and specific neuropathologic lesions associated with each compound is not clear and it is thought that there may be other dietary and infectious factors interacting (Gilbert et al., 1981). However, a recent trial has shown 3-nitro to cause selective, central, and peripheral axonal degeneration (Rice et al., 1985), (Kennedy et al., 1986). Most likely, both compounds can result in a subacute ataxia and tetraparesis (Keenan, 1973), (Rice et al., 1980), (Rice et al., 1985), (Gilbert et al., 1981) from which mildly affected animals can recover following withdrawal of the intoxicating feed (Rice et al., 1980), (Keenan, 1973), (Harding et al., 1968). Relapses may still occur (Gilbert et al., 1981).

4. **Organomercury**

In cattle and horses a predominantly cerebellar syndrome results from chronic organomercury toxicity (also Problem 9). In swine alkylmercurial poisoning produces weakness and ataxia. Usually the syndrome progresses to include head signs, including blindness, wandering, and recumbency. Cerebral neuronal necrosis, endothelial proliferation, and peripheral axonal degeneration account for the clinical signs (Charlton, 1974), (Tryphonas et al., 1973).

5. **Cystitis and Ataxia Associated with *Sorghum* Spp Ingestion (see Table 14–2).**

Signalment. Horses of all ages are affected; cattle are less often

Table 14–2. Examples of Several Poisonous Plants of Domestic Herbivores That Can Cause Degrees of Paraparesis, Tetraparesis, or Recumbency

Plant (Ref)	Species Affected	Neurologic Signs (Syndrome)	Pathophysiology	Neural Lesions	Treatment*	Prognosis
Birdsville indigo, *Indigofera linnaei* (Rose et al., 1951; Seawright, 1982)	Horses	Weight loss, ataxia, weakness (Birdsville disease)	Arginine antagonist alkaloids: indospicine, canavanine	None	Arginine-rich feeds (gelatin, lucerne)	Good
Cycad palms (Hall, 1987; Mason et al., 1968; Hooper et al., 1974)	Cattle, sheep, goats, horses	Ataxia, recumbency (wobbles, rickets)	Possibly toxic glycosides, cycasin, and macrozamin	Spinal cord fiber degeneration	—	Bad
Coyotillo, *Karwinskia humboldtiana* (Charlton et al., 1971)	Goats, sheep, cattle	Hypersensitivity, tremor, marked hypermetria, weakness (Coyotillo poisoning)	Unknown	Peripheral neuropathy, central neuroaxonal dystrophy, myopathy	—	Bad
Melochia pyramidata (Palmer et al., 1975)	Cattle	Ataxia, recumbency (Derrengue)	Unknown	Spinal and nerve fiber degeneration	—	Bad
Carpet weed, *Kallstroemia hirsutissima* (Mathews, 1944)	Cattle, sheep, goats	Knuckling, weakness, recumbency	Unknown	Unknown	—	Good
Solanum esuriale (O'Sullivan, 1976)	Sheep	Exercise intolerance, weakness, arched back (humpyback)	Unknown (suspected toxin in *S. esuriale*)	Spinal cord fiber degeneration, myopathy	—	Bad
Sudan Grasses, *Sorghum* spp. (Adams et al., 1969; McKenzie et al., 1977)	Horses, cattle, sheep	Ataxia, bladder paralysis (Sudan paralysis)	Possibly HCN or lathyrogenic toxins	Neuronal fiber degeneration, spinal cord	—	Poor to fair
Yellow vine, *Tribulus micrococcus* (Bourke et al., 1985)	Sheep	Ataxia, knuckling, weakness	Unknown	Unknown	—	Very good
Cathead, *Tribulus terrestris* (Bourke, 1984, 1987)	Sheep	Asymmetric pelvic limb weakness (Coonabarabran Disease)	Suggested to be a nigrostriatial, dopaminergic receptor malfunction	None	—	Bad

*This also must include removal of toxic plant and catharsis.

affected; and sheep may be affected (Seawright, 1982), (Adams et al., 1969), (McKenzie et al., 1977). This disease is recorded in Southwestern and Western States, where *Sorghum* sp are used as fodder.

History. There should be a history of access to *Sorghum* spp, such as Sudan, Sorghum, and Johnson grass. There is incoordination of the pelvic limbs with dribbling of urine in about half the cases.

Physical Examination. Urinary incontinence and urine scald may be found; a distended urinary bladder with a thickened wall usually is palpable through the rectum.

Neurologic Examination. Symmetric ataxia of the pelvic limbs with some weakness and stiffness is present; this ultimately progresses to paraplegia. Hypalgesia, but not analgesia, of the perineum and hind quarters is reported.

Assessment. The primary lesion is neuronal fiber degeneration and possibly demyelination throughout the spinal cord, particularly in the thoracolumbar segments. Also a degenerative neuropathy of spinal nerves probably occurs. Urinary bladder paralysis results in secondary cystitis and ulceration. One suggested mechanism for this disease is that it is related to high hydrocyanide content of *Sorghum* sp grasses, although this is not proven (Seawright, 1982). Mares may deliver or abort foals with arthrogryposis (I.7 above). Signs stop progressing and may partially regress if animals are removed from *Sorghum* sp pastures.

Diagnosis. Primary cystitis should be ruled out if possible. Complete analgesia of the perineum and tail and a totally flaccid tail are rare in this disease, compared with neuritis of the cauda equina and fractured sacrum—both of which cause a more profound cauda equina syndrome (also Problem 12). No ancillary aids have been reported to be useful in confirming the diagnosis.

Therapy. There is no specific treatment. Removal from the pasture and treatment of cystitis are necessary if the animal is to survive.

Prognosis. Signs will improve with removal from pastures, although residual ataxia will remain in severe cases. For prevention, avoid *Sorghum* sp pastures.

6. **Miscellaneous Toxic Plants and Mycotoxins (Table 14–2)**

Many toxic plants and mycotoxins result in ataxia. See Table 14–2, Problems 1, 6, 8, and 9, and Blood et al. (1983) and Seawright (1982).

Astragalus, Halogeton, sweet pea (*Lathyrus* sp), Buckeye (*Aesculus* sp), and *Melochia pyramidata* (El Salvador) have been associated with syndromes of ataxia and paraparesis, especially in cattle. In most cases, signs of cerebral (Problems 1 and 2) or cerebellar (Problem 9) involvement also are seen. *Tribulus terrestris, Cycas media,* Wimmera grass, *Xanthorrhoea* sp, *Solanum esuriale, Echinopogon ovatus,* and *Ipomoea muelleri* are some plants associated with ataxia and weakness in Australian livestock (Blood et al., 1983). The neural lesions and suspected pathophysiology of some of these is given in Table 14–2. Of interest in this regard is Birdsville disease, which is seen in horses in Australia that consume *Indigofera* spp

(Birdsville indigo). Signs include weight loss, progressive ataxia, and weakness. Affected animals may collapse and show terminal convulsions. Complete recovery can occur but toe dragging may persist. The toxicity appears to be prevented by feeding arginine-rich feeds such as alfalfa (Rose et al., 1951).

V. Nutritional

1. Equine Degenerative Myeloencephalopathy (EDM)

Signalment. Young horses of most light breeds can be affected (Mayhew et al., 1977). A similar disorder has been seen in captive Przewalskii horses (Liu et al., 1983), in Grant zebras (Fig. 14–26) (Montali et al., 1974), and in a few ruminant species including wildebeest, llamas, and camels (Palmer et al., 1980). Usually signs begin before 6 months of age, with the oldest affected animal about 3 years of age. Some clusters of cases in related equids on single farms have been related to lack of access to green feed or to use of commercial (heated) pellets and sunbaked forages.

History. Ataxia and weakness, which may be quite sudden in onset according to owners, is reported. Generally signs are progressive, although they plateau by maturity.

Physical Examination. Affected young equids usually are in good health apart from neurologic signs.

Neurologic Examination. There is symmetric ataxia, paresis, and hypometria, usually affecting all four limbs. The relative ab-

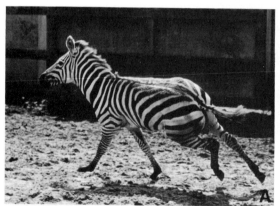
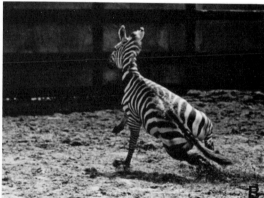
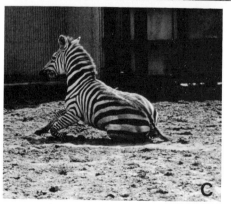

Figure 14–26. Degenerative myeloencephalopathy occurs in a variety of equid species including Grant zebras (A) and results in progressive ataxia and tetraparesis that often is profound in the pelvic limbs and mild in the thoracic limbs (B and C).

normality of gait in the limbs may not be consistent with a focal cervical compression. Thus, the thoracic limbs may be mildly affected while the pelvic limbs are profoundly affected (Fig. 14–26). In severe cases there is prominent hyporeflexia over the neck and trunk, specifically involving the slap test, local cervical, cervico-facial, and cutaneous trunci reflexes (Mayhew et al., 1987). Only rarely does the disease progress to recumbency.

Assessment. This is a diffuse degenerative disease of the brain-stem and particularly the spinal cord, which occurs in particular family lines (Mayhew et al., 1987), (Blythe, 1986). Dystrophic lesions are seen in several sensory (proprioceptive) relay nuclei in the me-dulla oblongata and spinal cord. This neuroaxonal dystrophy has been seen as the prominent lesion in Morgan horses having a similar, if not identical, disease that appears to be familial (Beech, 1984), (Beech et al., 1987). Neuronal fiber degeneration throughout the spinal cord is most prominent in the midthoracic region (Fig. 14–3B). The precise etiology is unknown, although it bears resem-blance to toxic, nutritional, and metabolic diseases in other species (Mayhew et al., 1977). Recent evidence strongly implicates a rela-tionship between the disease etiology and vitamin E deficiency (Mayhew et al., 1987), (Blythe LL, 1988, pers. comm.). Serum vi-tamin E concentrations in young, recently affected foals often are 0.2 to 0.8 µg/ml. Some herdmates, particularly within the same family, also have serum vitamin E concentrations below the accepted minimal normal of 1.0 µg/ml. (Most samples from normal horses eating green forage range from 1.5 to 3.0 µg/ml.) Supplementation with vitamin E at 1000 to 3000 units/day on many farms has in-creased serum vitamin E concentrations and reduced the true in-cidence of EDM from about 40% to 0%. On one of these particular farms no further cases have been reported in 3 years (Farm 1, as discussed in Mayhew et al., 1987).

This uncontrolled data supports the role of vitamin E deficiency, but does not prove that this is the sole etiologic factor. Indeed, there appears to be a strong familial component to the disease (Mayhew et al., 1987), (Blythe, 1986), (Blythe, 1988), (Blythe LL, 1988, pers. comm.), (Dyson S, 1988, pers. comm.), suggesting a heritable trait also is operative. In addition, the possibility of other nutritive and environmental factors being of importance must not be overlooked.

Diagnosis. Rule out other diseases. Normal serum vitamin E concentrations are expected to be greater than 1.5 µg/ml. Concen-trations less than 0.5 µg/ml and probably less than 1.0 µg/ml are consistent with a deficient state. Heat-treated pellets (made of mixed grains or alfalfa), stored oats, and sunbaked coastal Bermuda grass hay used on farms where EDM has occurred at high frequencies, all have had measured vitamin E contents of 0 to 5 units/kg dry weight.

Therapy. Vitamin E supplementation is certainly worth trying. Probably 1000 to 2000 units/day is useful, but better still, large amounts of fresh green forage with a vitamin E content of 500 to 1000 units/kg dry weight should be available.

Prognosis. The signs may progress but usually stabilize, particularly with vitamin E therapy. Supplementation at 2000 units/day did not seem to improve signs in several severe and chronic cases, but Blythe (1988, pers. comm.) has supplemented Appaloosa foals suspected to have EDM with 6000 units/day and seen improvement in the severity of signs from severe to mild in 6 months. A familial predisposition may exist and the owner should be so advised.

2. **Bracken Fern and Horsetail-Induced Thiamin Deficiency**

This is a rare syndrome of horses that follows prolonged ingestion of Bracken fern (*Pteridium equalinum*) (Evans et al., 1951), horsetail (*Equisetum arvense*), and unusually restricted, poor diets, such as turnips (Blood et al., 1983) and beet pulp; the syndrome responds to thiamin administration. Signs include ataxia, depression, weight loss, and bradycardia. Death can occur suddenly, probably resulting from the induced cardiopathy. The neurologic lesions are not well-defined. Treatment of affected horses includes removing them from abnormal diets and systemic administration of grams of thiamin.

Amprolium-induced thiamin deficiency in horses has resulted in bradycardia, arrhythmia, ataxia, muscle fasciculations, and peripheral hypothermia—with blindness and weight loss seen in some experimental cases (Cymbaluk et al., 1978).

A similar syndrome may be seen in pigs and possibly in ruminants (Blood et al., 1983).

The syndrome of thiamin-responsive polioencephalomalacia in ruminants is described in Problem 1.

3. **Enzootic Ataxia—Swayback—Copper Deficiency**

Signalment. Congenital swayback occurs in newborn lambs (Chalmers, 1974) that show weakness, recumbency, and blindness (Problem 1). Growing, 3 to 12-week-old kids, lambs, and possibly piglets show enzootic ataxia or delayed swayback consisting of ataxia of the pelvic limbs progressing to tetraplegia (Chalmers, 1974), (Barlow et al., 1966), (Wouda et al., 1986), (McGavin et al., 1962). A form of ataxia in adolescent captive deer appears to be the same disorder (Barlow et al., 1964), (Terlecki et al., 1964), (Wilson et al., 1979).

Clinical Findings. Other copper deficiency syndromes, such as steely wool, diarrhea, white hair coats, spontaneous long bone fractures, epiphysitis, or sudden death may occur on the farm. Progressive paraparesis of young sheep, goats, and deer usually first becomes evident when animals trail behind the mob and drag the pelvic limbs when moved. Lower motor neuron involvement (LMN)—with flaccid paralysis of the limbs, hypotonia, hyporeflexia, and muscle atrophy—is particularly evident in growing kids that are affected and is of considerable help in arriving at a clinical diagnosis (Wouda et al., 1986). Occasionally goats with the disease demonstrate mild signs of cerebellar involvement (Wouda et al., 1986), (Cordy et al., 1978). Piglets suspected of having copper deficiency may have a rapidly progressive syndrome of ataxia, weak-

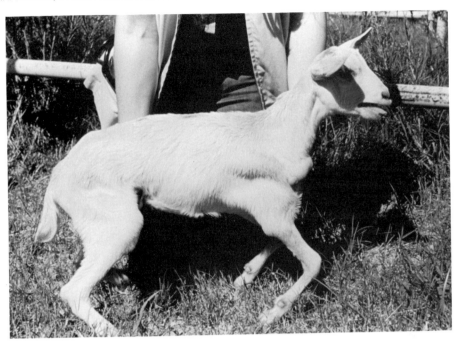

Figure 14–27. This 2-month-old alpine-cross goat showed progressive tetraparesis and muscle atrophy with spinal hyporeflexia. Histologic lesions consistent with enzootic ataxia (copper deficiency) were found at postmortem examination. The blood copper concentrations of this kid and its dam were 0.49 and 0.33 ppm, respectively. (From Brewer, B.D. Neurologic disease of sheep and goats. Vet Clin North Am 1983; 5(3):695.)

ness, nystagmus, recumbency, and paddling, with death in 3 to 5 days from onset of signs (Pletcher et al., 1983).

Newborn lambs with congenital swayback (Chalmers, 1974) often show head signs of obtundation, blindness, and head tremor (also Problem 1).

Assessment. Copper deficiency may cause hypomyelinogenesis and porencephaly in utero, which is probably the result of a primary neuroaxonal defect.

Delayed forms of copper deficiency appear to result from some defect in maintenance of neuroaxonal function, which may begin in utero (Smith et al., 1977) (Smith et al., 1978). There is axonal loss with associated myelin depletion and neuronal cell body swelling caused by filamentous accumulations (Wouda et al., 1986). It is generally accepted that in enzootic ataxia a defect in the neuroaxon results in myelin degradation and finally is reflected in degenerative changes in the neuronal cell body (Wouda et al., 1987), (Patterson et al., 1974), (Smith et al., 1978). Central axonal and myelin degeneration can occur in the fetus and may be most florid when maximal axonal growth and myelination are occurring (Smith et al., 1977). The disease affects central and peripheral fibers, thus LMN signs (EMG changes and neurogenic muscle atrophy) is to be expected

(Wouda et al., 1986). There may be a familial aspect to the disease, at least in sheep and goats (Wouda et al., 1986).

The fact that copper deficiency alone is the cause of enzootic ataxia is not well documented. Interpretation of blood and liver copper concentrations and their relationship to the presence and severity of clinical signs is obscure, notably in the syndromes in goats and deer (Wilson et al., 1970), (Wouda et al., 1986), (Cordy et al., 1978).

Piglets suspected of dying of copper deficiency with fulminant neurologic signs also frequently had intimal hemorrhages in the great vessels (Pletcher et al., 1983).

Diagnosis. Blood and tissue copper levels of affected and un-affected (older) animals indicates if a low copper status exists on a farm. Unaffected herdmates of affected kids and fawns may have low copper status (Wouda et al., 1986), (Wilson et al., 1979).

Treatment and Prevention. Copper supplementation is recom-mended. Topdressing pastures with copper salts can be expensive and can cause blood copper concentrations in stock to rise errati-cally. Injections with copper glycinate (50 to 120 mg) has been used successfully in ruminants but needs to be repeated frequently (De-land et al., 1986), (Wilson et al., 1979).

Using orally administered oxidized copper wire (Deland et al., 1986) or cupric oxide particles in gelatin boluses for cattle and sheep (Suttle, 1987a,b) results in more sustained blood copper status and probably is the preferred treatment and prophylactic regimen.

Prognosis. Affected growing lambs and kids can improve with therapy, but residual neurologic deficits are most likely.

VI. Neoplastic

Neoplastic spinal cord disease in large animals is extremely rare except for epidural lymphosarcoma, which is infrequent in dairy cattle (Fig. 14–28). Often there is an acute onset of paraparesis or recumbency. Usually other evidence of bovine leukosis is evident,

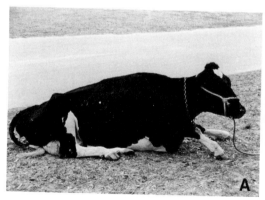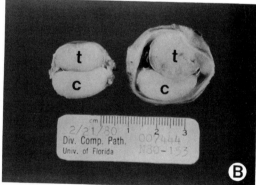

Figure 14–28. Epidural, and less frequently subdural (B), lymphosarcoma in cattle is the most common neoplasm affecting the CNS in large animal practice. Surprisingly, there is often a sudden onset of recumbency or paraparesis/paraplegia. It occurred in this case (A) even though a large tumor mass (t) compressed the spinal cord (c) which is shown in B.

although the epidural space may be regarded as a primary site for the disease because it contains histologic aggregates of lymphoid nodules. Trauma, osteomyelitis, and parasite migration are primary differentials. Rare cases of numerous other tumors result in progressive para or tetraparesis in large animals and are summarized in Table 14–3. Signs can begin suddenly and even progress rapidly. These are most likely associated with sudden decompensation of blood supply to the nervous tissue involved (Fig. 14–28).

VII. Idiopathic

1. Premature Synostosis of Thoracolumbar Vertebrae in Angus Calves

Development of a dwarf-like appearance, bowleggedness, and progressive paraparesis, which characterizes this syndrome, occurred in all 10 Angus calves in a Canadian herd (Orr et al., 1981). The signs were associated with premature bony fusion across thoracolumbar, vertebral, epiphyseal growth-plates, resulting in vertebral canal stenosis. Other growth plates, especially of the basicranium, were affected. Etiologic possibilities included teratogenic plants, chemical toxins, mineral deficiencies, and particularly hypervitaminosis A.

2. Poliomyelomalacia of Sheep, Goats, and Calves

Symmetric poliomyelomalacia occurs in lambs (Innes et al., 1955b), adult sheep (Bonniwell et al., 1985), kid goats (Cordy et al.,

Table 14–3. A Classification of Many of the Reported* Neoplasms (Tumors) Involving the Central Nervous System in Large Animals That Can Cause Degrees of Tetraparesis

Cell Type/Tumor	Predilection Site	Species Affected
Tumors of Nerve Cells		
Ganglioneuroma	Spinal	Horse, cow
Hamartoma	Spinal	Foal
Tumors of Neuroepithelium		
Ependymoma	Ependymal surfaces	Horse, cow
Plexus papilloma	Fourth ventricle	Horse, cow
Tumors of Glia		
Astrocytoma	Brainstem, spinal cord	Cow, sheep
Oligodendroglioma	Spinal cord	Cow
Undifferentiated glioma	Spinal cord	Horse, cow, sheep, pig
Glioblastoma	Spinal cord	Cow, pig
Medulloblastoma	Foramen magnuum	Cow, pig
Tumors of Meninges, Vessels, Etc.		
Meningioma	Variable	Horse, cow, sheep
Angioma/blastoma	Variable	Horse, cow, pig
Sarcoma	Meninges	Horse, cow, sheep
Tumors of Nerve Sheaths		
Schwannoma; neurofibroma; neurofibrosarcoma	Spinal	Horse, cow, pig, sheep
Tumors from Surrounding Tissues		
Lymphosarcoma	Spinal, foramen magnuum	Horse, cow, goat
Other: Hemangiosarcoma, adenocarcinoma; osteosarcoma; malignant melanoma	Spinal	Cow, horse, goat, sheep

*Based on data from Baker et al. (1980); Braund (1987); Cho et al. (1979); Cimprich et al. (1975); Craig et al. (1986); de Lahunta (1983); Gilmour et al. (1977); Helfer et al. (1978); Kannegieter et al. (1987); Kirker-Head et al. (1985); Livesey et al. (1986); Mayhew et al. (1982); Palmer et al. (1960); Rebhun et al. (1984); Roth et al. (1987); Sullivan (1985); Sutton et al. (1982); Whitwell (1980).

1984), and in Ayreshire calves (Palmer et al., 1986) with resulting para- or more frequently tetraplegia. There is necrosis of ventral gray matter with hyporeflexia and flaccid paralysis, particularly of the cervicothoracic region. Gray matter areas in the brainstem also can be affected (Bonniwell et al., 1985).

There is no treatment and the cause is unknown. Possibly this clinicopathologic syndrome represents more than one etiology. Similarities exist between it and selenium toxicity (Fig. 14–23) and experimental nicotinic acid deficiency in swine (see IV.1), focal symmetric leukoencephalomalacia-edema disease (Problem 1), and postanesthetic hemorrhagic myelopathy in horses (VII.3). Because of similarities to other diseases it would be valuable to evaluate the diet of affected animals and determine the copper, selenium, nicotinic acid, and other nutrient concentrations and the presence of possible toxins. The possibility of clostridial and other biologic toxins also should be considered when evaluating cases.

3. Postanesthetic Hemorrhagic Myelopathy

Signalment. This rare complication of general anesthesia, seen only after dorsal recumbency, has been seen in at least six young horses of both sexes (Schartzmann et al., 1979), (Blakemore et al., 1984), (Zink, 1985), (Brearley et al., 1986), (Yovich et al., 1986).

Clinical Syndrome. A diffuse thoracolumbar hemorrhage of gray matter results in degrees of paraplegia, areflexia, hypotonia, and analgesia involving the trunk, pelvic limbs, perineum, tail, and anus. At the time of recovery from anesthesia or soon thereafter (Brearley et al., 1986), the horse usually does not regain its footing.

Assessment. The syndrome has occurred in heavy (300 to 470 kg) but young (6 to 24 month) horses after 40 to 95 minutes in dorsal recumbency; they were under gas anesthesia for routine surgical procedures. The lesion most often occurs in the thoracolumbar region but was at C_6-T_8 in one case (Yovich et al., 1986).

Congestion, hemorrhage, and necrosis involve the dorsal and particularly the ventral gray matter, suggesting interference with venous drainage in the dorsal and ventral spinal veins (Fig. 14–29). Compartmentalization of blood flow and local or systemic blood pressure alterations (Zink, 1985), (Brearley et al., 1986), associated with recumbency and anesthesia, may play roles in the genesis of the lesion. A tenable hypothesis is that degrees of hypotension and vena caval and aortic compression result in congestion, hemorrhage, and tissue necrosis in the thoracolumbar spinal cord (Blakemore et al., 1984).

A clinically indistinguishable bilateral femoral paralysis and paraplegia, associated with hemorrhage along both femoral nerves, has been seen postanesthetically (Dyson et al., 1988). Such lesions have been seen as postfoaling paralysis. Two of three affected horses have survived, although the precise lesions were not defined in survivors (see Postfoaling Paralysis, B.II.3).

Treatment. Aggressive, anti-inflammatory medical therapy, es-

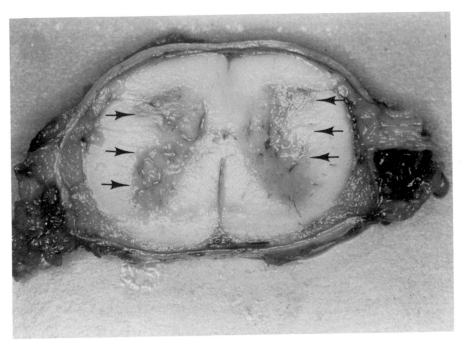

Figure 14–29. Postanesthetic myelopathy with poliomyelomalacia (arrows) is seen here in a segment of thoracolumbar spinal cord from a 6-month-old Shire horse that had undergone elective surgical procedure positioned in dorsal recumbency. (Courtesy of WL Blakemore, Cambridge, UK.)

pecially with systemic DMSO, could be undertaken, but residual deficits would be expected.

Prevention. Heavy horses, which require dorsal recumbency for surgery, should be positioned on a slight angle off the perpendicular and attempts should be made to maintain adequate blood pressure.

4. Vascular Malformations

Various vascular malformations, such as aneurysms, hematomata, arteriovenous malformations, and thromboses have been recognized as causing ataxia in horses and cattle (Miller et al., 1985), (Cho et al., 1979), (Gilmour et al., 1977). They usually occur in young-adult animals. In one study, three of these were in the cerebellomedullary region of the brainstem and resulted in a progressive wobbler syndrome without any detectable cranial nerve deficits (Miller et al., 1985). Some of these anomalies are possibly neoplastic (Palmer et al., 1960).

5. Thoracolumbar Spondylosis Deformans and Osteoarthrosis (See also Problem 10B, VII.1)

Signalment. This is a common condition involving the vertebral column, usually in adult bulls and pigs (Jubb et al., 1985), (Doige, 1979), (Weisbrode et al., 1982). Less commonly is it a problem in horses (Fig. 14–35).

Primary Complaint. Stiffness of gait with variable lameness is the major presenting complaint. Degrees of ataxia and paraparesis are less commonly seen.

History. A slowly progressive stiff gait and minor pelvic limb weakness occurs. Signs can fluctuate markedly with time. A sudden onset of paralysis or paraparesis may occur, particularly in breeding bulls (Weisbrode et al., 1982). Excessive calcium in the diet (e.g., alfalfa) may be of etiologic significance (Krook et al., 1970). Reluctance to jump fences may be reported in horses.

Physical Examination. This usually is unremarkable, although some disuse atrophy in the hind quarters may be present. Stiffness and lameness in the pelvic limbs, often with a characteristic, intermittent, flexion motion without stepping, is seen in horses with lumbar osteoarthrosis. True back pain with poor movement of the lumbar vertebrae into lordosis or kyphosis may be demonstrated. There may be excessive wear of the toes (shoes) in horses.

Neurologic Examination. In addition to signs resulting from pain and restricted vertebral movement, the neurologic deficit depends on the degree and location of any nerve root or spinal cord encroachment. There can be weakness and stiffness in the rear limbs, hyperesthesia along the lumbar paravertebral region, and difficulty mounting to breed.

Assessment. The primary lesion in cattle and pigs is believed to be degeneration of the annulus fibrosis allowing abnormal movement of vertebrae and secondary osteophyte production, which is particularly prominent ventrally (Jubb et al., 1985). It has been suggested that proliferation of bony spurs around the vertebral bodies (spondylosis) and articular processes (arthrosis) is associated with hypercalcitoninism induced by a prolonged high calcium diet, at least in bulls (Krook et al., 1970). Although this process is evident in old horses, particularly in the thoracolumbar region, it rarely causes neurologic signs (Townsend et al., 1986). Some degree of back stiffness sometimes appears to be associated with degenerative changes in dorsal intervertebral articulations. In individual cases, the possibility of hypervitaminosis D and some 2,4-dihydroxycholecalciferol-like toxin-containing plants should be given consideration.

Diagnosis. Radiography of lumbar vertebrae is difficult but helpful. Local anesthesia of affected vertebral bodies or articular surfaces for more definite diagnosis is extremely difficult to achieve.

Therapy. Aspirin, phenylbutazone, and glucocorticosteroids are useful on "bad" days. Most cases are generalized and this is only symptomatic medical therapy. Rest is indicated but may be impracticable.

Prognosis. The outlook is poor, as signs will slowly progress. In bulls, there is hope for possible stabilization if the diet is corrected.

6. Neurofibrillary Degenerations

Syndromes of tetraparesis progressing to tetraplegia, sometimes with evidence of a weak neck with the head held low, have occasionally been seen in young stock. Affected animals have included Yorkshire piglets (Higgins et al., 1983), Afrikaner cattle (vonMaltitz et al., 1969), and Zebra foals (Higgins et al., 1977). Widespread neurofibrillary accumulations within neurons and degrees of spinal neuronal fiber degeneration have been present. Whether these syndromes are related to copper deficiency, other nutritional or toxic disorders, or are familial, is not known at present.

Neurofilamentous accumulation is a prominent component of enzootic ataxia—swayback in goats, sheep, and deer (see V.3 above).

7. Embolic Myelopathy

Although acute, single, spinal cord infarcts have been suspected clinically and seen pathologically, in horses at least, usually no proof of the cause is evident (Whitwell, 1980). Rarely, fibrocartilaginous material has been found in blood vessels adjacent to such lesions in horses (Taylor et al., 1977), (Whitwell, 1980), and weaner pigs, although this is rare (Tessaro et al., 1983). One adult, pregnant sow with fractures of the fifth lumbar vertebra and a degenerate disc at L_{5-6} had infarction of the lumbar spinal cord associated with intra-arteriolar fibrocartilaginous material (Pass, 1978). These emboli are assumed to arise from intervertebral disc material. Parasites such as *Strongylus vulgaris* cause vasculitis and embolic episodes and may be regarded as other potential etiologic agents.

Problem 10B.

Neuromuscular Diseases

Considered herein are diseases diffusely affecting lower motor neurons (LMN), notably multiple peripheral nerves, neuromuscular junctions, muscles, and combinations thereof. Thus, demonstration of LMN involvement is important in the diagnosis of these disorders. Clinically, widespread, symmetrical and diffuse weakness of limbs (and other body parts) characterize these diseases. Consequently, degrees of paraparesis and tetraparesis leading to recumbency are seen.

The rapid development of muscle atrophy, elevated, circulating muscle enzyme activities, and electromyographic evidence of LMN disease are consistent markers.

A few of these processes involve diffuse "irritation" or stimulation of LMNs, notably in the early stage of some diseases, with subsequent stiffness and muscle contraction occurring.

Interestingly, any process that causes decreased movement in utero, especially diseases affecting any part of the LMN, can result in arthrogryposis at birth because of the rapid fibrous contracture of muscles and fixation of joints that occur in the fetus.

Widespread polyneuritis with typical, acute onset of tetraparesis/plegia and stabilization and improvement does not seem to occur often in large animals, although a case of polyradiculoneuritis in a goat has been reported (MacLachlan et al., 1982).

For a fuller review of myopathies in large animals the reader is directed to Bradley (1981), Cardinet and Holliday (1979), and Goedegebuure (1987).

Categories of Disease and Differential Diagnosis
*NOTE: Only those diseases marked * are discussed in this problem.*

I. Congenital and Familial
   *1. Myotonia
   *2. Ovine Progressive Muscular Dystrophy
   *3. Congenital Myopathy in Lambs
   *4. Kyphosis in Jersey Cattle
   *5. Pietrain Creeper Syndrome
   6. Porcine Stress Syndrome—Malignant Hyperthermia (see II.4 below)
   7. Arthrogryposis (see A.I.7 above)
   8. Hyperkalemic Periodic Paralysis (Problem 8B)

II. Physical
   *1. Exertional Rhabdomyolysis and Capture Myopathy
   *2. Postanesthetic Myoneuropathy
   *3. Postcalving and Postfoaling Paralyses (also Problem 11)
   *4. Porcine Stress Syndrome—Malignant Hyperthermia

III. Infectious, Inflammatory, Immune
   *1. Polymyositis

IV. Metabolic
   *1. Acute Azotemia, Hypocalcemia, Hypomagnesemia

V. Toxic
   *1. Tick Paralysis
   *2. Botulism—Shaker Foal Syndrome
   *3. Postanesthetic Myasthenic Syndrome
   *4. *Cassia* spp
   *5. Monensin and Lasalocid
   *6. Ivermectin
   *7. Methyl Bromide
   8. Tetanus (Problem 8A)

VI. Nutritional
   *1. Nutritional Myodegeneration—White Muscle Disease— Myodegeneration and Steatitis

VII. Idiopathic
   *1. Vague Neuromusculoskeletal Lameness and Back Problems (also A. VII.5 above)
   *2. Aortic-Iliac Thrombosis—Ischemic Neuromyopathy

I. Congenital and Familial
   1. Myotonia
       Signalment. This rare disease of large animals appears to be

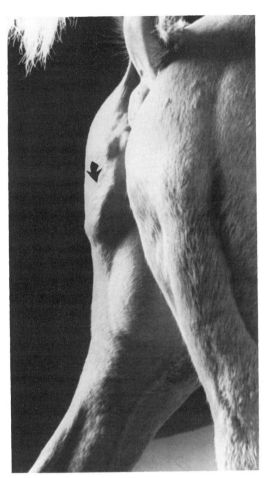

Figure 14–30. This 18-month-old thoroughbred colt had myotonia since birth. Muscles of the hind quarters were prominent and prolonged contraction, as shown in the semimembranous muscle (arrow), occurred with percussion of these muscles.

familial in goats and Shropshire lambs (Goedegebuure, 1987). It also has been seen in thoroughbred (Fig. 14–30), standardbred, Swedish halfbred, Appaloosa, and quarterhorse foals, and in a Welsh pony and calf. Heritability has not been proven in any of these cases (Goedegebuure, 1987), (Andrews et al., 1986), (McKerrell, 1987), (Jamison et al., 1987), (Steinberg et al., 1962).

Clinical Signs. Muscles of the hind quarters are most severely affected and usually are prominent (Fig. 14–30). The gait is stiff, especially after resting for a while. The clinical diagnosis can be made by seeing and feeling a prominent and prolonged muscle contraction with "knotting" following mechanical (finger-flick) percussion (Jamison et al., 1987). Affected animals do not appear to be debilitated by the disorder, although limb deformity with contracture may occur.

Diagnosis. Clinical diagnosis is confirmed by electromyographic (EMG) examination. Needle EMG studies reveal bizarre, spontaneous electrical discharges from affected muscle membranes. These myotonic discharges metaphorically are referred to as sounding like a "dive bomber" or a "revving motor cycle." The former perhaps are best termed pseudomyotonic or myotonic-like discharges, and the latter are termed myotonic discharges. These spectacular potentials can be stimulated by voluntary movement, needle movement, percussion, and chemicals. Significantly, they do not disappear with depolarizing or nondepolarizing muscle relaxant drugs (Jamison et al., 1987). Usually, evidence of LMN disease with fibrillation potentials and positive sharp waves are detected between bizarre discharges (Andrews et al., 1986), (Jamison et al., 1987) (Fig. 14–31).

Assessment. A muscle membrane defect exists, rendering the cells hypersensitive to action potential discharge. Although a specific transmembrane, chloride conduction defect has been determined in man and goats, no specific defect has been found in other species. Indeed, there may well be multiple etiologies to the syndrome of myotonia in large animals.

Outcome. Some muscle relaxant drugs can alter the clinical signs, but the presumed muscle membrane defect and hypersensitivity to mechanical, electrical, and chemical stimulation remains. Phenytoin has not been beneficial in treating horses with myotonia (Beech, 1987), (Mayhew IG, de Lahunta A, pers. observ.).

2. Ovine Progressive Muscular Dystrophy

Signs of progressive stiffness in the pelvic limbs, thoracic limbs,

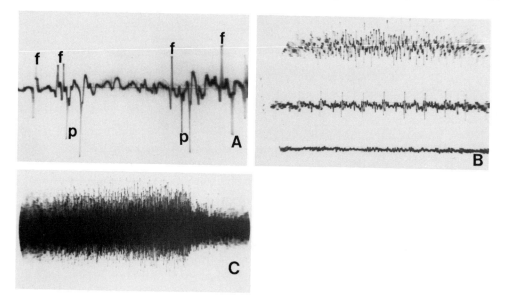

Figure 14–31. Needle EMG studies on a colt with myotonia (Fig. 14–30) reveal evidence of a myopathy with fibrillation potentials (f) and positive sharp waves (p) in A. Spontaneous and stimulated waxing and waning, bizarre, high-frequency discharges in B and C are heard on the EMG speaker as dive-bomber-like sounds. Scale as shown per cm: A 100 μv and 10 ms; B 200 μv and 50 ms; C 200 μv and 500 ms.

then neck begin in 3 to 4-week-old Merino lambs affected with this inherited disorder (Richards et al., 1986). Some sheep become crippled by a few years of age, others live to old age. Variable muscle fiber diameter, fiber splitting, and development of sarcoplasmic masses occur; they are similar to lesions of myotonic dystrophy in man. However, clinical myotonia did not develop and no myotonic discharges were detected in an affected ram on which electromyography was performed (Richards et al., 1986).

3. Congenital Myopathy in Lambs

Flexed limb joints and inability to raise the head and neck was seen in newborn Suffolk lambs in Scotland (Nisbet et al., 1961). A degenerative myopathy, particularly in the neck, was found. Several lambs recovered, while others developed rigid cervicothoracic kyphosis and wedge-shaped vertebrae, which are associated with fibrotic paraxial musculature. The cause is unknown, but may be a congenital form of nutritional myodegeneration (see VI.1).

4. Kyphosis in Jersey Calves

Four Jersey calves, sired by the same bull, were normal at birth but developed progressive thoracolumbar kyphosis, lumbosacral lordosis, and an abnormal gait beginning at 3 to 4 months of age (Jeffrey et al., 1985). The significant lesion was type II myofiber atrophy in lumbar muscles. The disorder is suspected to be inherited muscular dystrophy.

5. Pietrain Creeper Syndrome

This syndrome of progressive muscular weakness (beginning at 3 weeks of age and ending at about 3 months of age) with recumbency has been seen in two litters of Pietrain pigs (Bradley et al., 1986). Atrophy of type I myofibers and myofiber caliber variation is most prominent in proximal limb muscles. The disease is suspected to be inherited as an autosomal recessive trait.

II. Physical

1. Exertional Rhabdomyolysis and Capture Myopathy

Signalment. This disorder is also referred to as azoturia, paralytic myoglobinuria, tying-up, set fast, and Monday morning disease—each of which emphasizes a particular component of the syndrome. Horses of all ages are affected, particularly young, mature working and racing horses—especially 2-year-old fillies (Harris et al., 1986), (Hodgson, 1985), (Fraunfelder et al., 1986). In exotic and wild animals, capture myopathy is similar if not identical to exertional rhabdomyolysis in its pathophysiology (Bartsch et al., 1977), (Chalmers et al., 1977), (Haigh et al., 1977), (Lewis et al., 1977).

History. The horse may not be training as well as expected, or it may fade in races and become stiff and sore after a workout. Alternatively, the horse may suddenly stop after beginning strenuous exercise and refuse to move. Wild animals are affected under the stress of capture, and remain recumbent.

Physical Examination. The affected horse usually is in good physical condition but may be overweight. Discolored (brown) urine is present in severe cases. The horse is reluctant to move and experiences degrees of paraparesis and stiff pelvic limbs. Pain responses are induced on palpation of muscles, especially lumbar and sublumbar muscles, which may be swollen.

Neurologic Examination. Reluctance to move, a saw-horse posture, and a weak and stiff gait usually are present.

Assessment. A noninflammatory myonecrosis, preferentially affecting type II fibers occurs (McEwen et al., 1986). Muscles used most during exercise and work are affected. Altered glycogen storage, hypokalemia, other electrolyte disturbances, induced anerobic metabolism in the contracting muscles, and other metabolic alterations may initiate the myolysis. Myoglobin is released and excreted in the urine. Myoglobin nephrosis and azotemia may result. With recovery, severe muscle atrophy may occur.

A nonspecific finding of loosely coupled myofiber mitochondria has been detected in two affected standardbred mares (Van den Hoven et al., 1986). Altered total body electrolyte status, detected in affected horses by determining the relative loss of electrolytes in the urine (see Diagnostic Aids), may be of some significance (Harris et al., 1988). Low intraerythrocytic K^+ concentrations have been detected in affected horses in training compared with unaffected horses in training (Bain FT and Merritt AM, pers. comm.). Also, the role of sex hormones and thyroid hormones have been discussed (Harris et al., 1986). Finally, the status of vitamin E and glutathione peroxidase activity of affected horses appear adequate (Roneus, 1985). The role of these factors and many others in the pathogenesis of this syndrome is not known.

In wild animals with capture myopathy, hyperthermia and metabolic disturbances are recognized as significant clinical factors. The disease has been likened to porcine stress syndrome (See II.4 below).

Acute myopathy with azoturia has occurred in grazing horses without being associated with exercise (Hosie et al., 1986).

Diagnostic Aids. Muscle damage is evidenced by increased serum muscle enzyme activities, such as CPK of 500 to 50,000 IU/L, SGOT of 1000 to 20,000 IU/L, and LDH of 500 to 2000 IU/L. It should be realized that CPK activity in serum of horses in training may fluctuate widely and average 100 to 500 IU/L (Fraunfelder et al., 1986).

In subtle cases, a CPK-exercise test can be done (McEwen et al., 1986). Serum CPK activity is determined (baseline) before, then 4 to 8 hours after and 12 to 24 hours after moderate (e.g., 20 minutes lunging) exercise. Normally the serum CPK activity may rise to approximately 200 to 600 IU/L (or higher in an unfit horse), but will fall after 12 to 24 hours to no more than twice the base-line. With myolysis, the CPK activity peaks within 4 to 8 hours at levels of several thousand IU/L and remains elevated for 12 to 48 hours (McEwen et al., 1986).

Acid-base and electrolyte imbalances are variable and alkalosis and hypokalemia may occur, both of which may be significant in the pathogenesis of the disease (Carlson et al., 1976). Wild animals with capture myopathy usually become acidotic, which can be contributed to by degrees of heat exhaustion.

Recent work on electrolyte (x) fractional urinary excretion ratios (FE_x) has revealed some abnormalities in affected horses that may be significant (Harris, 1986), (Harris et al., 1988). For example, a FE_{Na} of 0.006 has been determined in affected animals, and with dietary sodium supplementation, the ratio rose to 0.27, with resolution of signs. In this context it has been suggested (Harris et al., 1986), (Harris et al., 1988) that clinical improvement, reportedly due to sodium bicarbonate supplementation of an affected filly's diet (Robb et al., 1986), may as likely be the result of a Na^+ effect as much as an alkalinizing effect.

Urinalysis, blood-urea nitrogen (BUN), and creatinine changes reflect degrees of myoglobin nephrosis and shock.

Therapy. Exercise should be stopped. Elevated body temperature should be lowered with alcohol baths and ice. Acid base and electrolyte imbalance require correction, but it should not be assumed that all cases are acidotic. Phenylbutazone and flunixin can be used sparingly for pain and swelling, but the animal should not be allowed to exercise; hydration must be maintained to minimize the possibility of renal disease resulting from myoglobin and from such drugs. Tranquilization may be necessary.

Dantrolene sodium, a muscle relaxant used to prevent and treat malignant hyperthermia (see II.4 below) may help alleviate attacks but this is still an experimental therapy (see Prevention). Methocarbamol at 20 mg/kg, QID has been suggested (Hodgson, 1985). Corticosteroids probably are not indicated. Most clinicians empirically administer vitamin E and selenium (600 mg vitamin E and 25 mg Selenium, IM), and some use thiamin (1–5 g, IM); the effectiveness of the three is unknown.

Prognosis. The serum CPK activity at the beginning of the disease gives some evaluation of total muscle damage. Horses die of azotemia and metabolic derangements, so these are worth assessing. If the animal is recumbent, the prognosis is bad.

Prevention. Preventing the disease can be difficult if the horse must be exercised strenuously. Changes in feed (energy) intake should not be drastic, but amounts fed should be changed based on activity levels. Exercise needs to be carefully regulated. Many practitioners try prophylactic vitamin E and selenium; others use prophylactic (pre- and postrace) mixed, balanced electrolyte solutions ("jugging"); and some use dantrolene sodium and thyroid extract, all with unknown results.

Dantrolene has been recommended at 2 mg/kg, PO, SID for 3 to 5 days, followed by 2 mg/kg every third day for a month (Hodgson, 1985). However, hepatocellular damage has been reported and it appears that much higher doses would be necessary to achieve blood concentrations regarded as therapeutic for humans (Court et al., 1987).

Recently Beech (1987) recommended phenytoin for prevention

of, what she termed, chronic intermittent rhabdomyolysis—perhaps based on the similarity of this syndrome to myotonia. A dose of 10 to 12 mg/kg, PO, BID was recommended; the clinician is cautioned to vary the dose according to clinical signs and to measure serum concentrations (which possibly should be 4 to 12 μg/ml, 4 hours postdosing) (Beech, 1987).

Detection of abnormal FE_x values allows rational correction of possible electrolyte deficiencies in the diet of affected horses (Harris et al., 1988). On the assumption that poor buffering capacity may be related to exertional rhabdomyolysis, dietary $NaHCO_3$ (2% of dry matter) has been added, supposedly with beneficial effects (Robb et al., 1986). As mentioned above, such supplementation also adds over 1500 mEq of Na per day to the horse's diet, which in itself may be of some consequence.

2. Postanesthetic Myoneuropathy

Signalment. Often this syndrome appears to occur in fit performance horses, but it does occur in any heavy, large animal after prolonged (usually) general anesthesia (Cox et al., 1982).

Examination. There are degrees of recumbency, tetra-, para-, or monoparesis/plegia following anesthesia. Pain and swelling are evident in groups of muscles, usually, but not always, on the dependent side (Trim et al., 1973), (White, 1982).

Some characteristics of neurapraxia, especially of the radial and peroneal nerves, complicate the syndrome of painful myopathy. Postanesthetic myelopathy (A.VII.3 above) and myasthenic syndrome (V. 3 below) initially can look remarkably similar (Dyson et al., 1988).

Assessment. The pathogenesis is thought to involve components of compartmental (muscle groups) pressure elevation, systemic hypotension, anerobic glycolysis, pressure-induced and ischemic myopathy, pressure-induced and perhaps ischemic neuropathy, blood supply noflow/reflow phenomenon with tissue-oxidant injury, and other factors. Malignant hyperthermia (II.4 below) may be involved (White, 1982), (White et al., 1986), (Lindsay et al., 1980), (Grandy et al., 1987), (Trim et al., 1973).

Diagnosis. Serum CPK, aldolase, SGOT (or AST), and LDH activities are excessively elevated and myoglobin often is found in the urine. Areas of analgesia corresponding to mono- and polyneuropathies (also Problem 11), and hyporeflexia in the absence of marked muscle swelling, indicate that degrees of neurapraxia also are present.

Treatment. If recumbent, the animal should rest in a sternal position or be supported in a sling if possible. Intravenous and oral fluids and electrolytes are necessary to correct any imbalances and to encourage diuresis if myoglobinuria is present. Phenylbutazone and flunixin are administered with caution because of potential renal toxicity. Many clinicians use vitamin E and selenium preparations empirically. Tranquilization may be necessary. Butorphanol, demerol, or morphine may be necessary for pain relief. Methocarbamol (10 to 20 mg/kg, IV, QID) for muscle relaxation has not been terribly helpful. Furosemide therapy is not indicated as it may exaggerate K^+ depletion. Also the resulting hypovolemia may exacerbate degrees of hypotension and reduce muscle blood flow, which probably are significant pathophysiologic factors (Lindsay et al., 1980), (Grandy et al., 1987). Topical or systemic (10%) DMSO is worth using in severe cases, but blood volume must be maintained because of the possibility of myoglobin and hemoglobin nephrosis. Massage and limb manipulations promote muscle blood flow and reduce the chance of decubital sores occurring. Good padding, turning the patient regularly, and attending to bowel and bladder evacuations are part of sensible nursing care for a recumbent patient. Glucocorticoids probably are not indicated unless there is impending cardiovascular and renal collapse. Dantrolene sodium given to reduce Ca^{++} release may be useful as therapy, on the assumption that a mechanism similar to that operative in malignant hyperthermia (see II.4 below) is operative in this syndrome. However, a dose of 2 mg/kg, IV probably gives effective blood concentrations for only 30 minutes (Court et al., 1987).

Prognosis. If the horse remains standing, the outlook is good to excellent, depending on the degree of muscle involvement. Nursing care is extremely important if the animal is recumbent. Loss of muscle mass can occur with recovery.

Prevention. Adequate padding of heavy animals under general anesthesia, positioning the dependent thoracic limb forward, and elevating and supporting the uppermost thoracic and pelvic limb reduces intracompartmental pressure (White et al., 1986). Almost certainly, prolonged, halothane-induced hypotension (mean arterial blood pressure 55 to 65 mm Hg) is a major factor in severe and generalized postanesthetic myopathy in the horse (Grandy et al., 1987). Therefore, minimizing the duration of anesthesia and supporting normotension, particularly with minimal concentrations of volatile anesthetic agents, are important to achieve.

Prophylactic doses of dantrolene sodium at 10 mg/kg intragastrically, about 1 hour prior to general anesthesia, has been suggested to prevent malignant hyperthermia (Court et al., 1987). However, the effectiveness of this regimen in preventing postanesthetic myoneuropathy is unknown.

3. Postcalving and Postfoaling Paralyses

Signalment. Most often this syndrome is seen when a small cow delivers a large calf. Often it is an assisted delivery when it is termed calving paralysis (Fig. 14–32). The syndrome also occurs in high-producing dairy cows postpartum as a consequence of recumbency due to metabolic disorders such as hypocalcemia or milk fever. Both syndromes are part of the Downer Cow Syndrome. Various muscle ruptures occur during attempts to rise, which complicates the clinical picture (Roussel, 1986). Muscle ruptures are rare in horses. Also, femoral paralysis in calves and various pelvic limb muscle ruptures in foals (also Problem 11) occur under similar circumstances.

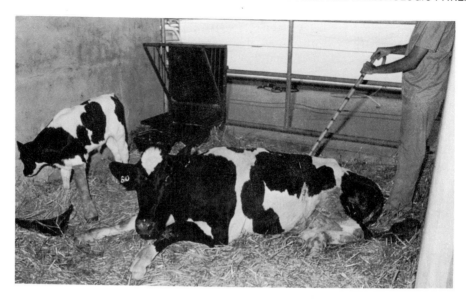

Figure 14–32.   A typical situation for postcalving paralysis is shown here. During assisted delivery of a large calf, the calf sustained a fractured metacarpus. The dam remained bright and alert but had difficulty rising. The pelvic limb flexor reflexes were poor. With nursing care, the cow returned to normal following this presumed neurapraxia of the last ventral lumbar roots.

History. There is an onset of stiffness to paraplegia after delivery, sometimes with signs progressing over hours to days. Metabolic disorders such as milk fever and evidence of trauma are sometimes also reported.

Physical Examination. Sometimes soft tissue, intrapelvic, and even bony pelvis damage is palpable. Other causes of the Downer Cow Syndrome, such as exhaustion, persistent milk fever, displaced abomasum, and pyometra, can be detected.

Neurologic Examination. With classic calving paralysis, mild cases may show unilateral obturator paresis (abduction of one limb upon rising) with a normal gait. Typically, an affected cow can dog-sit and has paresis in the pelvic limbs, flexor hyporeflexia, and mild degrees of limb hypalgesia with intact tail and anal function (Fig. 14–32). Patellar hyporeflexia suggests quadriceps recumbency myopathy or femoral nerve involvement.

Assessment. Recumbency following calving (Downer Cow Syndrome) can be associated with many metabolic, infectious, traumatic, toxic, and nutritional disorders (Cox, 1981). The specific neuromuscular syndromes discussed here can be divided into two forms. The first is primary calving paralysis, which is seen in bright and alert cows that cannot rise on their pelvic limbs or that have degrees of para/monparesis. This is most often associated with compression of the ventral branch of L_6 (less often L_5 and S_1) against the ventral ridge of the wing of the sacrum during delivery of a large calf (Cox et al., 1975). Degrees of neurapraxia, axonotmesis, and neurotmesis occur. Ischemic and hemorrhagic myopathy and neuropathy due to recumbency results in more profound paraplegia and even tetraplegia. The second form is seen as degrees of recumbency-induced myoneuropathy subsequent to recumbency induced by some other perinatal factor(s), which may be no more than prolonged labor (Cox et al., 1982), (Cox, 1981). The pathophysiologic mechanism for this is similar to postanesthetic myoneuropathy (Cox et al., 1982), (II.2 above). Degrees of pressure-induced neurapraxia (Onapito et al., 1986) and ruptured muscles (Roussel, 1986) complicate the picture.

Some cases of postfoaling paralysis in mares may be the result of ventral branch L_5-S_1 nerve root compression as in the cow, but this has not been proven. Occasionally in mares there has been hemorrhage in and around the femoral nerves, resulting in extensor weakness, patellar hyporeflexia, and medial thigh (saphenous nerve) analgesia (Fig. 14–33).

Therapy. The nerve roots usually are not severed, but contused. Phenylbutazone, flunixin, or aspirin probably are beneficial, at least initially. Surgical and gynecologic care is essential. Glucocorticoids may promote complications in periparturient animals. Intravenous DMSO (10%), as for spinal cord trauma, has been used in mares. Nursing care of a recumbent dam and support of newborn, are major undertakings, but are vital to successful therapy (Cox, 1981).

Prognosis. The prognosis for survival probably is about 50% with neuromuscular syndromes.

Recumbency for up to 2 weeks has occurred in cows that have survived. The degree of rise in serum CPK activity and the elevation

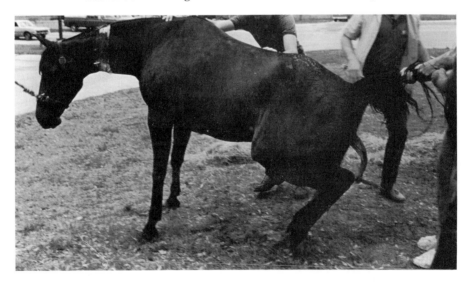

Figure 14–33. Postfoaling paralysis is far less frequent than postcalving paralysis. This mare became recumbent following foaling and here is demonstrating the extensor weakness typical of bilateral femoral paresis. While recumbent, normal flexor reflexes could be obtained. However, the patellar reflexes were poor and bilateral areas of analgesia were present on the medial thigh regions. Postmortem examination showed that hemorrhage had occurred in and around the sacroiliac joints and extended ventrally to encompass both femoral nerves.

of BUN and creatinine concentrations can indicate the degree of myonecrosis and renal and prerenal azotemia, respectively. These indicators may help determine a prognosis.

4. **Porcine Stress Syndrome (PSS)—Malignant Hyperthermia (MH)**

Signalment. Certain strains of German and Belgian Landrace pigs, Dutch and German Pietrain pigs, and Poland China pigs are particularly (68 to 94%) affected by PSS (O'Brien, 1987), (Chambers et al., 1987). Possibly MH has been seen in horses during anesthesia and may be associated with postanesthetic myopathy syndrome (II.2 above) (O'Brien, 1987).

Syndrome. Stiffness, hyperventilation, patchy skin vasodilation, and reluctance to move occurs with forced exercise in susceptible swine. Sudden death occurs. In certain families of susceptible pigs, the syndrome is associated with pale exudative pork and back muscle necrosis seen in meat plants.

Assessment. Malignant hyperthermia is a hypermetabolic myopathy triggered in genetically susceptible patients by potent volatile anesthetic agents and muscle relaxants. In pigs it is referred to as PSS because it is triggered by these inciters as well as by exertional, thermal, and mechanical stressors (O'Brien, 1987). Muscle hyperactivity occurs because of a hypersensitive calcium-release mechanism present in the sarcoplasmic reticulum. Resulting thermogenesis produces hyperthermia and a cascade of metabolic events, including lactic acidosis, hypoxemia, and hyperkalemia leading to rapid death (Chambers et al., 1987), (O'Brien, 1987).

Treatment. This is a fatal disease. Dantrolene sodium at blood concentrations of 2 to 4 µg/ml are protective and therapeutic. In horses, an oral dose of 10 mg/kg is required to achieve such concentrations for about 2 to 3 hours (Court et al., 1987).

Prevention. Reducing stress during transportation and routine management practices, along with genetic selection and culling to dilute the prevalence of the MH gene, are the primary means of reducing the disease incidence in swine (Chambers et al., 1987).

III. **Infectious, Inflammatory, Immune**

1. **Polymyositis**

Acute forms of polymyositis often are caused by *Clostridium chauvoei* (blackleg), less often *Cl septicum, Cl novyi, Cl sordelli*, and *Cl perfringens* (malignant edema) (Blood et al., 1983), (Goedegebuure, 1987). Cattle, sheep, goats, horses, and swine all are susceptible to these organisms, although clinical disease most often is seen in young ruminants. Usually sudden deaths signal the beginning of an outbreak. Some animals may be seen with degrees of mono-, para-, or tetraparesis and with painful, swollen muscles. These anerobic organisms grow in sites of mildly (bruising) or significantly (wound) damaged tissue and produce potent necrotizing exotoxins.

Penicillin is the drug of choice for treatment, and vaccination schedules are mandatory in endemic areas. Texts on large animal medicine and on veterinary microbiology should be consulted for full descriptions of these syndromes.

Only rarely has primary noninfectious (presumed to be immune-mediated) polymyositis been seen in horses.

IV. Metabolic

1. Azotemia, Hypocalcemia, and Hypomagnesemia

Acute azotemia, hypocalcemia, hypomagnesemia, and possibly other derangements have been associated with ataxia and stiff, almost hypermetric (goose-stepping) gaits, which resolve with correction of the metabolic alterations. These syndromes have been noted particularly often in horses.

V. Toxic

1. Tick Paralysis

Effects of tick neurotoxins depend on the size of the host, therefore signs of intoxication are rare in large animals. Progressive, ascending, flaccid paralysis (mimicking botulism) can occur in smaller patients. Offending ticks include *Dermacentor variabilis* and *D. andersoni* in the USA and *Ixodes holocyclus* in Australia.

2. Botulism and the Shaker-Foal Syndrome

Signalment. Botulism is seen in adult horses, cattle, and sheep worldwide (Whitlock et al., 1985), (Blood et al., 1983), (Mayhew et al., 1982). The Shaker Foal Syndrome is frequently seen in Kentucky and other eastern states of the USA (Swerczek, 1980a). It generally occurs in 1 to 3-month-old foals. Outbreaks of botulism can be devastating (Abbitt et al., 1984). The disease is much less common in pigs (Beiers et al., 1967).

Primary Complaint. This consists of flaccid tetraparesis leading to tetraplegia, dysphagia, and muscle tremor—usually with an abrupt onset.

History. Often only sudden deaths are observed at the onset of an outbreak. Otherwise there is an abrupt onset of flaccid tetraparesis/plegia with no associated illness or trauma. Sometimes mild dysphagia and depression are evident in the prodromal phase. Suckling foals typically show repeated episodes of trembling just before becoming recumbent.

A change in feedstuffs may have occurred. New batches of oat, rye, and corn silage (Whitlock et al., 1985), (Divers et al., 1986), big bale grass silage (Ricketts et al., 1984), and even grain (Mitchell et al., 1939) have been associated with outbreaks.

Physical Examination. There may be dyspnea and cyanosis. Initially, muscle atrophy is not present. Muscle trembling (weakness) may be prominent. Ileus may be prominent; tachycardia and urinary incontinence have been reported in cattle.

Neurologic Examination. Flaccid tetraplegia is characteristic of botulism. Horses tremble violently from weakness before becoming recumbent. There is normal sensation with depressed reflexes. Pupillary dilation, urine retention, and ileus and constipation may be evident. Intercostal and phrenic nerve paralysis may result in dyspnea, and pharyngeal paralysis is often seen in adults (Fig. 14–34).

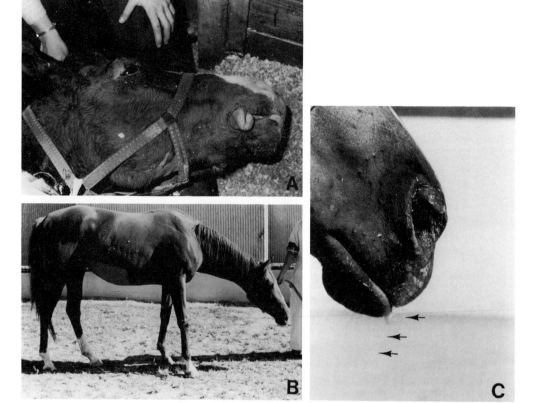

Figure 14–34. This horse suffered from a postanesthetic, myasthenic syndrome that mimics botulism. Typical of both disorders, there was flaccid tetraplegia with sluggish pupillary light, facial muscle, and tongue withdrawal reflexes (A). During recovery, which began in a few days, residual tetraparesis with low head carriage (B) and mild dysphagia (C) with drooling of saliva (arrows) (also characteristic of both disorders) was seen.

Assessment. In a suitable anaerobic environment, different strains of *Clostridium botulinum* organisms can produce one of eight serologically distinct neurotoxins (types A, B, C_α, C_β, D, E, F, G), which block exocytosis of acetylcholine at the presynaptic membrane of the neuromuscular junction. The toxin usually is preformed and ingested by the animal. It may be preformed in carrion or in feedstuffs (Mitchell et al., 1939), (Mayhew et al., 1982), (Whitlock et al., 1985), (Blood et al., 1983). Forage poisoning is the term used for the syndrome having identical signs but no isolated toxin, therefore it is only a presumptive diagnosis of botulism. There can be wound contamination with *Cl botulinum,* (Bernard et al., 1987). The shaker foal syndrome in suckling foals, especially in Kentucky, is a toxico-infectious form of botulism associated with *Cl botulinum* type B, which grows in ingesta (as in infant botulism in humans), in wounds, in gastric ulcers, or in liver abscesses (Lewis et al., 1981), (Swerczek, 1980a,b). The bacterial and toxin type varies in different areas and in different countries, but usually is types B, C, or D in large animals.

Diagnostic Aids. The needle EMG may be characterized by brief, small amplitude and abundant action potentials—there is more activity than expected for the amount of muscle contraction occurring (Volpe, 1987). On nerve stimulation small action potentials occur, which usually do not decrement with repeated (5 to 10 Hz) stimulation, but which may be augmented by tetanic (50 Hz) stimulation (Divers et al., 1986)—a characteristic of presynaptic blockade (Swift, 1981). Such EMG characteristics of infantile botulism (Volpe, 1987) have been detected in the shaker foal syndrome and could be useful in supporting a clinical diagnosis and in monitoring improvement in the disease. Detection of circulating toxin by mouse inoculation is possible, but often too little toxin is circulating in large animals, particularly in horses that are extremely sensitive to botulism toxin (Ricketts et al., 1984), (MacKay et al., 1982), (Whitlock et al., 1985). Isolation of *Cl botulinum* from grain, silage, carrion-contaminated feedstuffs, the patient's feces, or from lesions or wounds in the patient is strong circumstantial evidence of disease (Whitlock et al., 1985), (Bernard et al., 1987), (Swerczek, 1980a,b), (Mayhew et al., 1982).

Therapy. Botulism antitoxin is expensive (in 1987 type B antitoxin costed $1000/250 ml from R.H. Whitlock, University of Pennsylvania, New Bolten Center, Kennett Square, PA), and the specific type is required. Penicillin (not procaine) should be used systemically. It should be given orally as well if toxicoinfectious (alimentary) botulism is suspected in shaker foals and in isolated cases of forage poisoning. Nursing care is paramount; some foals have survived after assisted ventilation has been required for several weeks.

Prognosis. The outlook is poor to guarded with or without antitoxin, unless intensive, prolonged, and diligent nursing care is feasible. Forage poisoning is usually fatal in adult horses, unless the patient remains standing. Cases in which signs do not rapidly progress to recumbency have a better prognosis than those that show fulminant tetraplegia (Blood et al., 1983), (MacKay et al., 1982), (Rickettts et al., 1984). Vaccinating mares with *Cl botulinum* type B toxoid twice in the last trimester of pregnancy is practiced in some areas where the shaker-foal syndrome is common, and it appears to be successful in preventing the disease (Lewis et al., 1981).

3. Postanesthetic Myasthenic Syndrome

This rare clinical syndrome is identical to forage poisoning (botulism) and tick paralysis and is seen in horses that remain in a state of flaccid paralysis following anesthesia (Fig. 14–34A). Usually combinations of aminoglycoside or tetracycline antibiotics, and halothane and succinylcholine were used. Hypocalcemia, complicated surgeries (e.g., ovarian tumor removal), and drug combinations may play a role in the diffuse neuromuscular blockade that is evident. Facial, tongue, pharyngeal, body, and limb musculature is affected. Calcium salts and neostigmine are worth trying, but nursing care (as for botulism) is most important. Three animals recovered with nursing care and were able to walk in 5 to 7 days; they were totally normal within 4 weeks (see Fig. 14–34).

4. *Cassia occidentalis*

Coffee senna (*Cassia occidentalis*) is indigenous to the Southeastern USA. When ingested by cattle the plant, especially the seeds, cause weakness, ataxia, stumbling, reluctance to move, recumbency, and rapid death. Extensive myodegeneration occurs, particularly involving the limbs and heart, with elevated serum CPK activity and myoglobinemia detectable (O'Hara et al., 1969), (Mercer et al., 1967). The syndrome resembles nutritional myodegeneration (white muscle disease—VI.1 below).

5. **Monensin and Lasolocid**

Monensin and lasolocid are polyether antibiotics used in feedstuffs for cattle, swine, and chickens as growth promotants and coccidiostats. All large animals, particularly horses, are susceptible to poisoning with these carboxylic ionophores, which interfere with metal ion transfer across biomembranes (Amend et al., 1980), (Hanson et al., 1981), (Van Vleet et al., 1987).

Acute intoxication can result in hypovolemic shock and rapid death. Less severe intoxication causes degrees of ataxia, weakness, and recumbency with hyporeflexia. Evidence of myonecrosis, heart failure, and renal failure are variably present (Van Vleet et al., 1987), (Amend et al., 1980). In horses, ataxia and paraparesis may persist for several weeks and signs of chronic heart failure may become apparent (Amend et al., 1980), (Hanson et al., 1981). Experimental intoxication in horses and swine has caused early signs of hypermetric ataxia, which may result from an ionophore interfering with peripheral neurotransmitters (Van Vleet et al., 1987), (Amend et al., 1980). Vitamin E and selenium may ameliorate some of the toxic effects of these compounds; other antibiotics, such as tiamulin (used to prevent swine dysentery), may exacerbate the toxicity—at least in swine (Van Vleet et al., 1987).

6. **Ivermectin**

This macrocyclic lactone is used widely as an antiparasitic agent in all large animals (Campbell et al., 1984). Its effectiveness results because it interferes with gamma-amiobutyric acid neurotransmission in parasitic arthropods and nematodes. Ivermectin is a safe drug, but ataxia has been reported in cattle, sheep, and swine with overdosing. Horses have shown temporary blindness and ataxia when they received 10 times the recommended dose, which is 0.2 mg/kg (Campbell et al., 1984), (Bennett, 1986).

7. **Methyl Bromide**

Methyl bromide is used as a plant and soil fumigant, particularly prior to planting grapes. Hay harvested from ground treated with it has resulted in ataxia and depression in horses, goats, and cattle (Knight et al., 1977). Signs are seen when serum bromide concentrations reach about 30 mEq/L. Spurious laboratory results of chloride estimations might be expected with methyl bromide intoxication.

VI. Nutritional

1. **Nutritional Myodegeneration—White Muscle Disease—Myodegeneration and Steatitis**

Signalment. This condition is frequently seen in young ruminants; less frequently seen in swine; and infrequently seen in goats, foals, horses, and ponies (Goedegebuure, 1987), (Dill, et al., 1985), Foreman et al., 1986), (Maas et al., 1984), (Owen et al., 1977), (Bradley, 1981). Yearling and adult cattle sometimes are affected in outbreaks (Anderson et al., 1976), (Chalmers et al., 1979), (Linklater et al., 1977).

History. There is progressive to peracute weakness and stiffness of the limbs or neck. Some are presented for treatment because of tachypnea and occasionally may be found dead. Exercise, inclement weather, or transport may precipitate and exacerbate the signs (Kennedy et al., 1987).

Examination. Palpably swollen and painful muscle masses may be found. In foals and ponies the base of the tail, the tissues beneath the mane, and the tongue and submandibular area may appear to be painful on palpation (Dill and Rebhun, 1985). Reluctance to move and a stiff, sometimes weak gait are evident. This can mimic diseases such as pleuritis, acute pneumonia, laminitis, and polyarthritis. Reflexes are normal or slightly depressed, and sensation is intact. The syndrome can be difficult to distinguish from spinal cord disease in an individual, lamb, or calf. Myoglobinuria may be found in the severe syndrome, particularly in adult cattle (Anderson et al., 1976).

Assessment. Muscle degeneration and necrosis (Bradley, 1981), (Anderson et al., 1977), and fat necrosis in horses (Foreman et al., 1986), (Platt et al., 1971), (Sandersleben et al., 1977) and donkeys (Vanselow et al., 1981) are present; the syndromes are usually related to low vitamin E or selenium status. Fibrinoid degeneration and sometimes mineralization may be present in subacute and chronic stages.

In most cases, low vitamin E or selenium status can be confirmed. A period of exercise, a change in feed, transportation, or other stressors, appear to trigger signs of widespread myodegeneration in susceptible patients. Experimentally, elevated muscle enzyme activity in serum and subclinical myopathy can be achieved with vitamin E and selenium depletion. However, factors like the addition of polyunsaturated fatty acids, such as linolenic acid (protected linseed oil), appear necessary to trigger the typical clinical syndrome (Kennedy et al., 1987).

Involvement of muscles of the head occasionally occurs in horses (Kroneman et al., 1968) and is discussed in Problem 6C.

Diagnostic Aids. Elevated serum muscle enzyme activities and detection of myopathic potentials on needle EMG examination help to confirm the presence of a myopathy. Low serum vitamin E concentration and more often low serum and tissue selenium concentrations and depressed serum glutathion peroxidase activity help incriminate low vitamin E and selenium status as a factor in the myodegeneration.

Therapy. Rest, phenylbutazone, and vitamin E and selenium are particularly useful in treatment. Some spectacular responses can be seen.

Prognosis. This is bad if the heart or respiratory musculature are affected and permanent muscle atrophy may occur with recovery. Treatment of foals with steatitis and myodegeneration has not been particularly successful (Foreman et al., 1986), (Kroneman et al., 1968).

VII. Idiopathic

1. Vague Neuromusculoskeletal Lameness and Diseases of the Back (also Problem 10A, VII.5)

Many horses with subtle gait abnormalities, in the pelvic limbs in particular, show some evidence of ataxia, weakness, or dysmetria, with no proof of a specific neurologic disorder. Many of these patients are referred to as having back, hip, or stifle problems or as being "tail wringers" or "daisy cutters." Occasionally, evidence of polyneuropathy or myelitis becomes evident on a thorough evaluation, but usually a complete workup is inconclusive.

An animal with osteochondrosis involving the proximal limb joints and particularly the intervertebral joints can present with degrees of reluctance to move and a stiff, apparently weak gait—which mimics spinal cord or peripheral nerve disease. Osteochondrosis most often occurs in young feeder pigs and in horses. A thorough physical examination and a lameness examination should reveal the cause of such pseudoneurologic gait abnormalities (Fig. 14–35).

Back problems in horses are a clinical enigma. With the exclusion of fractures and overt exercise-associated rhabdomyolysis, definitive etiologic and morphologic diagnoses are the exception rather than the rule. One major reason for this is the wide range of biomechanical and pathologic changes that can be detected in apparently normal horses (Townsend et al., 1986). A procedure for examining horses suspected of having a (non-neurologic) back problem has been suggested by Jeffcott (1985a). Such a procedure allows cases to be classified into suspected causes (Jeffcott, 1985b). However, additional detailed studies of normal horses and clinical cases, using ultrasound, infrared thermography, nuclear scintigraphy and computer-assisted radiographic imaging, and electrophysiologic testing, should provide a more precise definition of etiopathologic syndromes.

Remarkable claims have been made for the curative effects of acupuncture therapy on horses with chronic back pain (Martin et al., 1987), and for chiropractic manipulations. If such regimens of therapy do no harm, and appear to relieve the clinical syndrome, their use may be justified.

2. Aortic-Iliac Thrombosis, Ischemic Neuromyopathy

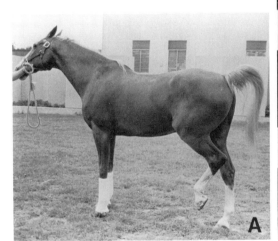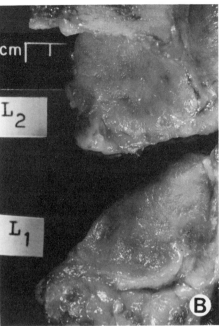

Figure 14–35. Vague back problems in horses are difficult to diagnose successfully. This horse had evidence of "back pain" because prominent lordosis resulted from lumbar manipulation. The horse had a stiff gait in the pelvic limbs and would elevate the tail and flex the pelvic limbs while standing still (A) and particularly when beginning to walk. Significantly, the flexion does not involve digital extension with the toe brought cranial as in stringhalt (Problem 8). Radiographs revealed significant lumbar osteoarthrosis, which was confirmed at postmortem examination. The irregular dorsal articular surfaces of L1-2, devoid of articular cartilage, are shown in B.

Signalment. Usually this is seen in adult racing and performance horses (Maxie et al., 1985).

History. This varies from stiffness in the hind limbs and slowing near the end of a race, to acute paraplegia (Reef et al., 1987).

Examinations. In mild cases there is a decreased arterial pulse pressure in the pelvic limbs and slow saphenous vein refill following exercise. Severely affected animals are paraplegic, with cold pelvic limbs and areflexia and analgesia that is clearly demarcated. A weak pulse in, or thrombosis and occlusion of, the terminal aorta or iliac arteries may be palpated through the rectum. Rectal ultrasonography can be used to define the thrombosis (Tithof et al., 1985), (Reef et al., 1987).

Assessment. Degrees of hypoxic-ischemic neuromyopathy result from major vessel occlusion. Associations with equine infectious anemia, *Strongylus vulgaris* arteritis, thrombotic diseases and cardiomyopathy in various cases have been suggested; none of which are substantiated (Maxie et al., 1985).

Therapy. Clinicians have tried combinations of heparin, anthelmintics, phenylbutazone, calcium gluconate, ivermectin, and glucocorticoids with unknown results. Heroic surgical treatment is feasible, but the prognosis for improvement is bad.

Problem 10C.

Episodic Weakness

True episodic weakness, epitomized by myasthenia gravis, with the patient being completely normal between episodes, is rare in large animals. Mild and perhaps transient cases of several familial, inflammatory, toxic, and metabolic disorders discussed in this and other Problems may be interpreted as episodic weakness.

Categories of Disease and Differential Diagnosis
NOTE: Only those diseases marked * are discussed in this problem.

   I. Congenital and Familial
      1. Myasthenia Gravis (Not proven to occur in large animals)
      2. Hyperkalemic Periodic Paralysis (Problem 8B)
      3. Narcolepsy—Cataplexy (Problem 4)
  II. Physical
     *1. Sunburn in Swine
 III. Infectious, Inflammatory, Immune
      1. Polymyositis (Problem 10B, above)
  IV. Metabolic
      1. Cardiopulmonary Collapse—Syncope
      2. Hypoglycemia (Problem 2)
      3. Electrolyte Derangements (Problems 2, 8)

   I. Inflammatory
     1. Sunburn in swine
       Although not likely to be misdiagnosed as a neurologic disease, this syndrome has been so baffling as to warrant inclusion.
       Affected pale-skinned swine, which stand in the sun usually to eat, periodically drop to the ground on their pelvic limbs, thoracic limbs, or on all four limbs. The degree of cutaneous erythema and ultimate blistering may appear minimal.

REFERENCES

Abbitt B, Murphy MJ, Ray AC, et al. Catastrophic death losses in a dairy herd attributed to type D botulism. J Am Vet Med Assoc 1984; 185:798–801.

Abbott LC, Finnell RH, Chernoff GF, et al. Crooked calf disease: A histological and histochemical examination of eight affected calves. Vet Pathol 1986; 23:734–740.

Adams LG, Dollahite JW, Romane WM, et al. Cystitis and ataxia associated with sorghum ingestion by horses. J Am Vet Med Assoc 1969; 155:518–524.

Adams DS, Klevjer-Anderson P, Carlson JL, et al. Transmission and control of caprine arthritis-encephalitis virus. Am J Vet Res 1983; 44:1670–1675.

Adams SB, Steckel R, Blevins W. Diskospondylitis in five horses. J Am Vet Med Assoc 1985; *168*:270–272.

Adcock JL, Hibler CP. Vascular and Neuro-ophthalmic pathology of elaeophorosis in elk. Vet Pathol 1969; *6*:185–213.

Alden C, Woodson F, Mohan R, Miller S. Cerebrospinal nematodiasis in sheep. J Am Vet Med Assoc 1975; *166*:784–786.

Alitalo I, Karkkainen M. Osteochondrotic changes in the vertebrae of four ataxic horses suffering from cervical vertebral malformation. Nord Vet Med 1983; *35*:468–474.

Allen GP, Bryans JT. Molecular epizootiology, pathogenesis, and prophylaxis of equine herpesvirus-1 infections. Prog Vet Microbiol Immun 1986; 78–144.

Amend JF, Mallon FM, Wren WB, et al. Equine monensin toxicosis: Some experimental clinico-pathologic observations. Comp Cont Ed Pract Vet 1980; S173–S182.

Anderson PH, Berrett S, Patterson DSP. Some observations on "paralytic myoglobinuria" of cattle in Britain. Vet Rec 1976; *99*:316–318.

Anderson PH, Bradley R, Berrett S, Patterson DSP. The sequence of myodegeneration in nutritional myopathy of the older calf. Br Vet J 1977; *133*:160–165.

Andrews AH. Abnormal reactions and their frequency in cattle following the use of organophosphorus warble fly dressings. Vet Rec 1981; *109*:171–175.

Andrews FM, Spurgeon TL, Reed SM. Histochemical changes in skeletal muscles of four male horses with neuromuscular disease. Am J Vet Res 1986; *47*:2078–2083.

Baker JR, Kippax IS. An oligodendroglioma in a bull. Vet Rec 1980; *107*:42.

Baker NF, Tucker EM, Stormont C, et al. Neurotoxicity of haloxon and its relationship to blood esterases of sheep. Am J Vet Res 1970; *31*:865–870.

Bartsch RC, McConnell EE, Imes GD, et al. A review of exertional rhabdomyolysis in wild and domestic animals and man. Vet Pathol 1977; *14*:314–324.

Barlow RM, Cancilla PA. Structural changes of the central nervous system in swayback (enzootic ataxia) of lambs. I. Light microscopy using phosphatases as organelle markers. Acta Neuro-pathol 1966; *6*:175–180.

Barlow RM, Greig A. Kangaroo gait in ewes. Vet Rec 1986; *119*:174–175.

Barlow RM, Butler EJ, Purves D. An ataxic condition in red deer (*Cervus elaphus*). J Comp Pathol 1964; *74*:519–529.

Barrett DS, Oehme FW, Kruckenberg SM. A review of organophosphorus ester-induced delayed neurotoxicity. Vet Hum Toxicol 1985: *27*:22–37.

Beck BE, Wood CD, Whenham GR. Triaryl phosphate poisoning in cattle. Vet Pathol 1977; *14*:128–137.

Beech J, Fletcher JE, Johnston J, et al. Use of phenytoin in horses with chronic intermittent rhabdomyolysis and myotonia. Proc 33rd Annu Conv Am Assoc Equine Pract 1987: pp 375–380.

Beech J. Discussion of the papers given in the seminar. Proc 31st Annu Conf Am Assoc Equine Pract 1985; 97–103.

Beech J. Neuroaxonal dystrophy of the accessory cuneate nucleus in horses. Vet Pathol 1984; *21*:384–393.

Beech J. Metrizamide myelography in the horse. J Am Vet Rad Soc 1979; *20*:22–31.

Beech J. Equine protozoal myeloencephalitis. Vet Med Small Anim Clin 1974; *69*:1562–1566.

Beech J. Dodd DC. Toxoplasma-like encephalomyelitis in the horse. Vet Pathol 1974; *11*:87–96.

Beech J, Haskins M. Genetic studies of neuroaxonal dystrophy in the Morgan. Am J Vet Res 1987; *48*:109–113.

Beiers PR, Simmons GC. Botulism in pigs. Aust Vet J 1967; *43*:270–271.

Belton DJ, Robins JH, Greening JO. Progressive spinal myelopathy in Murray grey cattle. NZ Vet J 1987; *35*:179–180.

Bennett DG. Clinical pharmacology of ivermectin. J Am Vet Med Assoc 1986; *189*:100–104.

Bernard W, Divers TJ, Whitlock RH, et al. Botulism as a sequel to open castration in a horse. J Am Vet Med Assoc 1987; *191*:73–74.

Blakemore WF, Jefferies A, White RAS, et al. Spinal cord malacia following general anaesthesia in the horse. Vet Rec 1984; *114*:569–570.

Blakemore WF, Palmer AC, Barlow RM. Progressive ataxia of Charolais cattle associated with disordered myelin. Acta Neuropathol (Berl) 1974; *29*:127–139.

Blood DC, Radostits OM, Henderson JA. *Veterinary Medicine*. 6th Ed. London: Bailliere Tindal, 1983. pp 536–556, 1163–1193, 1193–1195, 1195, 1267–1271.

Blunden AS, Khalil LF, Webbon PM. *Halicephalobus deletrix* infection in a horse. Equine Vet J 1987; *19*:255–260.

Blythe LL. Vitamin E in the horse. Proc Annu Meet West Can Assoc Equine Pract. January 1988; 130–136.

Blythe LL. Can wobbler disease be a family affair? [Abstract] Eastern States Vet Conf. February 1986; *1*:160.

Bonniwell MA, Barlow RM. Ataxia/paresis syndrome of sheep in West Africa associated with bilateral multifocal cerebrospinal poliomalacia. Vet Rec 1985; *116*:94–97.

Bourke CA. A novel nigrostriatal dopaminergic disorder in sheep affected by *Tribulus terrestris* staggers. Vet Sci 1987; *43*:347–350.

Bourke CA. Staggers in sheep associated with the ingestion of *Tribulus terrestris*. Aust Vet J 1984; *61*:360–363.

Bourke CA, MacFarlane JA. A transient ataxia of sheep associated with the ingestion of *Tribulus micrococcus* (yellow vine). Aust Vet J 1985; *62*:282.

Boyd JS. Congenital deformities in two Clydesdale foals. Equine Vet J 1976; *8*:161–164.

Boyd JS, McNeil PE. Atlanto-occipital fusion and ataxia in the calf. Vet Rec 1987; *120*:34–37.

Bradley R. Skeletal muscle in health and disease. In Practice 1981; *3*:5–13.

Bradley R, Done JT. Nervous and muscular systems. In: *Disease of Swine*. 6th Ed. Leman AD, Straw B, Glock RD, et al, eds. Ames: Iowa State University Press, 1986: pp 58–81.

Brearley JC, Jones RS, Kelly DF, et al. Spinal cord degeneration following general anesthesia in a Shire horse. Equine Vet J 1986; *18*:222–224.

Braun U, Ehrensperger F, Bracher V. Das Weaver-Syndrom beim Rind. Tierarztl Prax 1987; *15*:139–144.

Braund KG. Neoplasia. In: *Veterinary Neurology*. Oliver JE, Hoerlein BF, Mayhew IG, eds. Philadelphia: WB Saunders, 1987. Ch 9. pp 278–284.

Brewer BD. Therapeutic strategies involving antimicrobial treatment of the central nervous system in large animals. J Am Vet Med Assoc 1984; *185*:1217–1221.

Brown TT, Patton CS. Protozoal encephalomyelitis in horses. (Letter). J Am Vet Med Assoc 1977; *171*:492.

Campbell WC, Benz GW. Ivermectin: A review of efficacy and safety. J Vet Pharmacol Therap 1984; *7*:1–16.

Cardinet III GH, Holliday TA. Neuromuscular disease of domestic animals: A summary of muscle biopsies from 159 cases. Ann NY Acad Sci 1979; *317*:290–313.

Carlson GP, Nelson T. Exercise-related muscle problems in endurance horses. Proc 22nd Annu Conv Am Assoc Equine Pract 1976; 223–228.

Carroll CL, Westbury HA. Isolation of equine herpesvirus 1 from the brain of a horse affected with paresis. Aust Vet J 1985; *62*:345–346.

Casteel SW, Osweiler GD, Cook WO, et al. Selenium toxicosis in swine. J Am Vet Med Assoc 1985; *186*:1084–1085.

Chaldek DW, Ruth GR. Isolation of *Actinobacillus lignieresi* from an epidural abscess in a horse with progressive paralysis. J Am Vet Med Assoc 1976; *168*:64–66.

Chalmers GA. Swayback (enzootic ataxia) in Alberta lambs. Can J Comp Med 1974; *38*:111–117.

Chalmers GA, Barrett MW. Capture myopathy in pronghorns in Alberta, Canada. J Am Vet Med Assoc 1977; *171*:918–923.

Chalmers GA, Decaire MK, Zachar CJ, et al. Myopathy and myoglobinuria in feedlot cattle. Case Report. Can Vet J 1979; *20*:105–108.

Chambers J, Hall RR. Porcine malignant hyperthermia (porcine stress syndrome). Comp Cont Ed Pract Vet 1987; *9*:F317–F326.

Charlton KM. Experimental alkylmercurial poisoning in swine. Lesions in the peripheral and central nervous systems. Can J Comp Med 1974; *38*:75–81.

Charlton KM, Mitchell D, Girard A, et al. Meningoencephalomyelitis in horses associated with equine herpesvirus 1 infection. Vet Pathol 1976; *13*:59–68.

Charlton KM, Claborn LD, Pierce KR. A neuropathy in goats caused by experimental coyotillo (*Karwinskia humboltiana*) poisoning: Clinical and neurophysiologic studies. Am J Vet Res 1971; *32*:1381–1389.

Chiapetta JR, Baker JC, Feeney DA. Vertebral fracture, extensor hypertonia of thoracic limbs, and paralysis of pelvic limbs (Schiff-Sherrington syndrome) in an Arabian foal. J Am Vet Med Assoc 1985; *186*:387–388.

Child G, Higgins RJ, Cuddon PA. Acquired scoliosis associated with hydromyelia and syringomyelia in two dogs. J Am Vet Med Assoc 1986; *189*:909–912.

Cho CY, Cook JE, Leipold HW. Angiomatous vascular malformation in the spinal cord of a Hereford calf. Vet Pathol 1979; *16*:613–616.

Cho DY, Leipold HW. Syringomyelia in a Thoroughbred foal. Equine Vet J 1977a; *9*:195–197.

Cho DY, Leipold HW. Spina bifida and spinal dysraphism in calves. Zbl Vet Med A 1977b; *24*:680–695.

Cimprich R, Ardington P. Spinal ganglioneuroma in a steer. Vet Pathol 1975; *12*:59–60.

Clark EG, Townsend HGG, McKenzie NT. Equine protozoal myeloencephalitis: A report of two cases from Western Canada. Can Vet J 1981; *22*:140–144.

Clemmons RM, Meyer DJ, Sundlof SF, et al. Correction of organophosphate-induced neuromuscular blockade by diphenhydramine. Am J Vet Res 1984; *45*:2167–2169.

Cordy DR. Progressive ataxia of Charolais cattle—an oligodendroglial dysplasia. Vet Pathol 1986; *23*:78–80.

Cordy DR, East NE, Lowenstine LJ. Caprine encephalomyelomalacia. Vet Pathol 1984; *21*:269–273.

Cordy DR, Knight HD. California goats with a disease resembling enzootic ataxia or swayback. Vet Pathol 1978; *15*:179–185.

Cordy DR, Richards WPC, Bradford GE. Systemic neuroaxonal dystrophy in Suffolk sheep. Acta Neuropathol 1967; *8*:133–140.

Cork LC. Differential diagnosis of viral leukoencephalomyelitis of goats. J Am Vet Med Assoc 1976; *169*:1303–1306.

Cork LC, Hadlow WJ, Crawford TB, et al. Infectious leukoencephalomyelitis of young goats. J Infect Dis 1974; *129*:134–141.

Court MH, Engelking LR, Dodman NH, et al. Pharmacokinetics of dantrolene sodium in horses. J Vet Pharmacol Therap 1987; *10*:218–226.

Cox VS. Understanding the downer cow syndrome. Comp Cont Ed Pract Vet 1981; 3:S472–S478.

Cox VS, Breazile JE, Hoover TR. Surgical and anatomic study of calving paralysis. Am J Vet Res 1975; *36*:427–430.

Cox VS, McGrath CJ, Jorgensen SE. The role of pressure damage in pathogenesis of the downer cow syndrome. Am J Vet Res 1982; *43*:26–31.

Craig DR, Roth L, Smith MC. Lymphosarcoma in goats. Comp Cont Ed Pract Vet 1986; *8*:S190–S198.

Crawford TB, Adams DS. Caprine arthritis-encephalitis: Clinical features and presence of antibody in selected goat populations. J Am Vet Med Assoc 1981; *178*:713–719.

Crawshaw GJ, Mould KL. Repair of a cervical fracture. Vet Med Small Anim Clin 1982; *77*:233–236.

Crowhurst FA, Dickinson G, Burrows R. An outbreak of paresis in mares and geldings associated with equid herpesvirus 1. Vet Rec 1981; *109*:527–528.

Cusick PK, Sells DM, Hamilton DP, et al. Toxoplasmosis in two horses. J Am Vet Med Assoc 1974; *164*:77–80.

Cutlip RC, Jackson TA, Lehmkuhl HD. Lesions of ovine progressive pneumonia: Interstitial pneumonitis and encephalitis. Am J Vet Res 1979; *40*:1370–1374.

Cymbaluk NF, Fretz PB, Loew FM. Amprolium-induced thiamine deficiency in horses: Clinical features. Am J Vet Res 1978; *39*:255–261.

DeBowes RM, Grant BD, Bagby GW, et al. Cervical vertebral interbody fusion in the horse: A comparative study of bovine xenografts and autografts supported by stainless steel baskets. Am J Vet Res 1984; *45*:191–199.

de Lahunta A. *Veterinary Neuroanatomy and Clinical Neurology.* 2nd Ed. Philadelphia: WB Saunders, 1983. pp 227, 233.

Deland MPB, Lewis D, Cunningham PR, et al. Use of orally administered oxidised copper wire particles for copper therapy in cattle. Aust Vet J 1986; *63*:1–2.

Dill SG, Rebhun WC. White muscle disease in foals. Comp Cont Ed Pract Vet 1985; *7*:S627–S635.

Divers TJ, Bartholomew RC, Messick JB, et al. *Clostridium botulinum* type B toxicosis in a herd of cattle and a group of mules. J Am Vet Med Assoc 1986; *188*:382–386.

Dickson J, Hopkins DL, Rasili DP. Torticollis in goats. Vet Rec 1986; 162–163.

Dodd DC, Cordes DO. Spinal abscess and cord compression syndrome in lambs. NZ Vet J 1964; *12*:1–5.

Doige CE. Pathological findings associated with locomotory disturbances in lactating and recently weaned sows. Can J Comp Med 1982; *46*:1–6.

Doige CE. Discospondylitis in swine. Can J Comp Med 1980; *44*:121–128.

Doige CE. Pathological changes in the lumbar spine of pigs: Gross findings. Can J Comp Med 1979; *43*:142–150.

Done JT. Congenital nervous diseases of pigs: A review. Lab Anim 1968; *2*:207–217.

Dorr TE, Higgins RJ, Dangler CA, et al. Protozoal myeloencephalitis in horses in California. J Am Vet Med Assoc 1984; *185*:801–802.

Drachman DB, Weiner LP, Price DL, et al. Experimental arthrogryposis caused by viral myopathy. Arch Neurol 1976; *33*:362–367.

Drudge JH, Lyons ET, Swerczek TW, et al. Cambendazole for strongyle control in a pony band: Selection of a drug-resistant population of small strongyles and teratologic implications. Am J Vet Res 1983; *44*:110–114.

Dubey JP. Toxoplasmosis in horses. (Letter). J Am Vet Med Assoc 1974; *165*:668.

Dubey JP, Davis GW, Koestner A, et al. Equine encephalomyelitis due to a protozoan parasite resembling *Toxoplasma gondii.* J Am Vet Med Assoc 1974; *165*:249–255.

Dubey JP, Miller S. Equine protozoal myeloencephalitis in a pony. J Am Vet Med Assoc 1986; *188*:1311–1312.

Duffell SJ, Wells AH, Winkler CE. Kangaroo gait in ewes: A peripheral neuropathy. Vet Rec 1986; *118*:296–298.

Dyson SJ, Taylor PM, Whitwell K. Femoral nerve paralysis after general anaesthesia. Equine Vet J 1988; 20:376–379.

Edington N, Bridges CG, Huckle A. Experimental reactivation of equid herpesvirus 1 (EHV 1) following the administration of corticosteroids. Equine Vet J 1985; *17*:369–372.

Edwards MJ. Congenital defects due to hyperthermia. Adv Vet Sci Comp Med 1978; *22*:29–52.

Ellis J, DeMartini JC. Retroviral diseases in small ruminants: Ovine progressive pneumonia and caprine arthritis-encephalitis. Comp Cont Ed Pract Vet 1983; *4*:S173–S181.

Evans ETR, Evans WC, Roberts HE. Studies on bracken poisoning in the horse. Brit Vet J 1951; *107*:364–371, 399–411.

Eyre P, Boulard C, Deline T. Local and systemic reactions in cattle to *Hypoderma lineatum* larval toxin: Protection by phenylbutazone. Am J Vet Res 1981; *432*:25.

Faden AI, Jacobs TP, Smith MT, et al. Comparison of thyrotropin-releasing hormone (TRH), naloxone, and dexamethasone treatments in experimental spinal injury. Neurology 1983; *33*:673–678.

Falco MJ, Whitwell K, Palmer AC. An investigation into the genetics of 'Wobbler disease' in Thoroughbred horses in Britain. Equine Vet J 1976; *8*:165–169.

Fayer R, Dubey JP. Comparative epidemiology of coccidia: Clues to the etiology of equine protozoal myeloencephalitis. Parasitiology: Quo vadit? Australian Academy of Science; Proc 6th Int Congr Parasitol, August 1986; 615–633.

Finly CG. A survey of vertebral abscesses in domestic animals in Ontario. Can Vet J 1975; *16*:114–117.

Fisher LF, Bowman KF, MacHarg MA. Spinal ataxia in a horse caused by a synovial cyst. Vet Pathol 1981; *18*:407–410.

Foley JP, Gatlin SJ, Selcer BA. Standing myelography in six adult horses. Vet Radiol 1986; *27*:54–57.

Foss RR, Gentzky RM, Riedesel EA, et al. Cervical intervertebral disc protrusion in two horses. Case report. Can Vet J 1983; *24*:188–191.

Frauenfelder HC, Kazacos KR, Lichtenfels JR. Cerebrospinal nematodiasis caused by a filariid in a horse. J Am Vet Med Assoc 1980; *177*:59–362.

Frauenfelder HC, Rossdale PD, Ricketts SW. Changes in serum muscle enzyme levels associated with training schedules and stage of the oestrous cycle in Thoroughbred racehorses. Equine Vet J 1986; *18*:371–374.

Foreman JH, Potter KA, Bayly W, et al. Generalized steatitis associated with selenium deficiency and normal vitamin E status in a foal. J Am Vet Med Assoc 1986; *189*:83–86.

Gerber VH, Fankauser R, Straub R, et al. Spinal ataxie beim pferd, verursacht durch synoviale Cysten in der halswirbelsaule. Schweiz Arch Tierheilk 1980; *122*:95–106.

Gilbert FR, Wells GAH, Gunning RF. 3-nitro-4-hydroxyphenylarsonic acid toxicity in pigs. Vet Rec 1981; *190*:158–160.

Gilmour JS, Fraser JA. Ataxia in a Welsh cob filly due to a venous malformation in the thoracic spinal cord. Equine Vet J 1977; *9*:40–42.

Goedegebuure SA. Spontaneous primary myopathies in domestic mammals: A review. Vet Q 1987; *9*:1555–171.

Grandy JL, Steffey EP, Hodgson DS, et al. Arterial hypotention and the development of post-anesthetic myopathy in halothane-anesthetized horses. Am J Vet Res 1987; *48*:192–197.

Grant BD, Hoskinson JJ, Barbee DD, et al. Ventral stabilization for decompression of caudal cervical spinal cord compression in the horse. Proc 31st Annu Conv Am Assoc Equine Pract 1985a; 75–90.

Grant BD, Barbee DD, Wagner PC, et al. Long term results of surgery for equine cervical vertebral malformation. Proc 31st Annu Conv Am Assoc Equine Pract 1985b; 91–96.

Greene JH. Arthrogryposis. In: *Spontaneous Animal Models of Human Diseases. Part XV. Skeletal System. A. Developmental Abnormalities.* Andrews EJ, Wad BC, Altman NH, eds. New York: Academic Press, 1979. Vol II, Ch 254, pp 209–212.

Greenwood RES, Simson ARB. Clinical report of a paralytic syndrome affecting stallions, mares and foals on a Thoroughbred studfarm. Equine Vet J 1980; *12*:113–117.

Grewal AS, Greenwood PE, Burton RW, et al. Caprine retrovirus infection in New South Wales: Virus isolations, clinical and histopathological findings and prevalence of antibody. Aust Vet J 1986; *63*:245.

Guffy MM. Coffman JR, Strafuss AC. Atlantoaxial luxation in a foal. J Am Vet Med Assoc 1969; *155*:754–757.

Gunn HM. Morphological aspects of the deep digital flexor muscle in horses having rigid flexion of their distal forelimb joints at birth. Ir Vet J 1976; *30*:145–151.

Hadlow WJ, Ward JK, Krinsky WL. Intracranial myiasis by *Hypoderma bovis* (linnaeus) in a horse. Cornell Vet 1977; *67*:272–281.

Haigh JC, Stewart RR, Wobeser G, et al. Capture myopathy in a moose. J Am Vet Med Assoc 1977; *171*:924–926.

Hall WTK. Cycad (zamia) poisoning in Australia. Aust Vet J 1987; *64*:149–151.

Handler M, Ho V, Whelan M, et al. Intracerebral toxoplasmosis in patients with acquired immune deficiency syndrome. J Neurosurg 1983; *59*:994–1001.

Hanson LJ, Eisenbeis HG, Givens SV. Toxic effects of lasalocid in horses. Am J Vet Res 1981; *42*:456–461.

Harding JDJ, Lewis G, Done JT. Experimental arsanilic acid poisoning in pigs. Vet Rec 1968; *83*:560–564.

Harper PAW, Duncan DW, Plant JW, et al. Cerebellar abiotrophy and segmental axonopathy: Two syndromes of progressive ataxia in Merino sheep. Aust Vet J 1986; *63*:18–21.

Harris P. Equine rhabdomyolysis—the "tying-up" syndrome. The 25th Ann Congr Brit Equine Vet Assoc (Warwick, UK) 1986.

Harris P, Colles C. The use of creatinine clearance ratios in the prevention of equine rhabdomyolysis: A report of four cases. Equine Vet J 1988; *20*:459–463.

Harris P, Snow DH. Tying up the loose ends of equine rhabdomyolysis. Equine Vet J 1986; *18*:346–348.

Harrison LH, Colvin BM, Stuart BP, et al. Paralysis in swine due to focal symmetrical poliomalacia: Possible selenium toxicosis. Vet Pathol 1983; *20*:265–273.

Hartley WJ, Kater JC. Observations on diseases of the central nervous system of sheep in New Zealand. NZ Vet J 1962; *10*:128–142.

Healy PJ, Sewell CA, Neiper RE, et al. Control of generalized glycogenosis in a Brahman herd. Aust Vet J 1987; *64*:278–280.

Helfer DH, Stevens DR. Spinal neurofibroma in a sheep. Vet Pathol 1978; *15*:784–786.

Henninger RW, Sigler RE. Spinal dysraphism in a calf. Case Report. Comp Cont Ed Pract Vet 1983; *5*:S488–492.

Higgins RJ, Vandevelde M, Hoff EJ, et al. Neurofibrillary accumulation in the zebra (*Equus burchelli*). Acta Neuropathol (Berl) 1977; *37*:1–5.

Higgins RJ, Rings DM, Fenner WR, et al. Spontaneous lower motor neuron disease with neurofibrillary accumulation in young pigs. Acta Neuropathol (Berl) 1983; *59*:288–294.

Hodgson DR. Myopathies in the athletic horse. Comp Cont Ed Pract Vet 1985; *7*:S551–S555.

Hooper PT, Best SM, Campbell A. Axonal dystrophy in the spinal cords of cattle consuming the cycad palm, *Cycas media*. Aust Vet J 1974; *50*:146–149.

Hosie BD, Gould PW, Hunter AR, et al. Acute myopathy in horses at grass in east and south east Scotland. Vet Rec 1986; *119*:444–449.

Howard JR. Bovine "knuckler" syndrome; nervous system degeneration. Proc XIIX World Vet Congress (Mexico) 1971; 176–180.

Howell JMcC, Dorling PR, Cook RD, et al. Infantile and late onset form of generalised glycogenosis type II in cattle. J Pathol 1981; *134*:267–277.

Innes JRM, Pillai CP. Kumri—so-called lumbar paralysis—of horses in Ceylon (India and Burma), and its identification with cerebrospinal nematodiasis. Brit Vet J 1955a; *3*:223–235.

Innes JRM, Plowright W. Focal symmetrical poliomalacia of sheep in Kenya. J Neuropathol Exp Neurol 1955b; *14*:185–197.

Ishizuka MM, Miguel O, Brogliato DF. Prevalence of antitoxoplasma antibodies in normal thoroughbred horses. Rev Fac Med Vet Zootec Univ São Paulo 1975; *12*:289–292.

Jackson TA, Osburn BI, Cordy DR, et al. Equine herpesvirus 1 infection of horses: Studies on the experimentally induced neurologic disease. Am J Vet Res 1977; *38*:709–719.

Jamison JM, Baird JD, Smith-Maxie LL, et al. A congenital form of myotonia with dystrophic changes in a Quarterhorse. Equine Vet J 1987; *19*:353–358.

Jeffcott LB. The examination of a horse with a potential back problem. Proc 31st Annu Meet Am Assoc Equine Pract 1985a; 271–284.

Jeffcott LB. Conditions causing thoracolumbar pain and dysfunction in horses. Proc 31st Annu Meet Am Assoc Equine Pract 1985b; 285–296.

Jeffrey M, Hopper SA, Bradley R. Kyphosis in Jersey calves. Vet Rec 1985; *117*:608–610.

Jubb KVF, Kennedy PC, Palmer N. *Pathology of Domestic Animals*. 3rd Ed. Orlando: Academic Press. 1985: Vol 1, Ch 1, pp 103–104.

Kannegieter NJ, Alley MR. Ataxia due to lymphosarcoma in a young horse. Aust Vet J 1987; *64*:377–379.

Keeler RF, Shupe JL, Crowe MW, et al. *Nicotiana glauca*-induced congenital deformities in calves: Clinical and pathologic aspects. Am J Vet Res 1981; *42*:1231–1234.

Keenan DM. Acute arsanilic acid intoxication in pigs. Aust Vet J 1973; *49*:229–231.

Kelley WR, Collins JD, Farrelly BT, et al. Vertebral osteomyelitis in a horse associated with *Mycobacterium tuberculosis var bovis* (*M. bovis*) infection. J Am Vet Rad Soc 1972; *13*:59–69.

Kennedy S, Rice DA, Davidson WB. Experimental myopathy in vitamin E- and selenium-depleted calves with and without added dietary polyunsaturated fatty acids as a model for nutritional degenerative myopathy in ruminant cattle. Res Vet Sci 1987; *43*:384–394.

Kennedy S, Rice DA, Cush PF. Neuropathology of experimental 3-nitro-4-hydroxyphenylarsonic acid toxicosis in pigs. Vet Pathol 1986; *23*:454–461.

Khan MA. Significance of 'spinal-stage' *Hypoderma* larvae in systemic insecticide toxicity. Res Vet Sci 1969; *10*:355–360.

Kirker-Head CA, Loeffler D, Held J-P. Pelvic limb lameness due to malignant melanoma in a horse. J Am Vet Med Assoc 1985; *186*:1215–1218.

Knight AP, Jokinen MP. Caprine arthritis-encephalitis. Comp Cont Ed Pract Vet 1982; *4*:S263–S270.

Knight DA, Gabel A, Reed SM, et al. Correlation of dietary mineral to incidence and severity of metabolic bone disease in Ohio and Kentucky. Proc 31st Annu Meet Am Assoc Equine Pract 1985; 445–461.

Knight DA, Reed SM. Developmental orthopedic disease of horses. Proc Vet Int Med Forum (San Diego), 1987; 495–505.

Knight HD, Reina-Guerra M. Intoxication of cattle with sodium bromide-contaminated feed. Am J Vet Res 1977; *38*:407–409.

Kohn CW, Fenner WR. Equine herpes myeloencephalopathy. Vet Clin Nth Am: Equine Pract 1987; *3*:405–419.

Konno S, Nakagana M. Akabane disease in cattle: Congenital abnormalities caused by viral infection. Experimental disease. Vet Pathol 1982; *19*:267–279.

Krogdahl DW, Thilsted JP, Olsen SK. Ataxia and hypermetria caused by *Parelaphostrongylus tenuis* infection in llamas. J Am Vet Med Assoc 1987; *190*:191–193.

Kroneman J, Wensvoort P. Muscular dystrophy and yellow fat disease in Shetland pony foals. Neth J Vet Sci 1968; *1*:42–49.

Krook L, Lutwak L, McEntee K, et al. Nutritional hypercalcitoninism in bulls. Cornell Vet 1970; 625–639.

Kruckenberg M, Strafuss AC, Marsland WP, et al. Posterior paresis in swine due to dermal absorption of the neurotoxic organophosphate tri-o-tolyl phosphate. Am J Vet Res 1973; *34*:403–404.

Kummeneje K. Encephalomyelitis and neuritis in acute cerebrospinal nematodiasis in Reindeer calves. Nord Vet Med 1974; *26*:456–458.

Leipold HW, Oehme FW, Cook JE. Congenital arthrogryposis associated with ingestion of Jimsonweed by pregnant sows. J Am Vet Med Assoc 1973a; *162*:1059–1060.

Leipold HW, Blaugh B, Huston K, et al. Weaver syndrome in Brown Swiss cattle: Clinical signs and pathology. Vet Med Small Anim Clin 1973b; 645–647.

Lewis GE, Kulinski SS, Fallon EH, et al. Evaluation of a *Clostridium botulinum* toxoid, type B, for the prevention of shaker foal syndrome. Proc 27th Annu Meet Am Assoc Equine Pract 1981; 233–237.

Lewis RJ, Chalmers GA, Barrett MW, et al. Capture myopathy in elk in Alberta, Canada: A report of three cases. J Am Vet Med Assoc 1977; *171*:927–932.

Lindsay WA, McDonell W, Bignell W. Equine postanesthetic forelimb lameness: Intracompartmental muscle pressure changes and biochemical patterns. Am J Vet Res 1980; *41*:1919–1924.

Linklater KA, McTaggart HS, Wain EB. Acute myopathy in outwintered cattle. Vet Rec 1977; *100*:312–314.

Little PB. Cerebrospinal nematodiasis of equidae. J Am Vet Med Assoc 1972; *160*:1407.

Little PB, Thorsen J. Disseminated necrotizing myeloencephalitis: A herpes-associated neurological disease of horses. Vet Pathol 1976; *13*:161–171.

Little PB, Lwin US, Fretz P. Verminous encephalitis of horses: Experimental induction with *Strongylus vulgaris* larvae. Am J Vet Res 1974; *35*:1501–1510.

Liu S-K, Dolensek EP, Adams CR, et al. Myelopathy and vitamin E deficiency in six Mongolian wild horses. J Am Vet Med Assoc 1983; *183*:1266–1268.

Liu IKM, Castleman W. Equine posterior paresis associated with equine herpesvirus 1 vaccine in California: A preliminary report. J Equine Med Surg 1977; *12*:397–410.

Livesey MA, Wilkie IW. Focal and multifocal osteosarcoma in two foals. Equine Vet J 1986; 18:407–410.

Maas J, Bulgin MS, Anderson BC, Frye TM. Nutritional myodegeneration associated with vitamin E deficiency and normal selenium status in lambs. J Am Vet Med Assoc 1984; *184*:201–204.

Macruz R, Lenci O, Ishizuka MM, et al. Toxoplasmosis in the equine. Serological evaluation. Rev Fac Med Vet Zootec Univ São Paulo 1975; *12*:277–282.

Madigan JE, Higgins RJ. Equine protozoal myeloencephalitis. Vet Clin North Am [Equine Pract] 1987; *3*:397–403.

Manktelow BW, Hartley WJ. Generalized glycogen storage disease in sheep. J Comp Path 1975; *85*:139–145.

Markel MD, Madigan JE, Lichtensteiger CA, et al. Vertebral body osteomyelitis in the horse. J Am Vet Med Assoc 1986; *188*:632–634.

Martin Jr BB, Klide AM. Treatment of chronic back pain in horses. Stimulation of acupuncture points with a low powered infrared laser. Vet Surg 1987; *16*:106–110.

Mason JE. A case of spinal cord compression causing paraplegia of a foal. Equine Vet J 1971; *3*:155–157.

Mason MM, Whiting MG, Usphs O. Caudal motor weakness and ataxia in cattle in the Caribbean area following ingestion of cycads. Cornell Vet 1968; *58*:541–554.

Mathews FP. The toxicity of *Kallstroemia hirsutissima* (carpet weed) for cattle, sheep, and goats. J Am Vet Assoc 1944; 152–155.

May SA, Wyn-Jones G, Church S. Iopamidol myelography in the horse. Equine Vet J 1986; *18*:199–202.

Mayhew IG. Neuromuscular arthrogryposis multiplex congenita in a Thoroughbred foal. Vet Pathol 1984; *21*:187–192.

Mayhew IG, Brewer BD, Reinhard MK, Greiner EC. Verminous (*Strongylus vulgaris*) myelitis in a donkey. Cornell Vet 1984; *74*:30–37.

Mayhew IG, Brown CM, Stowe HD, et al. Equine degenerative myeloencephalopathy: A vitamin E deficiency that may be familial. J Vet Int Med 1987; *1*:45–50.

Mayhew IG, de Lahunta A, Georgi JR, Aspros DG. Naturally occurring cerebrospinal parelapho-strongylosis. Cornell Vet 1976; *66*:56–72.

Mayhew IG, de Lahunta A, Whitlock RH, Geary JC. Equine degenerative myeloencephalopathy. J Am Vet Med Assoc 1977; *170*:195–201.

Mayhew IG, de Lahunta A, Whitlock RH, et al. Spinal cord disease in the horse. Cornell Vet 1978a; *68 (Suppl 6)*:1–208.

Mayhew IG, Fayer R, Simpson CF. Clinical, pathologic and edpidemiologic observations on equine protozoal myeloencephalitis (Abstract). In: Proc Ann Meet Am Assoc Parasitol, 1981.

Mayhew IG, Lichtenfels JR, Greiner EC, et al. Migration of a spiruroid nematode through the brain of a horse. J Am Vet Med Assoc 1982; *180*:1306–1311.

Mayhew IG, MacKay RJ. The Nervous System. In: *Equine Medicine and Surgery.* 3rd Ed. Mansmann RA, McAllister ES, Pratt PW, eds. Santa Barbara: American Veterinary Publications, 1982: Vol II, Ch 21, pp 1159–1252.

Mayhew IG, Watson AG, Heissan JA. Congenital occipitoatlantoaxial malformation in the horse. Equine Vet J 1978b; *10*:103–113.

Maxie MG. The Urinary System. In: *Pathology of Domestic Animals.* Jubb KVF, Kennedy PC, Palmer N, eds. 3rd Ed. Orlando: Academic Press, 1985; Vol 2, p 385.

Maxie MG, Physick-Sheard PW. Aortic-iliac thrombosis in horses. Vet Pathol 1985; *22*:238–249.

Mercer HD, Neal FC, Himes JA, et al. *Cassia occidentalis* toxicosis in cattle. J Am Vet Med Assoc 1967; *151*:735–741.

Miller LM, Reed SM, Gallina AM, et al. Ataxia and weakness associated with fourth ventricle vascular anomalies in two horses. J Am Vet Med Assoc 1985; *186*:601–604.

Mitchell CA, Walker RVL, McKercher DG. Isolation of *Cl. botulinum* from oat grain. Can J Comp Med 1939; *3*:245–247.

Montali RJ, Allen GP, Bryans JT, et al. Equine herpesvirus type 1 abortion in an onager and suspected herpesvirus myelitis in a zebra. J Am Vet Med Assoc 1985; *187*:1248–1249.

Montali RJ, Bush M, Sauer RM, et al. Spinal ataxia in zebras. Comparison with the Wobbler syndrome of horses. Vet Pathol 1974; *11*:68–78.

Mumford JA. Equid herpesvirus 1 (EHV 1) latency: More questions than answers. Equine Vet J 1985; *17*:340–341.

Mumford JA, Edington N. EHV 1 and equine paresis. Vet Rec 1980; 277.

McClintock AE, O'Neil JA. A possible case of inherited abnormalities in the central nervous system of calves by an AI sire. Vet Rec 1974; *94*:382–383.

McCoy DJ, Shires PK, Beadle R. Ventral approach for stabilization of atlantoaxial subluxation secondary to odontoid fracture in a foal. J Am Vet Med Assoc 1984; *185*:545–550.

McEwen SA, Hulland TJ. Histochemical and morphometric evaluation of skeletal muscle from horses with exertional rhabdomyolysis (tying-up). Vet Pathol 1986; *23*:400–410.

McGavin MD, Ranby PD, Tammemagi L. Demyelination associated with low liver copper levels in pigs. Aust Vet J 1962; *38*:8–14.

McGrath JT. Some nervous disorders of the horse. Proc 8th Annu Conv Am Assoc Equine Pract 1962; 157–163.

McIlwraith CW, James LF. Limb deformities in foals associated with ingestion of locoweed by mares. J Am Vet Med Assoc 1982; *181*:255–258.

McKelvey WAC, Owen RapR: Acquired torticollis in eleven horses. J Am Vet Med Assoc 1979; *175*:295–297.

McKenzie RA, McMicking LI. Ataxia and urinary incontinence in cattle grazing sorghum. Aust Vet J 1977; *53*:496–497.

McKerrell RE. Myotonia in man and animals: Confusing comparisons. Equine Vet J 1987: 266–267.

MacLachlan NJ, Gribble DH, East NE. Polyradiculoneuritis in a goat. J Am Vet Med Assoc 1982; *180*:166–167.

McLaughlin BG, Doige CE, McLaughlin PS. Thyroid hormone levels in foals with congenital musculoskeletal lesions. Can Vet J 1986; *27*:264–267.

Nisbet DI, Renwick CC. Congenital myopathy in lambs. J Comp Pathol 1961; *71*:177–182.

Nixon AJ, Stashak TS. Surgical therapy for spinal cord disease in the horse. Proc 31st Annu Conv Am Assoc Equine Pract 1985; 61–74.

Nixon Aj, Stashak TS. Dorsal laminectomy in the horse. I. Review of the literature and description of a new procedure. Vet Surg 1983; *12*:172–176.

Nixon AJ, Stashak TS, Ingram JT, et al. Dorsal laminectomy in the horse. II. Evaluation in the normal horse. Vet Surg 1983a; *12*:177–183.

Nixon AJ, Stashak TS, Ingram JT. Dorsal laminectomy in the horse. III. Results in horses with cervical vertebral malformation. Vet Surg 1983b; *12*:184–188.

Norman S, Smith MC. Caprine arthritis-encephalitis: Review of the neurologic form in 30 cases. J Am Vet Med Assoc 1983; *182*:1341–1345.

Nyland TG, Blythe LL, Pool RR, Helphrey MG. Metrizamide myelography in the horse: Clinical, radiographic, and pathologic changes. Am J Vet Res 1980; *41*:204–211.

O'Brien PJ. Etiopathogenetic defect of malignant hyperthermia: Hypersensitive calcium-release channel of skeletal muscle sarcoplasmic reticulum. Vet Res Comm 1987; *11*:527–559.

O'Hara, Pierce KR, Ready WK. Degenerative myopathy associated with ingestion of *Cassia occidentalis* L.: Clinical and pathologic features of the experimentally induced disease. Am J Vet Res 1969; *30*:2173–2180.

Onapito JS, Raffe MR, Cox VS. Pressure-induced changes in fibular motor nerve conduction velocity and fibularis (peroneus) tertius muscle-evoked potentials in a goat model of the downer cow syndrome. Am J Vet Res 1986; *47*:1747–1750.

Orr JP, McKenzie GC. Unusual skeletal deformities in calves in a Saskatchewan beef herd. Case Report. Can Vet J 1981; *22*:121–125.

O'Sullivan BM. Humpy back of sheep. Clinical and pathological observations. Aust Vet J 1976; *52*:414–433.

O'Sullivan BM, Blakemore WF. Acute nicotinamide deficiency in the pig induced by 6-amino-nicotinamide. Vet Pathol 1980; *17*:748–758.

O'Sullivan BM, Healy PJ, Fraser IR, et al. Generalised glycogenosis in Brahman cattle. Aust Vet J 1981; *57*:227–229.

Owen RapR, Smith-Maxie LL. Repair of fractured dens of the axis in a foal. J Am Vet Med Assoc 1978; *173*:854–856.

Owen RapR, Moore JN, Hopkins JB, Arthur D. Dystrophic myodegeneration in adult horses. J Am Vet Med Assoc 1977; *171*:343–349.

Palmer AC, Blakemore WF. Progressive ataxia of Charolais cattle. Bovine Pract 1975; *10*:84–86.

Palmer AC, Blakemore WF, O'Sullivan B, et al. Ataxia and spinal cord degeneration in llama, widebeeste and camel. Vet Rec 1980; *107*:10–11.

Palmer AC, Hickman J. Treatment of quadriplegia in a ram due to pressure on the spinal cord by an abscess involving the cervical vertebrae. Vet Rec 1963; *75*:213–215.

Palmer AC, Hickman J. Ataxia in a horse due to an angioma of the spinal cord. Vet Rec 1960; *72*:611–613.

Palmer AC, Kelly WR, Ryde PS. Stenosis of the cervical vertebral canal in a yearling ram. Vet Rec 1981; *109*:53–55.

Palmer AC, Lamont MH, Wallace ME. Focal symmetrical poliomalacia of the spinal cord in Ayrshire calves. Vet Pathol 1986; *23*:506–509.

Palmer AC, Woodham CB. Derrengue, a paralysis of cattle in El Salvador ascribed to ingestion of *Melochia pyramidata*. Vet Rec 1975; *96*:547–548.

Panter KE, Keeler RF, Buck WB. Congenital skeletal malformations induced by maternal ingestion of *Conium maculatum* (poison hemlock) in newborn pigs. Am J Vet Res 1985; *46*:2064–2066.

Pass DA. Posterior paralysis in a sow due to fibrocartilagenous emboli in the spinal cord. Aust Vet J 1978; *54*:100–101.

Patterson DSP, Foulkes JA, Sweasey D, et al. A neurochemical study of field cases of the delayed spinal form of swayback (enzootic ataxia) in lambs. J Neurochem 1974; *23*:1245–1253.

Perdrizet JA, Cummings JF, de Lahunta A. Presumptive organophosphate-induced delayed neurotoxicity in a paralyzed bull. Cornell Vet 1985; *75*:401–410.

Petursson G, Nathanson N, Palsson PA, et al. Immunopathogenesis of visna. A slow virus disease of the central nervous system. Acta Neurol Scand 1978; Suppl 67, *57*:205–219.

Platt H, Singh H, Whitwell KE. Pathological observations on an outbreak of paralysis in broodmares. Equine Vet J 1980; *12*:118–126.

Platt H, Whitwell KE. Clinical and pathological observations on generalized steatitis in foals. J Comp Path 1971; *81*:499–506.

Pletcher JM, Banting LF. Copper deficiency in piglets characterized by spongy myelopathy and degenerative lesions in the great blood vessels. J S Afr Vet Assoc 1983; *54*:43–46.

Powers RD, Benz GW. *Micronema deletrix* in the central nervous system of a horse. J Am Vet Med Assoc 1977; *170*:175–177.

Prichard JT, Voss JL. Fetal ankylosis in horses associated with hybrid sudan pasture. J Am Vet Med Assoc 1967; *150*:871–873.

Prickett ME. Equine spinal ataxia. Proc 14th Annu Conv Am Assoc Equine Pract 1968; 147–158.

Pritchard DH, Napthine DV, Sinclair AJ. Globoid cell leucodystrophy in polled Dorset sheep. Vet Pathol 1980; *17*:399–405.

Pursell AR, Sangster LT, Byars TD, et al. Neurologic disease induced by equine herpesvirus 1. J Am Vet Med Assoc 1979; *175*:473–474.

Rantanen NW, Gavin PR, Barbee DD, et al. Ataxia and paresis in horses. Part II. Radiographic and myelographic examination of the cervical vertebral column. Comp Cont Ed Pract Vet 1981; *3*:S161–S171.

Rebhun WC, de Lahunta A, Baum KH, et al. Compressive neoplasms affecting the bovine spinal cord. Comp Cont Ed Pract Vet 1984; *6*:S396–S400.

Reed SM, Bayly WM, Traub TL, et al. Ataxia and paresis in horses. Part I. Differential diagnosis. Comp Cont Ed Pract Vet 1981; *3*:S88–S99.

Reef VB, Roby KAW, Richardson DW, et al. Use of ultrasonography for the detection of aortic-iliac thrombosis in horses. J Am Vet Med Assoc 1987; *190*:286–288.

Rendano VT, Quick CB. Equine radiology—the cervical spine. Mod Vet Pract 1978; *53*:921–929.

Rice DA, Kennedy S, McMurray CH, et al. Experimental 3-nitro-4-hydroxyphenylarsonic acid toxicosis in pigs. Res Vet Sci 1985; *39*:47–51.

Rice DA, McMurray CH, McCracken RM, et al. A field case of poisoning caused by 3-nitro-4-hydroxy phenyl arsonic acid in pigs. Vet Rec 1980; *106*:312–313.

Richards RB, Edwards JR. A progressive spinal myelinopathy in beef cattle. Vet Pathol 1986; *23*:35–41.

Richards RB, Passmore IK, Bretag AH, et al. Ovine congenital progressive muscular dystrophy: Clinical syndrome and distribution of lesions. Aust Vet J 1986; *63*:396–401.

Richardson DW. *Eikenella corrodens* osteomyelitis of the axis in a foal. J Am Vet Med Assoc 1986; *188*:298–299.

Ricketts SW, Greet TRC, Glyn PJ, et al. Thirteen cases of botulism in horses fed big bale silage. Equine Vet J 1984; *16*:515–518.

Robb EJ, Kronfeld DS. Dietary sodium bicarbonate as a treatment of exertional rhabdomyolysis in a horse. J Am Vet Med Assoc 1986; *188*:602–607.

Robinson WF, Ellis TM. Caprine arthritis-encephalitis virus infection: From recognition to eradication. Aust Vet J 1986; *63*:237–241.

Roneus B, Hakkarainen J. Vitamin E in serum and skeletal muscle tissue and blood glutathione peroxidase activity from horses with the azoturia-tying-up syndrome. Acta Vet Scand 1985; *26*:425–427.

Rook JS, Spaulding K, Coe P, et al. The spider syndrome: A report on one purebred flock. Comp Cont Ed Pract Vet 1986; *8*:S402–S405.

Rooney JR. Contracted foals. Cornell Vet 1966; *56*:172–187.

Rooney JR. The vertebral column. In: *Biomechanics of Lameness in the Horse*. Baltimore: Williams & Wilkins, 1969: pp 90–253.

Rooney JR, Prickett ME, Delaney FM, et al. Focal myelitis-encephalitis in horses. Cornell Vet 1970; *60*:494–501.

Rose AL, Banks AW, McConnell JD. Birdsville disease in the northern territory. Aust Vet J 1951; *27*:189–196.

Roth L, Scarratt WK, Shipley CF, et al. Ganglioglioma of the spinal cord in a calf. Vet Pathol 1987; *24*:188–189.

Rousseaux CG, Wenger BS. Are pesticides involved in arthrogryposis? Can Vet J 1985; *26*:257–258.

Roussel Jr AJ. Downer cow syndrome. Agri Pract 1986; *7*:31–35.

Rubin HL, Woodard JC. Equine infection with *Micronema deletrix*. J Am Vet Med Assoc 1974; *165*:256–258.

Rudert CP, Lawrence JA, Foggin C, et al. A rigid lamb syndrome in sheep in Rhodesia. Vet Rec 1978; *102*:374–377.

Russell RG, Doige CE, Oteruelo FT, et al. Variability in limb malformations and possible significance in the pathogenesis of an inherited congenital neuromuscular disease of charolais cattle (syndrome of arthrogryposis and palatoschisis). Vet Pathol 1985; *22*:2–12.

Sanders DE, de Lahunta A, Cumming JF, et al. Progressive paresis in sheep due to delayed neurotoxicity of triarylphosphates. Cornell Vet 1985; *75*:493–504.

Sandersleben JV, Schlotke B. Muscular dystrophy in foals, apparently a disease with increasing incidence. Dtsch Tierärztl Wschr 1977; *84*:105–107.

Saperstein G, Leipold HW, Dennis SM. Congenital defects of sheep. J Am Vet Med Assoc 1975; *167*:314–322.

Schartzmann U, Meister V, Fankhauser R. Akute Hamatomyelie nach Langerer Rukenlarge bein Pferd. Schweiz Arch Tierheilk 1979; *121*:149–155.

Schneider JE. Immobilizing cervical vertebral fractures. Proc 27th Annu Conv Assoc Equine Pract 1981; 253–256.

Seaman JT, Smeal MG, Wright JC. The possible association of a sorghum (*Sorghum sudanese*) hybrid as a cause of developmental defects in calves. Aust Vet J 1981; *57*:351–352.

Seawright AA. *Animal Health in Australia.* Vol 2, *Chemical and Plant Poisons.* Canberra, Australia: Australian Government Publishing Service, 1982; pp 1–290.

Sheffield WD, Narayan O, Strandberg JD, et al. Visna-maedi-like disease associated with an ovine retrovirus infection in a Corriedale sheep. Vet Pathol 1980; *17*:544–552.

Sherman DM, Ames TR. Vertebral body abscesses in cattle: A review of five cases. J Am Vet Med Assoc 1986; *188*:608–611.

Shoho C. Prophylaxis and therapy in epizootic cerebrospinal nematodiasis of animals by 1-diethylcarbamyl-4-methyl-piperazine dihydrogen citrate: Report of a second field trial. Vet Med 1954; *49*:459–464.

Simpson CF, Mayhew IG. Evidence for *Sarcocystis* as the etiologic agent of equine protozoal myeloencephalitis. J Protozool 1980; *27*:288–292.

Slone DE, Bergfeld WA, Walker TL. Surgical decompression for traumatic atlantoaxial subluxation in a weaning filly. J Am Vet Med Assoc 1979; *174*:1234–1236.

Smith RM, Fraser FJ, Robertson JS. Enzootic ataxia in lambs: Absence of detectable neuronal pathology in foetal and neonatal spinal cord. J Comp Pathol 1978; *88*:401–408.

Smith RM, Fraser FJ, Russel GR, et al. Enzootic ataxia in lambs: Appearance of lesions in the spinal cord during foetal development. J Comp Pathol 1977; *87*:119–128.

Smith KD, Miller CW. Dorsal laminectomy in a calf. J Am Vet Med Assoc 1984; *184*:1508–1510.

Sorjonen DC, Powe TA, West M, et al. Ventral surgical fixation and fusion for atlanto-occipital subluxation in a goat. Vet Surg 1983; *12*:127–129.

Stackhouse LL. Cerebral Nematodiasis in two New Hampshire moose. J Am Vet Med Assoc 1977; *171*:987–988.

Stashak TS, Mayhew IG. The Nervous System. In: *The Practice of Large Animal Surgery.* Jennings PB, ed. Philadelphia: WB Saunders, 1984. Vol II, Ch 17, pp 983–1041.

Steinberg S, Botelho S. Myotonia in a horse. Science 1962; *137*:979–980.

Stuart LD, Leipold HW. Lesions in bovine progressive degenerative myeloencephalopathy ("weaver") of Brown Swiss cattle. Vet Pathol 1985; *22*:13–23.

Stuart LD, Leipold HW. Bovine progressive degenerative myeloencephalopathy ("weaver") of Brown Swiss cattle I, II. Bovine Pract 1983; *18*:129–132, 133–146.

Sullivan ND. The Nervous System. In: *Pathology of Domestic Animals.* Jubb KVF, Kennedy PC, Palmer N, eds. 3rd Ed. Orlando: Academic Press, 1985. Vol 1, Ch. 3, pp 201–338.

Suttle NF. Safety and effectiveness of cupric oxide particles for increasing liver copper status in sheep. Res Vet Sci 1987a; *42*:219–223.

Suttle NF. Safety and efficacy of cupric oxide particles for increasing liver copper status in cattle. Res Vet Sci 1987b; *42*:224–227.

Sutton RH, McLennan MW. Hemangiosarcoma in a cow. Vet Pathol 1982; *19*:456–458.

Swift TR. Disorders of neuromuscular transmission other than myasthenia gravis. Muscle Nerve 1981; 334–353.

Swerczek TW. Toxicoinfectious botulism in foals and adult horses. J Am Vet Med Assoc 1980a; *176*:217–219.

Swerczek TW. Experimental induced toxicoinfectious botulism in horses and foals. Am J Vet Res 1980b; *41*:348–350.

Taylor HW, Vandevelde M, Firth EC. Ischemic myelopathy caused by fibrocartilagenous emboli in a horse. Vet Pathol 1977; *14*:479–481.

Terlecki S, Done JT, Clegg FG. Enzootic ataxic of red deer. Brit Vet J 1964; *120*:311–321.

Tessaro SV, Doige CE, Rhodes CS. Posterior paralysis due to fibrocartilaginous embolism in two weaner pigs. Can J Comp Med 1983; *47*:124–126.

Thornton RN, MacColl DJ. A suspected inherited neuromuscular disease in Dorset Down sheep. NZ Vet J 1985; *33*:172–173.

Tithof PK, Rebhun WC, Dietze AE. Ultrasonographic diagnosis of aortoiliac thrombosis. Cornell Vet 1985; *75*:540–544.

Torano ME, Oplistil M, Gomes A. Aetiology, therapy and prevention of the syndrome called "bovine paralysis" in Zebu cattle in Cuba. Acta Vet Brno 1975; *44*:197–202.

Townsend HGG, Leach DH, Doige CE, et al. Relationship between spinal biomechanics and pathological changes in the equine thoracolumbar spine. Equine Vet J 1986; *18*:107–112.

Traver DS, Coffman JR, Moore JN, et al. Protozoal myeloencephalitis in sibling horses. J Equine Med Surg 1978; *2*:425–428.

Trim CM, Mason J. Post-anaesthetic forelimb lameness in horses. Equine Vet J 1973; *5*:71–76.

Tryphonas L, Nielsen NO. Pathology of chronic alkylmercurial poisoning in swine. Am J Vet Res 1973; *34*:379–392.

Van den Hoven R. Breukink HJ, Wensing TH, et al. Loosely coupled skeletal muscle mitochondria in exertional rhabdomyolysis. Equine Vet J 1986; *18*:418–421.

Vandeplassche M. The pathogenesis of dystocia and fetal malformation in the horse. J Reprod Fert 1987; *Suppl 35*:547–552.

Vandeplassche M, Simoens P, Bouters R, et al. Aetiology and pathogenesis of congenital torticollis and head scoliosis in the equine foetus. Equine Vet J 1984; *16*:419–424.

Van Huffel X, DeMoor A. Congenital multiple arthrogryposis of the forelimbs in calves. Comp Cont Ed Pract Vet 1987; *9*:F333–F339.

Vanselow BA, McCausland IP. Steatitis in two donkey foals. Aust Vet J 1981; *57*:304–305.

Van Vleet JF, Runnels LJ, Cook JR, et al. Monensin toxicosis in swine: Potentiation by tiamulin administration and ameliorative effect of treatment with selenium and/or vitamin E. Am J Vet Res 1987; *48*:1520–1524.

Volpe JJ. *Neurology of the Newborn*. Philadelphia: WB Saunders, 1987. pp 500–502.

Von Maltitz L, Basson PA, van der Merwe JLde B. Suspected hereditary spinal ataxia in cattle. J S Afr Vet Med Assoc 1969; *40*:33–36.

Vos JH, Franken P, Wouda W, et al. Spinal nematodosis in a donkey with posterior paresis. Vet Q 1985; *7*:101–106.

Wagner PC. Large Animal Vertebral and Spinal Cord Surgery. In: *Veterinary Neurology.* Oliver JE, Hoerlein BF, Mayhew IG, eds. Philadephia: WB Saunders, 1987. Ch 17.3, pp 459–469.

Wagner PC, Grant BD, Gallina A, et al. Ataxia and paresis in horses. Part III. Surgical treatment of cervical spinal cord compression. Comp Cont Ed Pract Vet 1981; *3*:S192–S202.

Wagner PC, Bagby GW, Grant BD, et al. Surgical stabilization of the equine cervical spine. Vet Surg 1979; *8*:7–12.

Wagner PC, Grant BD, Watrous BJ, et al. A study of the heritability of cervical vertebral malformation in horses. Proc 31st Annu Conv Am Assoc Equine Pract 1985a; 43–50.

Wagner PC, Grant BD, DeBowes RM. Treatment of cervical vertebral instability by interbody fusion in the horse. Proc 31st Annu Conv Am Assoc Equine Pract 1985b; 51–59.

Wasserman C. Myelodysplasia in a calf. Mod Vet Pract 1986; 879–882.

Watson AG, Wilson JH, Cooley AJ, et al. Occipito-atlanto-axial malformation with atlanto-axial subluxation in an ataxic calf. J Am Vet Med Assoc 1985; *187*:740–742.

Watson AG, Mayhew IG. Familial congenital occipitoatlantoaxial malformation (OAAM) in the Arabian horse. Spine 1983; 334–339.

Weisbrode SE, Monke DR, Dodaro ST, et al. Osteochondrosis, degenerative joint disease, and vertebral osteophytosis in middle-aged bulls. J Am Vet Med Assoc 1982; *181*:700–705.

Wells GAH. Locomotor disorders of the pig. In Practice 1984; *6*:43–53.

White ME, Pennock PW, Seiler RJ. Atlanto-axial subluxation in five young cattle. Can Vet J 1978; *19*:79–82.

White NA. Postanesthetic recumbency myopathy in horses. Comp Cont Ed Pract Vet 1982; *4*:S44–S52.

White NA, Suarez M. Change in triceps muscle intracompartmental pressure with repositioning and padding of the lowermost thoracic limb of the horse. Am J Vet Res 1986; *47*:2257–2260.

Whitlock RH, Messick J, Divers T, et al. Botulism in cattle: Clinical and diagnostic approaches. Proc 18th Annu Meet Am Assoc Bov Pract 1985; *18*:164–167.

Whitwell KE. Causes of ataxia in horses. In Practice 1980; *2*:17–24.

Whitwell KE. Craniovertebral malformations in an Arab foal. Equine Vet J 1978; *10*:125–126.

Whitwell KE, Dyson S. Interpreting radiographs 8: Equine cervical vertebrae. Equine Vet J 1987; *19*:8–14.

Williams JF, Dade AW, Benne R. Posterior paralysis associated with anthelmintic treatment of sheep. J Am Vet Med Assoc 1976; *169*:1307–1309.

Wilson PR, Orr MB, Key EL. Enzootic ataxia in Red deer. NZ Vet J 1979; *27*:252–254.

Wilson TM, Hammerstedt RH, Palmer IS, et al. Porcine focal symmetrical poliomyelomalacia: Experimental reproduction with oral doses of encapsulated sodium selenite. Can J Vet Res 1988; *52*:83–88.

Wilson TM, Scholz RW, Drake TR. Selenium toxicity and porcine focal symmetrical poliomyelomalacia: Description of a field outbreak and experimental reproduction. Can J Comp Med 1983; *47*:412–421.

Wilson WD, Hughes SJ, Ghoshal NG, et al. Occipitoatlantoaxial malformation in two non-Arabian horses. J Am Vet Med Assoc 1985; *187*:36–40.

Wouda W, Borst GHA, Gruys E. Delayed swayback in goat kids, a study of 23 cases. Vet Q 1986; *8*:45–56.

Yamagiwa J, Yoshikawa T, Oyamada T. Pathological studies on equine ataxia in Japan. Jpn J Vet Sci 1980; *42*:681–694.

Yovich JV, LeCouteur RA, Stashak TS, et al. Postanesthetic hemorrhagic myelopathy in a horse. J Am Vet Med Assoc 1986; *188*:300–301.

Zink MC. Postanesthetic poliomyelomalacia in a horse. Case report. Can Vet J 1985; *26*:275–277.

Zink MC, Narayan O, Kennedy PGE, et al. Pathogenesis of visna/maedi and caprine arthritis-encephalitis: New leads on the mechanism of restricted virus replication and persistent inflammation. Vet Immunol Immunopathol 1987; *15*:167–180.

CHAPTER 15

Problem 11:
Paresis or Paralysis of One Limb

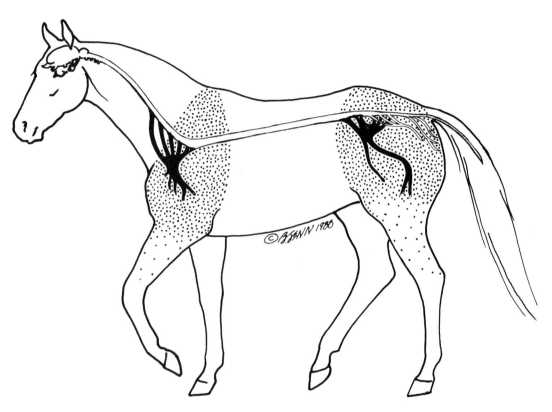

Locations of lesions resulting in paresis or paralysis of one limb: nerve roots and peripheral ganglia, plexuses and nerves of the limbs (blackened), and muscles of the limbs (stippled).

The term monoplegia can be used to describe the syndromes discussed in this problem that result from lesions in the ventral gray matter, nerve roots, brachial and lumbosacral plexuses, and peripheral nerves and muscles of the limbs. On occasion, a lesion involving just thoracolumbar white matter on one side results in degrees of ataxia, weakness, and dysmetria in only one pelvic limb. EPM in horses would be the best example of such a syndrome.

Monoplegia is a common problem in large animals, with trauma being the most frequent cause. Vague lamenesses occur frequently, but are difficult to evaluate and diagnose. In horses, EPM can produce such selective gray matter lesions that mimic syndromes of peripheral nerve disease (LMN).

Specific peripheral nerve paralyses do not, for the most part, result in precise gait abnormalities, detectable muscle atrophy, or particularly analgesic zones, as are seen in small animals (Mayhew et al., 1982), (Diesem et al., 1985), (Henry, 1976), (Vaughan, 1964), (Dyce et al., 1987). The precise zones of skin insensitivity that occur consistently with selective nerve ablations (autonomous zones) in the limbs of horses have recently been identified (Blythe et al., 1982), (Blythe, LL, 1987, pers. comm.). These relatively small zones are shown in Figure 15–1 and should be evaluated using a two-step, cutaneous pinch technique, as described in the neurologic examination (Chapter 2). Single supra-scapular, musculocutaneous, median, and ulnar nerve sections result in little, if any, permanent gait abnormalities (Henry, 1976). Horner's syndrome, associated with brachial plexus lesions, and focal areas of sweating due to local loss of the sympathetic supply to skin in the horse, can be findings that are helpful in localizing a lesion. Repeated, careful, documented, neurologic examination and repeated EMG studies are most helpful in evaluating these cases.

The functional and morphologic categories of neurapraxia, axonotmesis, and neurotmesis and the process of Wallerian degeneration and regeneration are pertinent to understanding diseases of peripheral nerves (see Chapter 4).

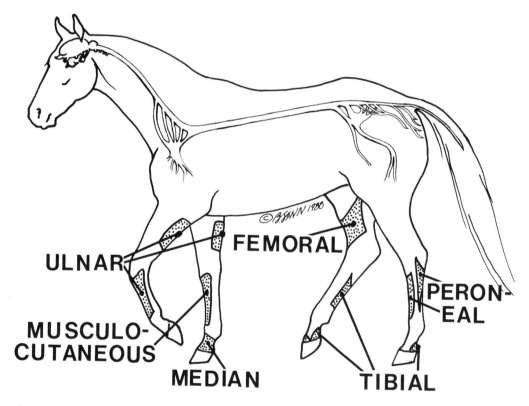

Figure 15–1. Areas of skin insensitivity (autonomous zones) can be expected to result from selective, singular sectioning of the major peripheral nerves to the limbs of the horse. The center of each autonomous zone (●) should be tested for sensation to determine sensory function of these nerves. (Modified from Blythe LL, Kitchell RL. Electrophysiologic studies of the horse. Am J Vet Res 1982; 43:1511–1524; and Blythe LL, 1987, pers. comm.)

Categories of Disease and Differential Diagnosis
NOTE: Only diseases marked * are discussed in this section.

I. Congenital and Familial
    1. Arthrogryposis (Problem 10)

II. Physical
    *1. Injury to Peripheral Nerves
    *2. Postcalving, Postfoaling Paralyses (Problem 10)
    3. Exertional Rhabdomyolysis and Capture Myopathy (Problem 10)
    4. Postanesthetic Myoneuropathy (Problem 10)

III. Infectious, Inflammatory, Immune
    *1. Rabies (Problem 1)
    2. Equine Protozoal Myeloencephalitis (Problems 1 and 10)
    3. Vertebral Osteomyelitis (Problem 10)
    4. Verminous Myelitis (Problems 1 and 10)
    5. Caprine Arthritis—Encephalomyelitis (Problem 10)
    6. Myositis (Problem 10)
    7. Miscellaneous Infections (Problem 1)

IV. Nutritional
    1. Nutritional Myodegeneration—White Muscle Disease— Myodegeneration and Steatitis (Problem 10)

V. Neoplastic
    *1. Peripheral Nerve Sheath Neoplasms
    *2. Lymphosarcoma

VI. Miscellaneous Disorders
    *1. Cervical Vertebral Osteoarthropathy
    2. Thoraco-Lumbar Osteoarthrosis (Problem 10)
    3. Vague Musculoskeletal Lamenesses (Problem 10)
    4. Stringhalt (Problem 8C)
    5. Embolic Myelopathy (Problem 10A)
    6. Aortic-Iliac Thrombosis, Ischemic Neuromyopathy (Problem 10)

I. Physical
  1. Injury to Peripheral Nerves
      Refer to Figure 15–1 for areas of cutaneous insensitivity likely to be encountered with specific peripheral nerve injury in the horse (Blythe et al., 1982), (Dyce et al., 1987), (Blythe LL, 1988, pers. comm.). The discussion below relates to specific peripheral nerves most frequently affected by external injury (Henry, 1976), (Mayhew et al., 1982), (Ciszewski et al., 1987), (Diesem et al., 1985), (Vaughan, 1964).
      a. *Suprascapular nerve.* This nerve is commonly damaged in horses colliding against objects. The syndrome called sweeney results, with eventual atrophy of supraspinatus and infraspinatus muscles (Fig. 15–2). Lateral subluxation (popping) of the shoulder upon weight bearing may be seen (Fig. 15–3). The latter might be caused by a lack of lateral collateral support (suprascapular muscles) or more likely by an additional involvement of the

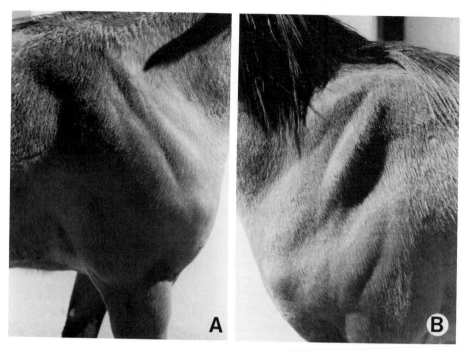

Figure 15–2. This yearling thoroughbred filly suddenly developed sweeney several weeks after injuring the left shoulder (B). Because entrapment neuropathy was suspected, the suprascapular nerve was surgically explored and the entrapping fibrous tissue was removed (MP Brown, University of Florida). Several months later the horse's owner reported that the muscle mass of the left shoulder had returned to its normal size (A).

pectoral nerve, the subscapular nerve, the caudal cervical nerve roots, the pectoral, subclavius, and subscapular muscles or other supporting structures of the shoulder (Dyson, 1986), (Henry, 1976), (Dyson S, 1987, pers. comm.).

The following general principles on management of suprascapular nerve trauma can be expanded to fit any large animal peripheral nerve injury case. As a basis, one must remember that no more than 12 in. of nerve regrowth (6 to 12 months) can be expected because of irreversible muscular fibrosis. Electromyographic examinations are helpful about 2 to 4 weeks after the damage occurs to detect involvement of other nerves of the brachial plexus that may be affected by injury to the shoulder. At this stage one may surgically explore and free the nerve from any entrapment (Fig. 15–2). Preferably, one should delay any decision for surgical exploration about 12 weeks. If the degree of atrophy (measured by tape or needle depth gauge) is then improving, it is reasonable to wait for up to 4 to 5 months. If atrophy is the same, then the nerve should be explored to relieve any entrapment or to perform anastomosis for neuroma-in-continuity. If, in show animals, the best cosmetic result is mandated, then

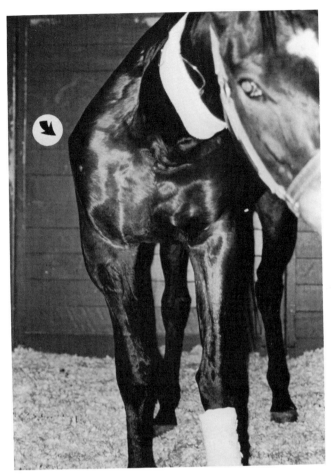

Figure 15–3. Injury to the shoulder often results in sweeney (Fig. 15–2) and additional signs that frequently include a lateral subluxation of the shoulder joint seen during weight bearing (arrow). This sign most likely is caused by tissue damage in addition to the suprascapular nerve.

exploring the area at an earlier time, say 2 to 6 weeks after injury occurs, may be justified (Schneider et al., 1985), (Duncan et al., 1985).

At the time of exploration and removal of any entrapping tissue, removal of a piece of bone from the cranial surface of the scapular has been suggested to relieve tension on the nerve that may occur postoperatively (Schneider et al., 1985), (Adams et al., 1985), (Duncan et al., 1985).

With axons regrowing at about 1 in. per month, there probably is time for reinervation of the suprascapular musculature before fibrous metaplasia occurs in the muscles.

Exercise should be maintained, and physiotherapy—such as passive range of motion maneuvers, faradic stimulation, and particularly swimming—all are useful. These exercises should not be attempted at the time of surgery.

b. *Radial nerve.* This nerve is not commonly damaged alone; it can be involved with humeral fractures (Rooney, 1963). The animal is unable to bear weight on its limb because of a lack of elbow extension. The shoulder is rested in an extended position, and the limb rests with the dorsum of the pastern on the ground. The limb may be thrust forward by the action of the proximal pectoral girdle muscles while the animal walks.

Although many pathophysiologic mechanisms for radial paralysis have been discussed (Rooney, 1963), most cases are probably like that described for brachial plexus damage (below).

Postrecumbency radial paralysis can be a prominent component of postanesthetic myoneuropathy (Problem 10).

c. *Brachial plexus.* Many cases of shoulder injury with signs of radial paralysis are probably caused by compression of the brachial plexus and radial nerve roots between the scapular and the ribs (Fig. 15–4). This often is accompanied by sweeney (Fig. 15–2). An EMG detects involvement of more than just the radial nerve. Sensory loss usually is equivocal. Some of these cases improve dramatically in 2 to 4 weeks (neurapraxia) (Fig. 15–5), otherwise the outlook is guarded. Nevertheless, a few have progressively improved over 6 to 18 months with physiotherapy such as swimming exercise. Even with degrees of residual triceps atrophy, some horses have returned to full performance and even gallop and race successfully (Fig. 15–6).

d. *Musculocutaneous nerve.* Paralysis is not common. Injury to this nerve probably would not alter the gait, although the elbow may be overextended. Ultimately the biceps and brachial muscles would atrophy, with hypalgesia on the median forearm.

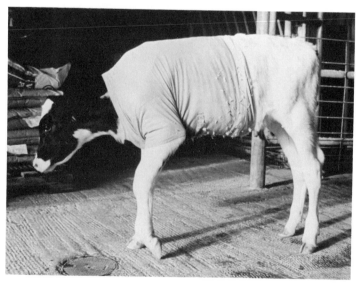

Figure 15–4. This Holstein calf suffered multiple injuries, including shoulder trauma and left brachial compression. As a result it was unable to support its weight (as shown) and had sensory loss up to the elbow. With careful nursing care the calf made a full recovery. (Courtesy JH Wilson, University of Florida.)

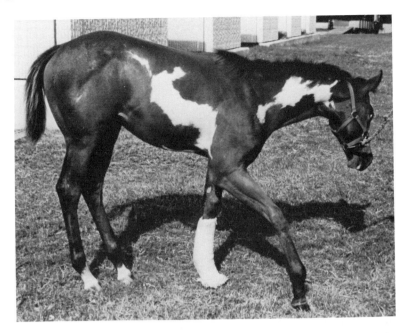

Figure 15–5. This 5-month-old Paint filly was thought to have sustained an injury to the right brachial plexus. It could not stand on the limb, had a dropped elbow, and only advanced the limb by flipping the whole brachial region forward. Within several weeks the filly was walking normally. (Courtesy JH Wilson, University of Florida.)

    e. *Median and ulnar nerves.* Paralysis in the calf and pony results in a stiff, goose-stepping gait, with hyperextension of the carpal, fetlock, and pastern joints. In the calf there may be cutaneous analgesia of the plantar and lateral surfaces of the limb from the elbow to the coronet (See Fig. 15–1 for autonomous zones of these nerves in the horse.) In the pony, within 3 months only an occasional toe drag may be evident with a total ulnar lesion; no gait abnormality can be detected without additional median nerve damage.

    f. *Femoral nerve.* This nerve is rarely affected by an external blow to the limb. Paralysis is seen as an inability to support weight on the limb as a result of lack of stifle extension (Paulsen et al., 1981). At a walk, the limb is advanced with difficulty and the length of stride is considerably reduced. The limb buckles when the animal attempts to bear weight on the limb. In the horse, the stifle collapses (flexes) and the hock and fetlock flex automatically. Thus, the horse rests with all the joints flexed in an affected limb. Atrophy of the quadriceps muscle is evident within one to two weeks, and the patellar reflex is absent. The sensory branch (the saphenous nerve) separates from the femoral nerve at the level of the iliopsoas muscle and innervates the medial leg from midthigh to the hock.

        Bilateral femoral paralysis has been seen in calves. This usually follows dystocia in a hip or stifle-lock position, which results

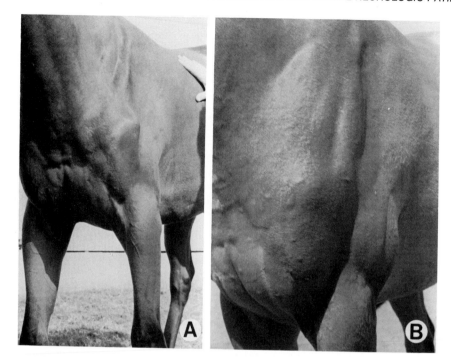

Figure 15–6. This 2-year-old thoroughbred colt had a left brachial injury, could not support weight on the limb, and had mild, diffuse hypalgesia of the distal limb. Six weeks after the injury, the colt could just bear weight on the limb and had profound atrophy of the shoulder, arm, and forearm musculature—all of which displayed denervation potentials on EMG examination (A). After 6 months, with much swimming exercise, the colt had a normal gait and mild suprascapular, triceps, and forearm muscle atrophy (B). Within one year the colt was racing successfully.

in stretching and compression of the femoral nerves and a compressive myopathy of the proximal limbs (see Post Calving Paralysis). This syndrome has also been reported in horses following general anesthesia (Dyson et al., 1988). One of these patients survived but the other showed evidence of hemorrhage around the femoral nerves. Such bilateral femoral paralysis, with perineural hemorrhage resulting from sacroiliac luxations, has been seen in mares after dystocia.

g. *Obturator nerve.* The L_6 ventral nerve roots, which form this nerve, commonly are injured during parturition in cows (see Postcalving Paralysis, Problem 10B). Paralysis results in a lack of adductor function because the obturator nerve supplies the adductor muscles of the pelvic limb. In the calf, some abduction of the pelvic limbs is evident with bilateral obturator neurectomy. This abduction is unnoticeable at rest and slightly evident at a walk; however it is obvious when the calf is running.

In the adult cow, signs of unilateral obturator paralysis are more evident, with abduction and circumduction of the limb while walking and difficulty standing because of lateral slipping of the affected limb. Bilateral obturator sectioning in the cow results in collapse of the pelvic limbs because of total abduction.

The syndrome of paraparesis and paraplegia in postparturient cattle (also Problem 10) occurs from damage to ventral, lumbar spinal nerve roots in the roof of the pelvic canal, as they form the lumbosacral plexus and divide into the peripheral nerves supplying the pelvic limbs. Such postcalving paralyses are the result of damage to more than just the obturator nerves, although pelvic limb abduction is often the most striking sign (Cox et al., 1975).

h. *Sciatic nerve.* Frequently this nerve is affected by various injuries. Paralysis results in poor limb flexion, with the stifle and hock extended and the fetlock flexed when the animal is not bearing weight on the limb. Weight can be supported on the limb if the digits are extended, otherwise weight is supported on the dorsal surface of the foot and the hock is overflexed (Fig. 15–7). Limb hypalgesia may occur from the stifle downward, except for

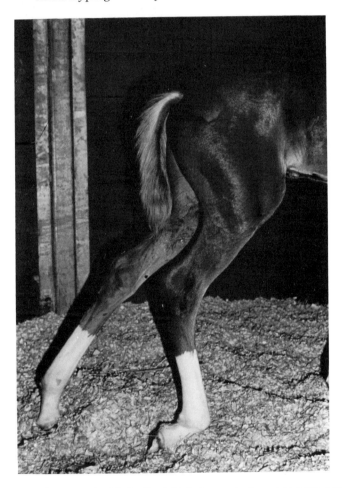

Figure 15–7. Sciatic paralysis in this foal's right limb was believed to have resulted from misplaced hypodermic injections. Inability to flex and advance the limb, but some weight support on the dorsum of the foot with hock flexion, all are characteristic of this syndrome. Mild, distal limb hypalgesia also was present.

the medial surface between the stifle and hock (also Fig. 15–1). Sciatic paralysis undoubtedly adds to the deficit seen with cox-ofemoral luxations and proximal femoral fractures in cattle. Sciatic paralysis, sometimes bilateral, has been observed with intramuscular injections into the caudal thigh in calves, kids, and foals; it may be expected in all species under these circumstances. Depending on the site of deposition of the drug, the resulting syndrome may resemble tibial or peroneal nerve involvement.

i. *Tibial nerve.* This nerve is probably affected less often than the peroneal branch of the sciatic nerve. Paralysis in the horse is reported to result in a hypermetric or stringhalt-like gait, with flexion of the hock (dropped hock) at rest. In the calf the hock is flexed at rest, and the fetlock is knuckled forward while the hooves remain flat on the ground. There is excessive, jerky, hock flexion when walking, and there is no dragging of the toes. Sensation is lost from the caudal aspect of the metatarsus in the calf and probably from areas of the caudal limb distal to the hock, including most of the caudal and medial coronet in the horse (Fig. 15–1). Tibial paralysis appears to be uncommon in large animals.

j. *Peroneal nerve.* Frequently, injury to this nerve is a component of sciatic injury. It is also damaged by a kick or by applying pressure to the lateral stifle. Paralysis results in an inability to flex the hock and extend the digits. In the acute phase in the horse and calf hyperextension of the hock and hyperflexion of the fetlock and interphalangeal joints causes the animal to drag the fetlock along the ground. The animal's stride has a shorter protraction phase and weight is taken when the dorsal surface of the foot is on the ground. If the foot is placed in a normal position, weight can be taken until the animal attempts to walk, at which time the fetlock again will knuckle. There is hypalgesia to the craniolateral portion of the limb from the level of the hock to the fetlock area.

Experimental peroneal sectioning in the pony results in these signs but within 3 months postoperatively, minimal, if any, gait abnormality is evident (Henry, 1976).

The peroneal nerve is subject to injury as it passes across the lateral surface of the tibia. Thus, peroneal paralysis is seen in adult cattle that are recumbent in the postpartum period (Cox et al., 1975b), in horses recumbent because of anesthesia, and in those receiving a kick to the lateral side of the pelvic limb.

k. *Cranial gluteal nerve.* Mostly this nerve is affected as a central lesion, with involvement of L_{5-6} ventral gray matter neurons. Paralysis results in little gait alteration. When turning away from the affected side, there may be a slight abduction or outward rotation of the stifle at the end of the propulsive phase of stride. Ultimately, atrophy of the gluteal region will occur, predominantly involving the middle gluteal muscle. The cranial gluteal nerve can be damaged as it traverses the shaft of the ilium when the pelvis is fractured, although this is rarely seen. Cranial gluteal nerve involvement and gluteal atrophy has been observed most frequently in American horses with protozoal myeloencephalitis when the lesion is confined to the ventral gray colums at L_6 (Fig. 14–21).

2. Postcalving, Postfoaling Paralyses (also Problem 10)

Signalment. In addition to the paralytic syndromes seen in post-parturient cows and mares (also Problem 10), the newborn calf or foal can suffer from unilateral or bilateral pelvic limb weakness progressing to paralysis (Fig. 15–8).

History. Usually there is a history of dystocia and an assisted delivery.

Examination. Luxated and fractured limb bones may be evident. Signs of femoral (Tryphonas et al., 1974) or sciatic-type paralysis are evident in one or both limbs. Swollen and torn muscles may be clearly evident (Sprinkle et al., 1985), (Schneider et al., 1986).

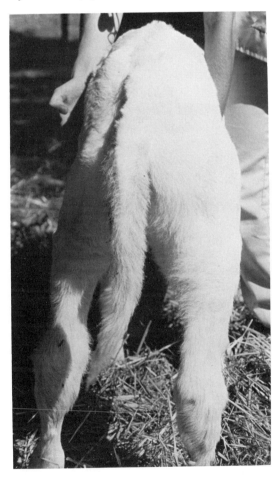

Figure 15–8. Following dystocia and an assisted delivery, this Charolais calf was weak on the pelvic limbs and developed left quadricep muscle atrophy as shown. This is typical of postcalving paralysis.

Assessment. Degrees of femoral nerve compression and stretching, with quadriceps muscle compression, can occur, resulting in inability to support weight. Hip-lock or stifle-lock dystocia most often will have occurred.

Combinations of ruptured extensor or flexor muscles of the hip, stifle, and hock result in obvious defects in limb function following dystocia, with or without assistance. Ruptured pelvic limb flexor muscles in foals probably occurs when one or both pelvic limbs are extended under the foal when it is delivered (Schneider et al., 1986). Occasionally, the mono- or paraparesis may only become evident when the newborn begins to move (several hours or days of age).

Outcome. Paraplegia with either syndrome warrants a bad prognosis. With time and nursing care, foals and calves with degrees of femoral or quadriceps paresis can recover (Tryphonas et al., 1974), (Paulsen et al., 1981). Muscle ruptures require specific surgical splinting and considerable nursing care.

II. Inflammatory, Infectious, Immune

    1. Rabies (also Problem 1)

Early in the course of rabies resulting from (presumably) a bite on a limb, progressive paralysis of one limb has occurred before signs of spinal cord or brainstem involvement occur. A syndrome believed to be vaccine-induced rabies in nine horses has been seen following use of a modified, live virus vaccine given in the neck musculature (should be given in the rump). Progressive hyperesthesia and lameness in the ipsilateral thoracic limb occurred prior to asymmetric tetraparesis; bulbar signs with some fatalities eventuated (Mayhew IG, Carlson GP, and Zent WW, unpublished observations).

III. Neoplastic

    1. Peripheral nerve sheath tumors

Neurofibromata are not common, but do occur in horses and cattle. Localized pain in association with nerve or nerve root (sometimes multiple) deficits are recognized when sensory nerves are affected (Bundza et al., 1986), (Doughty, 1977), (Hayes et al., 1975), (Mayhew et al., 1982).

    2. Lymphosarcoma

These tumors have been seen to encompass peripheral nerves in cattle and horses (Fankhauser et al., 1977), (Mayhew et al., 1982).

IV. Idiopathic

    1. Cervical vertebral osteoarthropathy

Degenerative bone and joint disease in the neck has been associated with some unusual forelimb gait abnormalities in horses. Whether there is a compressive radiculopathy (nerve root compression), dural irritation, painful arthrosis, or no correlation between these lesions and the clinical signs is unclear. Rest and neck braces have been empirically beneficial. A few syndromes have appeared to include such profound degrees of overt pain and disuse that they are worthy of comparison with causalgia in humans.

REFERENCES

Adams OR, Schneider RK, Bramlage LR, et al. A surgical approach to treatment of suprascapular nerve injury in the horse. J Am Vet Med Assoc 1985; *187*:1016–1018.

Blythe LL, Kitchell RL. Electrophysiologic studies of the thoracic limb of the horse. Am J Vet Res 1982; *43*:1511–1524.

Bundza A, Dukes TW, Stead RH. Peripheral nerve sheath neoplasms in Canadian slaughter cattle. Can Vet J 1986; *27*:268–271.

Ciszewski DK, Ames NK. Diseases of peripheral nerves. Vet Clin North Am: Food Anim Pract 1987; *3*:193–212.

Cox VS, Breazile JE, Hoover TR. Surgical and anatomic study of calving paralysis. Am J Vet Res 1975a; *36*:427–430.

Cox VS, Martin CE,. Peroneal nerve paralysis in a heifer. J Am Vet Med Assoc 1975b; *167*:142–144.

Diesem ChD, Hunter M, Rankin J. The effects on equine gait produced by neurectomies of the major nerves of the pelvic limb. Abstract. Anat Histol Embryol 1985; *14*:82–83.

Doughty FR. Incidence of neurofibroma in cattle in abattoirs in New South Wales. Aust Vet J 1977; *53*:280–281.

Duncan ID, Schneider RK. Equine suprascapular neuropathy (Sweeny): Clinical and pathologic observations. Proc 31st Annu Conv Am Assoc Equine Pract 1985; 415–428.

Dyce KM, Sack WO, Wensing CJG. *Textbook of Veterinary Anatomy*. Philadelphia: WB Saunders, 1987: pp 542–595, 697–728.

Dyson S. Shoulder lameness in horses: An analysis of 58 suspected cases. Equine Vet J 1986; *18*:29–36.

Dyson SJ, Taylor PM, Whitwell K. Femoral nerve paralysis after general anaesthesia. Equine Vet J. 1988; *20*:376–379.

Fankhauser VR, Bestetti G, Fatzer R, et al. Lymphosarcoma with peripheral nerve involvement in a horse. Dtsch Tierarztl Wschr 1977; *84*:81–124.

Hayes HM, Priester WA, Pendergrass TW. Occurrence of nervous tissue tumors in cattle, horses, cats and dogs. Int J Cancer 1975; *15*:39–47.

Henry RW. Gait alterations in the equine pectoral limb produced by neurectomies. Thesis, Ohio State University, 1976.

Mayhew IG, MacKay RJ. The Nervous System. In: *Equine Medicine and Surgery*, 3rd Ed. Mansmann RA, McAllister ES, Pratt PW, eds. Santa Barbara: American Veterinary Publications, 1982: Vol II, Ch 21, pp 1159–1252.

Paulsen DB, Noordsy JL, Leipold HW. Femoral nerve paralysis in cattle. Bov Pract 1981; *2*:14–26.

Rooney JR. Radial paralysis in the horse. Cornell Vet 1963; *53*:328–338.

Schneider JE., Guffy MM, Leipold HW. Ruptured flexor muscles in a neonatal foal. A case report. Equine Pract 1986; *8*:11–15.

Schneider JE, Adams OR, Easley KJ, et al. Scapular notch resection for suprascapular nerve decompression in 12 horses. J Am Vet Med Assoc 1985; *187*:1019–1020.

Sprinkle FP, Swerczek TW, Crowe MW. Gastrocnemius muscle rupture and hemorrhage in foals. Equine Pract 1985; *7*:10–17.

Tryphonas L, Hamilton GF, Rhoades CS. Perinatal femoral nerve degeneration and neurogenic atrophy of quadriceps femoris muscle in calves. J Am Vet Med Assoc 1974; *164*:801–807.

Vaughan LC. Peripheral nerve injuries: An experimental study in cattle. Vet Rec 1964; *76*:1293–1304.

CHAPTER 16

Problem 12:
Urinary Bladder Distention, Dilated Anus, and Atonic Tail: The Cauda Equina Syndrome

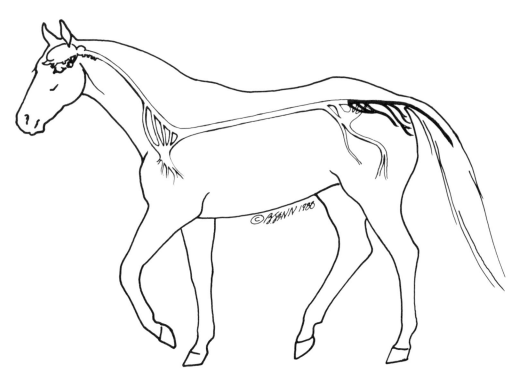

Locations of lesions resulting in degrees of the cauda equina syndrome: sacrococcygeal spinal cord segments, cauda equina, sacral plexus, and peripheral nerves to the bladder, rectum, anus, tail, and perineum (blackened).

This syndrome results from lesions involving the cauda equina; it is often present without any major gait abnormality because of minimal involvement of the lumbosacral nerve roots supplying the lumbosacral plexus. It consists of all degrees of hypotonia, hypalgesia, and hyporeflexia of the tail, anus, and perineal region; degrees of urinary bladder paresis and rectal dilatation are also present. This is a common problem in horses and most frequently results from fractures of the sacrum.

Recumbent large animals that have been assisted to stand by grasping or tying the tail often have poor tail and anal function. Heavy animals that dog-sit and those that receive multiple rectal examinations, also have poor tone and movement of the tail and anus. These animals also may have some degree of urinary and fecal retention without necessarily having sacrococcygeal segment or nerve lesions. Thus, distinguishing lower motor neuron paralysis of the bladder, tail, and anus from upper motor neuron weakness with urinary retention, and tail and anal contusion due to recumbency, is difficult—particularly in the horse.

Animals with even a prominent cauda equine syndrome can be maintained with nursing care, fecal softeners, frequent rectal examination, and attention to emptying the urinary bladder. Affected horses often get cystitis with mineral and purulent concretions accumulating in the bladder. Urinary pooling in the cranial vagina, and even in the uterus, may become a significant problem that inhibits reproductive capability. This is compounded by poor innervation of the caudal reproductive tract. The reproductive soundness of such mares is dubious at best. Stallions having even minor residual signs of sacral involvement have been rendered impotent because of incomplete erections and sterile because of urospermia (Asbury AC, Mayhew IG, unpublished).

Analysis of CSF collected from the lumbosacral space can be a useful ancillary aid in diagnosing the cause of this problem. This is partly because the CSF sample is collected close to the lesion. Needle electromyography has been useful in determining the extent of muscle denervation and can assist in monitoring the progress of a disease process, sometimes indicating that reinvervation is occurring. Measuring conduction velocity across the cauda equina has been undertaken under general anesthesia and can be considered for evaluating progress of a disease process. The conduction can be measured by using a stimulating electrode placed over the dura at the lumbosacral space, another in the sacrococcygeal cauda equina (with anode in adjacent shin), and recording electrodes in a ventral coccygeal muscle. No conduction early in a case of a fractured sacrum determines that the cauda equina is totally severed.

When evaluating horses with urinary incontinence only, consideration has to be given to cauda equina syndrome and to urinary tract and reproductive organ diseases. Included in these would be trypanosomiasis known variously as Dourine, Nagana, and Surra (Levine, 1985). Degrees of paralysis of the penis, bladder, and pelvic limbs can occur but the generalized signs of these venereal diseases are distinctive.

In this context, measuring the maximal bladder contraction pressure and maximal urethral closure pressure is a new technique (Clark et al., 1987), which should assist in better defining the site of a lesion and which should particularly assist in monitoring the use of drugs that can be used to treat patients suffering from urinary incontinence. Of note is the fact that there appears to be discrepancies in reported normal values (Clark et al., 1987), (Lavoie et al., 1987).

Categories of Disease and Differential Diagnosis
*NOTE: Only those diseases marked * are discussed in this problem*

I. Congenital and Familial
    *1. Miscellaneous Sacrococcygeal Vertebral and Spinal Cord Anomalies
II. Infectious, Inflammatory, Immune
    *1. Ascending Bacterial Empyema and Myelitis Associated with Tail Docking
    *2. Neuritis of the Cauda Equina/Polyneuritis Equi
    *3. Listeriosis
    4. Sacrococcygeal Vertebral Osteomyelitis (Problem 10)
    5. Equine Protozoal Myeloencephalitis (Problem 10)
    6. Equine Herpesvirus-1 Myelitis (Problem 10)
    7. Rabies (Problem 1)
    8. Cryptococcosis (Problem 1)
    9. Miscellaneous Infections (Problem 1)
III. Traumatic
    *1. Sacrococcygeal Fracture and Luxation
    *2. Avulsion of the Cauda Equina
IV. Toxic
    1. Cystitis and Ataxia Associated with *Sorghum* spp Ingestion (Problem 10)
V. Neoplastic
    *1. Lymphosarcoma, Neurofibroma, Melanosarcoma

I. Congenital and Familial
    1. Miscellaneous Sacrococcygeal Vertebral and Spinal Cord Anomalies

        These disorders occur sporadically in several breeds of cattle but are less common in other species. Ataxia, weakness to recumbency, and bilaterally-effective reflexes in the pelvic limbs usually occur; degrees of the cauda equina syndrome are less frequently present. Sacrococcygeal agenesis, spina bifida, myelocele, myelomeningocele, and other anomalies have been seen. In some cases, associated cranial anomalies such as hydrocephalus and the Arnold-Chiari malformation are present (Leipold et al., 1987).

II. Infectious, Inflammatory, Immune
    1. Ascending Bacterial Empyema and Myelitis Associated with Tail Docking and Tail Biting

        This disease occurs more often in lambs and piglets than in other species. Vertebral osteomyelitis and dissemination of the septic process elsewhere in the body can occur. It is seen in lambs and piglets following tail docking and in pigs involved with cannibalism (tail biting). The lesion may begin as a true ascending epidural empyema but may also begin as intervertebral arthritis (also Problem 10).

    2. Neuritis of the Cauda Equina/Polyneuritis Equi

        Signalment. Affected horses and ponies are of many breeds, both sexes, and of a wide age range—although this disease is not reported in foals and old horses (Fankhauser et al., 1975), (Scarratt et al., 1985), (Rousseaux et al., 1984), (Wright et al., 1987).

History. Urinary and fecal incontinence, possibly associated with colic or rubbing the tail head may be reported and usually there is an abrupt recognition of the signs by the owner. Occasionally, the horse is presented for signs of cranial nerve disease.

Physical Examination. Urine scald, obstipation, and broken tail-head hairs are likely to be found.

Neurologic Examination. There usually is analgesia, atonia, and areflexia of the tail, anus, perineum, rectum, bladder, and penis (not prepuce). A ring of hyperesthesia (hypersensitivity) frequently is evident surrounding the area of analgesia (Greenwood et al., 1973), (Scarratt et al., 1985), (Bilinski et al., 1977), (Cummings et al., 1979),

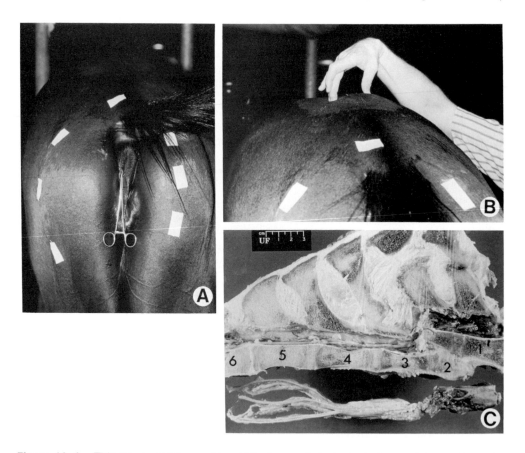

Figure 16–1. This 2-year-old thoroughbred filly demonstrated a typical, complete cauda equina syndrome. There was an atonic tail, atonic anus and vulva, anal areflexia, perineal analgesia within the area marked with tape, and a rim of hyperesthesia just above the tape markers (A). In addition the tubera sacrale were asymmetric, the left being lower than the right (B), and a fracture could be palpated per rectum at S_2. At postmortem examination, healed fractures of the sacral spines of S_1 and S_2 revealed that an injury to the sacrum had occurred several weeks earlier (C). An acute fracture-luxation of S_2, with acute cauda equina compression (C), was evident. The secondary luxation at S_2 was caused by the exertion of beginning a race. There was no external injury.

(Wright et al., 1987) (Fig. 16–1A). Pelvic limb gait abnormalities are subtle, if they are present at all. Cranial nerve signs, particularly involving the facial, vestibular, and trigeminal nerves, frequently are seen and can be asymmetric and fluctuating (Wright et al., 1987), (Cummings et al., 1979), (Fankhauser et al., 1975), (Bilinski et al., 1977).

Occasionally, involvement of nerve roots, other than those of the cauda equina, including cranial and other spinal nerves, is more prominent. The clinical syndromes of such cases of polyradiculoneuritis may thus be expressed as combinations of focal or multifocal muscle atrophy, pain, pruritus, sweating, and weakness of the affected part.

Assessment. There are well over 100 cases of polyneuritis equi documented from most parts of Europe and North America (Fankhauser et al., 1975), (Wright et al., 1987), (Cummings et al., 1979), (Greenwood et al., 1973), (Rousseaux et al., 1984), (Dahme et al., 1976), (Rimaila-Pärnänen, 1976).

The original lesion appears to be a demyelination that evolves into a granulomatous neuritis, perineuritis, and pachymeningitis involving the sacrococcygeal and lumbar roots (less often) of the cauda equina and some cranial nerves. The severe infiltrate can extend out into peripheral nerves (Cummings et al., 1979), (Wright et al., 1987). Sometimes there is diffuse involvement of many spinal nerve roots. Histologically, the latter stage is characterized by a severe, chronic, granulomatous inflammation involving lymphocytes, macrophages, eosinophils, fibroblasts, giant cells, and neutrophils. The early lesion resembles allergic neuritis with evidence of a demyelinating component (Cummings et al., 1979), (Wright et al., 1987), (Rousseaux et al., 1984), (Dahme et al., 1976). The lesion also affects the peripheral autonomic nervous system (Wright et al., 1987), although recognition of clinical signs resulting from this involvement, such as those of Horner's syndrome, is rare (White et al., 1984).

Affected horses have been found to have circulating antibodies against P_2-myelin protein (Kadlubowski et al., 1981). An enzyme-linked immunoabsorbant assay using P_2 preparations from bovine and equine myelin may be useful in identifying horses with this disease (Fordyce et al., 1987). Also, indirect immunofluorescence has demonstrated that cirulating IgG in affected horses has an affinity for myelin in the cauda equina (Edington et al., 1984). Thus, the evidence is mounting that this disease is an autoimmune polyneuritis. With the neuritogenic, immune-associated diseases Landry-Guillain-Barré syndrome in man and coonhound paralysis in dogs, exposure to an exogenous factor, such as influenza virus or raccoon saliva, respectively, may initiate an autoimmune attack on myelin (Braund, 1987), (Rousseaux et al., 1984), (Cummings et al., 1979), (Dahme et al., 1976), (Edington et al., 1984). Indeed, a history of recent vaccination or respiratory illness has been frequently mentioned in cases of neuritis of the cauda equina (Edington et al., 1984), (Wright et al., 1987), (Rousseaux et al., 1984), but by no means is this a constant finding (Cummings et al., 1979), (Greenwood et al., 1973). Thus, the role of viruses such as equine adenovirus (which was isolated from two of three cases of neuritis of the cauda equina by Edington et al., [1984]) in the pathogenesis of the disease is not known presently.

Diagnostic Aids. Clinically, the syndrome is typical if there is cauda equina and cranial nerve involvement. A thorough rectal examination and radiography are helpful to rule out a fractured sacrum, which usually is the most important differential diagnosis. Lumbosacral (and occasionally cisternal) CSF may be xanthochromic with moderately elevated protein content and prominent mononuclear pleocytosis, at least in the chronic stage (Cummings et al., 1979), (Rousseaux et al., 1984), (White et al., 1984); but it can be normal on analysis (Scarratt et al., 1985). A caudal epidural biopsy should provide a diagnosis. Denervation potentials in affected musculature of the tail and perineum are evident on needle electromyography.

Therapy. With nursing care and particular attention to bowel and urinary bladder evacuation horses have been maintained for up to a year (Wright et al., 1987). Systemic antibiotics and systemic and subarachnoid glucocorticosteroids do not appear to alter the disease course.

Prognosis. Signs may not progress rapidly but the horse becomes unacceptable to the owner. Valuable animals may be maintained for many months with intense nursing care; but with dense denervation of the genital tract, salvage for breeding purposes is not likely to be successful.

3. Listeriosis

Almost total cauda equina syndrome along with vestibular disease and facial paralysis in a working pony was caused by a suppurative myelomeningitis from which *Listeria monocytogenes* was isolated postmortem (Mayhew et al., 1982).

III. Trauma

1. Sacrococcygeal Fracture and Luxation

Signalment. This is most common in mature horses, less so in other animals.

History. Sometimes the horse has a history of rearing over backwards and sitting on its rump (Wagner et al., 1977). Occasionally it is seen in calves as an iatrogenic (malicious) injury and in cattle as a breeding-associated injury. The acute onset of neurologic signs has occurred in horses days to weeks after the primary sacral fracture occurred. This unusual pathogenesis has been determined to be caused by temporary but chronic stability of the sacral fracture, which becomes unstable with further injury or with the exertion of racing (see Fig. 16–1).

Neurologic Examination. Degrees of paresis to paralysis, hypalgesia to analgesia, and hypotonia to atonia around the tail and perineal region occur (Fig. 16–1). These signs generally are stable or they improve over weeks to months. Occasionally a callus will result and produce delayed and progressive signs.

Diagnosis. Careful palpation of the sacrum through the rectum

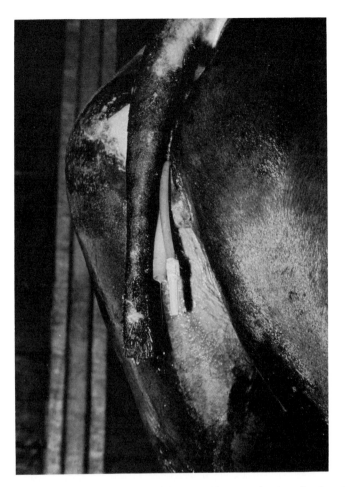

Figure 16–2. Mares with cauda equina syndrome (in this case due to a fractured S_2) suffer from urine scald (as shown), as well as fecal retention, urine pooling in the vagina, and cystitis. The outlook for breeding is bad.

often reveals a fracture site with or without callus formation. Repeated rectal examination, done on a flaccid rectum, must be performed with caution as mucosal tearing can easily result. Also, slight asymmetry of the ventral sacrum can be felt in normal horses. Radiographs of the area are possible, but they are difficult to undertake and to interpret. This is the case even with good evacuation of the rectum and even with rectally held x-ray film. Ultrasound examination of the sacrum through the rectum may be worth trying.

Therapy. Potentially, the area is accessible from a dorsal approach for exploratory surgery and removal of any tissues compressing the cauda equina. Conservative treatment usually is undertaken and signs are monitored as with any peripheral nerve disorder.

Prognosis. Without clinical improvement in 6 to 12 weeks, the prognosis for substantial long-term improvement is bad. As with neuritis of the cauda equina, genital denervation warrants a guarded prognosis for breeding (Fig. 16–2).

2. **Avulsion of the Cauda Equina**

This has occurred with heavy cattle and horses being assisted to stand with tail ropes. Excessive tail restraint may be a cause in cattle. The clinical syndrome is complicated by degrees of coccygeal traumatic myopathy.

The cauda equina nerve roots can be stretched or torn. If no luxation of the tail occurs, the neural lesion is most likely a neurapraxia with degrees of axonotmesis, which has been seen to improve and even resolve.

V. Neoplasia

1. **Lymphosarcoma, Neurofibroma, Melanosarcoma**

These neoplasms (and others) rarely encroach into the sacrococcygeal vertebral canal and entrap the cauda equina, which results in cauda equina syndrome with various degrees of gait abnormalities (Traver et al., 1977). Usually these neoplasms occur in older horses, although adult cattle of any age can have primary epidural lymphosarcoma at any site, including the cauda equina (also Problem 10).

REFERENCES

Bilinski J, Sprinkle T, Lee J. A case of cauda equina neuritis. Vet Med Small Anim Clin 1977; 72:597–598.
Braund KG. Diseases of Peripheral Nerves, Cranial Nerves and Muscle. In: *Veterinary Neurology.* Oliver JE, Hoerlein BF, Mayhew IG, eds. Philadelphia: WB Saunders, 1987. pp 353–392.
Clark ES, Semrad SD, Bichsel P, et al. Cystometrography and urethral pressure profiles in healthy horse and pony mares. Am J Vet Res 1987; 48:552–555.
Cummings JF, de Lahunta A, Timoney JF. Neuritis of the cauda equina, a chronic idiopathic polyradiculoneuritis in the horse. Acta Neuropathol (Berl) 1979; 46:17–24.
Dahme E, Deutschländer N. Die Neuritis der Cauda equina beim Pferd im elektronenmikroskopischen Bild. Beitrag zur weiteren Klärung der Pathogenese. Zbl Vet Med A 1976; 23:502–519.
Edington N, Wright JA, Patel JR, et al. Equine adenovirus 1 isolated from cauda equina neuritis. Res Vet Sci 1984; 37:252–254.
Fankhauser R, Gerber H, Cravero GC, et al. Klinik und Pathologie der Neuritis caudae equinae (NCE) des Pferdes. Schweiz Arch Tierheilk 1975; 117:675–699.
Fordyce PS, Edington N, Bridges GC, et al. Use of an ELISA in the differential diagnosis of cauda equina neuritis and other equine neuropathies. Equine Vet J 1987; 19:55–59.
Greenwood AG, Barker J, McLeish I. Neuritis of the cauda equina in a horse. Equine Vet J 1973; 5:111–115.
Kadlubowski M, Ingram PL. Circulating antibodies to the neuritogenic myelin protein, P_2, in neuritis of the cauda equina of the horse. Nature 1981; 293:299–300.
Lavoie J-P, Kay A. Urethral pressure profiles in mares. Proc 5th Annu Vet Med Forum 1987; Abstract No 29, 896.
Leipold HW, Dennis SM. Congenital defects of the bovine central nervous system. Vet Clin North Am [Food Anim Pract] 1987; 3:159–177.
Levine ND. *Veterinary Protozoology.* Ames: Iowa State University Press, 1985. pp 30–37.
Mayhew IG, MacKay R. The Nervous System. In: *Equine Medicine and Surgery,* 3rd Ed. Mansmann RA, McAlister ES, Pratt PW, eds. Santa Barbara: American Veterinary Publications, 1982; Vol 2, Ch 21, pp 1159–1304.
Rimaila-Pärnänen E. Neuritis of the cauda equina in a horse. Nord Vet Med 1976; 28:464–467.
Rousseaux CG, Futcher KG, Clark EG, et al. Cauda equina neuritis: A chronic idiopathic polyneuritis in two horses. Case report. Can Vet J 1984; 25:214–218.
Scarratt WK, Jortner BS. Neuritis of the cauda equina in a yearling filly. Case report. Comp Cont Ed Pract Vet 1985; 7:S197–S202.

Traver DS, Moore JN, Thornburg LP, et al. Epidural melanoma causing posterior paresis in a horse. J Am Vet Med Assoc 1977; *170*:1400–1403.

Wagner PC, Long GC, Chatburn CC, et al. Traumatic injury of the cauda equina in the horse: A case report. Equine Pract 1977; *1*:282–285.

White PL, Genetzky RM, Pohlenz JFL, et al. Neuritis of the cauda equina in a horse. Case report. Comp Cont Ed Pract Vet 1984; *6*:S217–S224.

Wright JA, Fordyce P, Edington N. Neuritis of the cauda equina in the horse. J Comp Pathol 1987; *97*:667–675.

CHAPTER 17

Problem 13:
Itching, Self-Mutilation, Head Shaking, and Miscellaneous Disorders

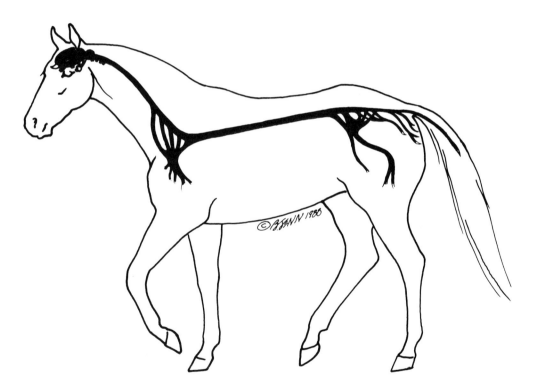

Locations of lesions resulting in itching, self-mutilation, head shaking, and miscellaneous disorders: diffuse and focal brain, spinal cord, and sensory peripheral nerves (blackened).

These are not common problems in large animals. However, when observed they can be spectacular. In the context of these problems it is assumed that there is itching, self-mutilation, or tail chasing without overt evidence of dermatologic disease (such as lice) or of more generalized or specific neurologic disease (with signs such as seizures, paralysis, or analgesia). One must still rule out dermatologic disorders and complete a careful neurologic evaluation.

Occasional episodes of bizarre, violent, and aggressive behavior—especially in horses—for which there often is no underlying neurologic explanation are reported by large animal clients. The possibility that these are isolated seizures does exist. A few unusual findings that have been thought to explain such occurrences include fright by the sight or smell of an offending animal or object, stinging nettle, fire ants, colic, and insects or objects in the external auditory canal.

A few adult beef and dairy cattle that frantically lick and chew on objects—to the point of self-inflicted mouth trauma—have been studied and were found to have neither evidence of metabolic derangement nor neurologic lesions accounting for the syndrome. Some affected cattle in one beef herd recovered spontaneously.

The so-called behavior problems that are discussed herein are those in which evidence or a strong suspicion of a neurologic lesion exists. This section does not attempt to cover stereotypic behavior or all forms of abnormal behavior for which there almost certainly is no morbid disease of the nervous system. The reader is referred to the following authors for excellent coverage of normal and abnormal behavior in farm animals: Houpt and Crowell-Davis, 1986; Price, 1987; Kiley-Worthington and Wood-Gush, 1987. Notwithstanding, if an animal with an acquired aggressive problem is euthanized, a thorough scrutinizing of the nervous system should be undertaken. The main reasons for this are the possibility of rabies (Probem 1), the possibility of a spongiform encephalopathy (Problem 1) and obscure but definitive neuropathologic lesions in the limbic system, which have at least been detected in the brains of aggressive dogs (Caldwell et al., 1980).

No inherited sensory neuropathies causing self-mutilation, with or without nociceptive (pain) deficits, appear to have been recognized in large animals.

Categories of Disease and Differential Diagnosis
*NOTE: Only those diseases marked * are discussed in this problem.*

   I. Congenital and Familial
         1. Mannosidosis (Problems 1 and 9)
  II. Physical
         *1. Peripheral Nerve Injury and Repair
 III. Infectious, Inflammatory, Immune
         *1. Rabies (Problem 1)
         *2. Pseudorabies (Problem 1)
         *3. Infectious Bovine Rhinotracheitis Encephalomyelitis
         *4. Scrapie (Problems 1 and 9)
          5. Bovine Spongiform Encephalopathy (Problem 1)
          6. Other Meningoencephalomyelitides (Problem 1)
  IV. Metabolic
         *1. Nervous Ketosis
   V. Toxic
          1. Locoweeds and *Swainsona* sp (Problems 1 and 9)

VI. *Nutritional
VII. Idiopathic
    *1. Self-Mutilation Syndrome
    *2. Head Nodding and Head Shaking
    *3. Head Rubbing

II. Physical
    1. Peripheral Nerve Trauma and Repair
        Although peripheral nerve injury and spinal cord injury are both common, the hyperesthetic or paresthetic (in humans "pins and needles") aspects of neuronal sprouting and repair appear to be clinically rare in large animal practice. Licking and rubbing at healing wounds is a common phenomenon, but extreme self-mutilation is not. The use of cobra venom injections and other untested drugs as therapy for such syndromes is noted but not recommended. Acupuncture and transcutaneous electrical nerve stimulation (TENS) seem to be sensible, probably harmless, modalities of therapy.
III. Infectious, Inflammatory, Immune
    1. Rabies (also Problems 1 and 11)
        Although this is uncommon, an affected animal may attack itself, particularly near the site of inoculation (Fig. 5–5). This has been observed with native virus and postvaccinally with modified live virus in the horse.
    2. Pseudorabies (also Problem 1)
        Signalment. All farm animals species, except the horse, have been affected by Aujeszky's disease.
        Clinical Signs. These are mild in adult pigs, but usually there is an acute fever with incoordination, seizures, and death in piglets. Pruritis is seen in other species, with violent licking, chewing, and rubbing of face, limbs, or trunk. Then maniacal behavior frequently develops with death occurring in 1 to 2 days (Braund et al., 1987), (Dow et al., 1962).
        Assessment. The virus enters abraded skin or the upper respiratory mucosa and spreads to the CNS through spinal and cranial nerves. Extensive neuronal loss with perivascular mononuclear cuffing and necrosis occurs and large intranuclear inclusions are seen.
        Treatment. No therapy is available. It is advisable to remove animals from association with swine. Confirmation of the diagnosis is by viral isolation. Vaccines are available for swine.
    3. Infectious Bovine Rhinotracheitis Encephalomyelitis
        This is a rare disease of young calves; it usually results in signs of diffuse encephalitis and death. However, one case is reported in a 3-year-old heifer that had signs of frenzied licking and attacking parts of the body (Beck, 1975). Other signs of encephalitis and myelitis were present and the disease was fatal. Hemorrhagic necrosis was scattered through the CNS with major lesions in the spinal cord

at the level of the pruritic sites. The virus can be isolated from the brain.

4. Scrapie (also Problems 1 and 9)

Profound pruritis with cerebellar ataxia and wasting characterize this rare disease of sheep and goats (Hadlow et al., 1982).

IV. Metabolic

1. Nervous Ketosis

Signalment. This syndrome occurs in cattle and sheep around the time of parturition and is most common in high-producing dairy cows at peak lactation time (Blood et al., 1979).

History. Diffuse nervous signs with constant licking of self or objects is one syndrome seen with ketosis. More frequent syndromes include anorexia, a drop in milk production, or wasting.

Physical Examination. A smell of ketones on the breath and the urine are likely to be detected. Urine and milk will give a positive test for ketones.

Neurologic Examination. Wandering, head pressing, ataxia, vigorous licking, depraved appetite, blindness and hyperesthesia may be present.

Assessment. Ketosis affects overweight animals using the energy stores in late pregnancy and early lactation, or animals receiving low levels of nutrition whose requirements (fetus, milk) are increasing. It may occur secondarily to other disease, such as a displaced abomasum (Blood et al., 1979).

Treatment. Cattle should receive dextrose IV and oral propylene glycol. Glucocorticosteroids may be effective because they reduce milk yield. Sheep are best treated with dextrose and alkalinizing fluids IV and force-feeding.

Prevention. Matching nutrient intake with requirements should be aimed for. Reducing silage (ketogenic) feeding can be helpful with cattle.

VI. Nutritional

Cattle with chronic phosphate deficiency and with sodium deficiency lick incessantly at anything that may contain these elements; this may include their own body parts. In addition, cattle with NaCl deficiency become polyuric and polydypsic (Blood et al., 1979).

VII. Idiopathic

1. Self-Mutilation Syndrome

Signalment. This syndrome usually involves mature, lightbred, stallions (Houpt, 1983), (Houpt, 1985), (Houpt et al., 1986); one mare and two geldings are known to have been affected.

History. The onset often follows a major change in the environment, the exercise program, or the breeding regimen—such as returning to stud from racing, or being taken into a new herd.

Physical Examination. Cutaneous lacerations with pieces of flesh missing are seen, particularly in the pectoral, flank, stifle, and thigh regions. Dermatologic and routine neurologic workups are essentially unremarkable.

Neurologic Examination. The horse shows spells of looking at

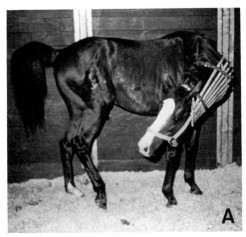 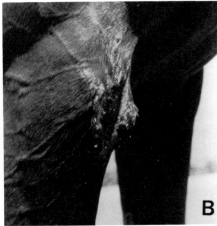

Figure 17–1. Self-mutilation syndrome in a thoroughbred stallion. The horse intermittently turns to bite at itself (A) while squealing and spinning. Pieces of skin and flesh may be removed, as on this horse's right forearm (B).

its flank, squealing, grunting, spinning, running in circles, kicking, and biting at its body (Fig. 17–1). The horse usually can be distracted with a whip. One gets the impression that it does not want to actually hurt itself; if it so desired it could completely devour the forelimbs.

Assessment. Considerations for pathogenesis include deviant behavior, focal seizures, myelitis, radiculitis, neuritis, and hormone imbalance. Breeding stallions require continued, hard exercise, which frequently is overlooked. This may be of some significance if the syndrome is one of stereotypic behavior stemming from boredom and the release of endogenous opioids afforded by performing the activity.

Treatment. If this is a profound form of stereotypic behavior, then as with other similar diseases (cribbing and weaving) prevention of the problem may induce more profound deviant behavior if the animal remains in the same environment (Houpt et al., 1986), (Kiley-Worthington et al., 1987). Thus, the best approach is to alter the environment, feeding practices, breeding management, and social contacts as appropriate to replace the vice with normal activity. In this regard, animal companionship with a goat, old barren mare, or placid gelding has been useful in reducing self-mutilation (Houpt, 1983), (Houpt, 1985). Castration has been relatively successful in preventing fighting among horses. It has been about 40 to 75% successful in this when performed after or before the onset of fighting, respectively (Line et al., 1985). Certainly castration can be tried in cases of self-mutilation syndrome, but it was not successful in one case. Once again, the general environment and management of the animal must be altered to expect a change in behavior.

Sedative drugs might exacerbate signs, although weekly to monthly doses of some unlicensed, long-term sedative such as reserpine (Serpasil, 1 mg IM or 4 mg PO), or fluphenazine enanthate

(Prolixin, 50 mg IM) may be tried. The owner should be cautioned that apparent "psychotic reactions" have been seen in horses treated with such drugs. Signs have included spinning in circles, a star-gazing attitude, snapping at imaginary flies, and total distraction and somnolence.

Narcotic agonist-antagonist drugs have been used to alter behavior in man and animals and have been said to be effective in suppressing stereotypic behavior in the dog (tail-chasing) (Brown et al., 1987) and in horses (crib-biting) (Dodman et al., 1987). Whether or not such regimens of treatment could benefit cases of self-mutilation is not known.

Various progestins have been used successfully to obviate aggressive and hypersexual behavior in horses (Roberts et al., 1987). Some regimens are: 0.4 mg/kg progesterone in oil, IM, daily; 0.044 mg/kg altrenogest (Regumate) PO, daily; 60 to 80 mg megestrol acetate (Ovaban) PO, per horse, daily; and 2000 mg repositol progesterone (Progesterone Injection Repository), IM, per horse, weekly.

Special chain muzzles often must be resorted to when this syndrome is severe, to prevent large wounds from developing.

2. Head Nodding and Head Shaking

Head nodding and head shaking in horses can occur at rest and while exercising but really only becomes a clinical problem when it occurs while a horse is being ridden. Head shaking may be instinctive and is part of normal sexual and avoidance behavior (Cook, 1979a). It may be regarded as stereotypic behavior (Kiley-Worthington, 1983) but has been associated with a few neurologic and several nonneurologic processes (Lane et al., 1987). The head movements may be continual or intermittent, mild or violent. They most often are on a vertical plane (nodding), but may be on a horizontal plane (shaking), or both. Extensive clinical workups (Cook, 1979a,b), (Cook, 1980a,b) are frequently undertaken, but specific findings are discovered only in a few cases (Fig. 17–2). Even if traumatic, inflammatory, or degenerative processes are defined in the region of the head, guttural pouches, pharynx, neck, or back, proving a causal relationship with the head nodding or head shaking is difficult. A review of 100 cases of head shaking revealed evidence of a possible cause in only 11 (Lane et al., 1987). These coincident findings included ear mites (three), otitis interna (one), vestibular and facial nerve paralysis (one), neck trauma (two), detached iris cysts or "aqueous floaters" (one), guttural pouch mycosis (one), periapical dental osteitis (one), and suspected Horner's syndrome and vasomotor rhinitis (one). These clinicians believed that allergic rhinitis would be the most likely cause of the majority of cases of idiopathic head shaking (Lane et al., 1987).

A clinical workup should be aimed at ruling out historical and clinical factors (ill-fitting gear and a fly-ridden environment [Cook, 1980a]) prior to expensive and invasive diagnostic testing, such as infraorbital nerve blocks, CSF collection, neck radiographs, and drug-therapy trials (Cook, 1980b), (Lane et al., 1987).

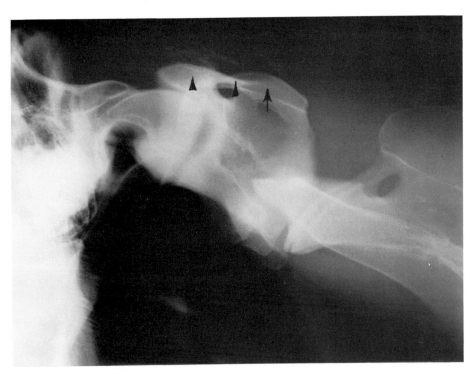

Figure 17–2. Even when mineralization in the region above the atlas (arrows) is found in a horse that began nodding its head while being ridden 4 weeks earlier, proving an association between head nodding and the lesion is almost impossible.

The long list of drugs that have been tried without documented success, reflects the idiopathic nature of the disorder.

3. Head Rubbing

This rare disorder may be behavioral, or some hypothesize that it is like *tic douloureux* in humans, which is purported to be caused by trigeminal neuritis. The affected horse rubs one or both sides of its head and face on objects, creating abrasions. Complete workups are lacking and prognosis is unpredictable. Occasionally, affected horses have evidence of other cranial nerve deficiencies, including facial paralysis and masseter atrophy, but the fact that signs resolved with time suggests that some patients have polyneuritis.

In a study of head shaking in 100 horses (Lane et al., 1987), rubbing the nose was seen in many animals, including two with ear mite infestation and one with Horner's syndrome and suspected vasomotor rhinitis.

REFERENCES

Beck BE. Infectious bovine rhinotracheitis encephalomyelitis in cattle and its differential diagnosis. Case report. Can Vet J 1975; *16*:269–271.
Blood DC, Henderson JA, Radostitis OM. *Veterinary Medicine,* 5th Ed. Philadelphia: Lea & Febiger, 1979. pp 849–858, 886–887; 906–910.

Braund KG, Brewer BD, Mayhew IG. Inflammatory, Infectious, Immune, Parasitic and Vascular Diseases. In: *Veterinary Neurology,* Oliver JE, Hoerlein BF, Mayhew IG, eds. Philadelphia: WB Saunders, 1987. Ch. 7, pp 216–254.

Brown SA, Crowell-Davis S, Malcolm T, et al. Naloxone-responsive compulsive tail chasing in a dog. J Am Vet Med Assoc 1987; 190:884–886.

Caldwell DS, Little PB. Aggression in dogs and associated neuropathology. Can Vet J 1980; 21:152–154.

Cook WR. Headshaking in horses. Part 1. Equine Pract 1979a; 1(5):9–17.

Cook WR. Headshaking in horses. Part 2. History and management tests. Equine Pract 1979b; 1(6):36–39.

Cook WR. Headshaking in horses. Part 3. Diagnostic tests. Equine Pract 1980a; 2(1):31–40.

Cook WR. Headshaking in horses. Part 4. Special diagnostic procedures. Equine Pract 1980b; 2(2):7–15.

Dodman NH, Shuster L, Court MH, et al. Investigation into the use of narcotic antagonists in the treatment of a stereotypic behavior pattern (crib-biting) in the horse. Am J Vet Res 1987; 48:311–319.

Dow C, McFerran JB. The pathology of Aujeszky's disease in cattle. J Comp Pathol 1962; 72:337–347.

Hadlow WJ, Kennedy RC, Race RE. Natural infection of Suffolk sheep with scrapie virus. J Infect Dis 1982; 146:657–664.

Houpt KA. Self-directed aggression: A stallion behavior problem. Equine Pract 1983; 5(2):6–8.

Houpt KA. Behavioral problems in horses. Proc 31st Annu Conv Am Assoc Equine Pract 1985; 113–123.

Houpt KA, Crowell-Davis SL (eds). Behavior. Vet Clin North Am [Equine Pract] 1986; 2:465–671.

Kiley-Worthington M. Stereotypes in horses. Cause, function and prevention. Equine Pract 1983; 5(1):33–40.

Kiley-Worthington M, Wood-Gush D. Stereotypic behavior. In: *Current Therapy in Equine Medicine–2.* Robinson NE, ed. Philadelphia: WB Saunders, 1987. pp 131–134.

Lane JG, Mair TS. Observations on headshaking in the horse. Equine Vet J 1987; 19:331–336.

Line SW, Hart BL, Sanders L. Effect of prepubertal versus postpubertal castration on sexual and aggressive behavior in male horses. J Am Vet Med Assoc 1985; 186:249–251.

Price EO (ed). Farm animal behavior. Vet Clin North Am [Food Animal Pract] 1987; 3:217–481.

Roberts SJ, Beaver BV. The use of progestins for aggressive and for hypersexual horses. In: *Current Therapy in Equine Medicine–2.* Robinson NE, ed. Philadelphia: WB Saunders, 1987. pp 129–131.

APPENDIX:
A Selection of Familial and Hereditary Neuromuscular Diseases of Large Animals*

Species	Disease	Breeds Affected	Problem Numbers
Cattle	1. Achondroplasia with hydrocephalus	Dexter Holstein Jersey Telemark	1
	2. Agenesis of corpus callosum	Murray Gray Others	1
	3. Arthrogryposis	Charolais Hereford	10
	4. Atlantoaxial luxation	Holstein	10
	5. Bovine progressive degenerative myeloencephalopathy	Brown Swiss	10
	6. Cerebellar abiotrophy	Holstein	9
	7. Cerebellar hypoplasia/degeneration	Angus-Shorthorn Ayreshire Guernsey Hereford Holstein Jersey Shorthorn	9
	8. Ceroid lipofuscinosis	Beemaster Hereford Devon	1
	9. Citrullinemia	Holstein	1
	10. Convulsions and ataxia	Aberdeen Angus	2, 9
	11. Epilepsy	Brown Swiss Swedish Red	2
	12. Gangliosidosis, GM_1	Holstein	1, 10
	13. Glycogenosis, generalized (Pompe's disease)	Shorthorn Brahman	10
	14. Hydrocephalus	Hereford Ayreshire Charolais Holstein Jersey Shorthorn	1
	15. Hypomyelinogenesis (congenital tremor)	Holstein Angus Santa Gertrudis Hereford Jersey Shorthorn	8

367

Species	Disease	Breeds Affected	Problem Numbers
Cattle *(Continued)*			
	16. Kyphosis	Jersey	10
	17. αMannosidosis	Angus	1, 9
		Murray Grey	
	18. Maple syrup urine disease	Hereford	8
	19. Myoclonia, congenital	Hereford	8
	20. Neurofibrillary degeneration	Afrikaner	10
	21. Nystagmus, pendular	Holstein	6
		Jersey	
		Ayreshire	
		Guernsey	
	22. Posterior paralysis	Norwegian Red Poll	10
		Red Danish	
	23. Premature vertebral synosteosis	Angus	1
	24. Progressive ataxia	Charolais	10
	25. Progressive myelinopathy	Murray Gray	10
	26. Retinal dysplasia	Hereford	3, 9
	27. Shaker calf syndrome	Horned Hereford	8
	28. Spastic paresis	All common breeds	8
	29. Spastic syndrome	Guernsey	8
		Holstein	
		Others	
	30. Strabismus, convergent	Holstein	5
		Shorthorn	
Horses			
	1. Cerebellar abiotrophy	Arabian	9
		Gotland Pony	
		Oldenburg	
	2. Cervical vertebral malformation	Thoroughbred	10
		All lightbreeds	
	3. Epilepsy, benign	Arabian	2
	4. Equine degenerative myeloencephalopathy	All lightbreeds	10
		Przewalskii	
		Grant Zebra	
	5. Hyperkalemic periodic paralysis	Quarterhorse	8
	6. Laryngeal hemiplegia	Thoroughbred	5
		Lightbreds	
		Draft breeds	
	7. Narcolepsy—cataplexy	Shetland	4
		Suffolk	
	8. Neurofibrillary degeneration	Zebra	10
	9. Night blindness (nyctalopia)	Appaloosa	3
	10. Occipitoatlantoaxial malformation	Arabian	10
	11. Shivering	Draft breeds	8
Sheep			
	1. Cerebellar abiotrophy	Merino	9
	2. Ceroid lipofuscinosis (Batten's disease)	South Hampshire	1
	3. Congenital myopathy	Suffolk	10
	4. Daft lambs (cerebellar atrophy)	Corredale	10
		Welsh Mountain	
	5. Globoid cell leukodystrophy (Krabbe's disease)	Polled Dorset	9
	6. Glucocerebrosidosis (Gaucher's disease)	Many	1
	7. Glycogenosis type II	Corredale	10
	8. Holoprosencephaly	Border Leicester	1
	9. Muscular dystrophy	Merino	10
	10. Myotonia	Shropshire	10

Species	Disease	Breeds Affected	Problem Numbers
Sheep *(Continued)*			
	11. Neuroaxonal dystrophy	Romney Suffolk	10
	12. Neuromuscular disease	Dorset Down	10
	13. Organophosphate (haloxon) toxicity, delayed	Suffolk and Crosses	10
	14. Rigid lamb syndrome	Dorper	10
	15. Spider syndrome	Suffolk	10
Goats			
	1. Ceroid lipofuscinosis	Nubian	1, 9
	2. βMannosidosis	Anglo-Nubian	1, 9
	3. Myotonia congenita (Thomson's disease)	Inbred strain	10
Swine			
	1. Cerebellar abiotrophy	Yorkshire	9
	2. Cerebellar hypoplasia/degeneration	Saddleback X Large White	9
	3. Creeper syndrome	Pietrain	10
	4. Gangliosidosis GM$_2$ (Tay-Sachs disease)	Yorkshire	1
	5. Glucocerebrosidosis (Gaucher's disease)	Many	1
	6. Hypomyelinogenesis	Wessex Saddleback Landrace	8
	7. Malignant hyperthermia— porcine stress syndrome	Landrace Pietrain Poland China	10
	8. Neurofibrillary degeneration	Yorkshire	11

*For references, see appropriate chapter in text and Oliver RE, Hoerlein BF, Mayhew IG. *Veterinary Neurology.* Appendix II. Philadelphia: WB Saunders, 1987: pp 525–535.

INDEX

Numerals in *italics* indicate a figure; "t" following a page number indicates tabular matter.

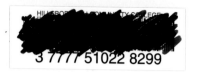
LINCC

Plant City